Physical Rehabilitation for Daily Living

EDITH BUCHWALD, M.A., A.R.P.T.

Director of Rehabilitation Courses for Physical Therapists
Institute of Physical Medicine and Rehabilitation
New York University—Bellevue Medical Center

IN COLLABORATION WITH

HOWARD A. RUSK, M.D.
Professor and Chairman
Department of Physical Medicine and Rehabilitation

GEORGE G. DEAVER, M.D.
Professor of Clinical Physical Medicine and Rehabilitation

DONALD A. COVALT, M.D.
Associate Professor
Physical Medicine and Rehabilitation

New York University—Bellevue Medical Center

THE BLAKISTON DIVISION
McGRAW-HILL BOOK COMPANY, INC.
NEW YORK TORONTO LONDON

PHYSICAL REHABILITATION FOR DAILY LIVING

Library of Congress Catalog Card Number: 51-12547

V

THE MAPLE PRESS COMPANY, YORK, PA.

FOREWORD

The purpose of this book is to outline teaching methods for a basic exercise and daily-activity program for patients with disabilities of the lower extremities. The book is directed to the members of the rehabilitation team who are concerned with teaching the patient the skills necessary for his physical independence, the foundation for his total rehabilitation.

Undoubtedly, much of the present growth of interest in extending rehabilitation opportunities and services to the handicapped has resulted both directly and indirectly from the Second World War. Such advances are not entirely due to the impetus of the war, however, as the growth of rehabilitation opportunities and services to the handicapped is part of a total pattern of an expanding national and community consciousness of social responsibility which is reflected by similar advances in all education, health, and social services.

More and more, we, in this nation, are beginning to adopt a progressive philosophy of the relationship of society and the individual. We, individually, are becoming more conscious of the fact that, in a democracy, society and government exist for the benefit of the individual and that it is the responsibility of society to see that every member of our social group shall have the opportunity, regardless of his circumstances, to become an effective, contributing member of society.

Physical medicine and rehabilitation offers the oldest therapeutic tools known to medicine; yet it is the newest medical specialty recognized by the Council of Medical Education and Hospitals of the American Medical Association. Because of the increasing knowledge of electronics and biophysics, a more comprehensive understanding of the biological and biomechanical principles involved in the pathological processes of the disabled and chronically ill, and more knowledge concerning the importance of the psychological, vocational, and social factors in the management of the disabled and chronically ill, this specialty has made more rapid strides in the past decade than in all time heretofore.

This is well, for paralleling the development of rehabilitation techniques and programs has been an even more rapid increase in the number of persons needing such services. The lack of a systematic approach requiring the reporting of cases of physical disability to a central agency, together with varying subjective interpretations of what constitutes a disability, makes it difficult to stake out the boundaries of the field of rehabilitation and services to the handicapped in any quantitative fashion.

Although a census of such conditions has been proposed on several occasions, there has never been a complete survey of the extent of physical disability in the United States. The most comprehensive source of information at present is the National Health Survey, conducted by the U.S. Public Health Service in 1935–1936. In this survey, 800,000 families in 83 cities and 23 rural areas of 19 states were studied. As the result of this survey, it was estimated at that time that there were some 23,000,000 persons in the United States who were handicapped to some extent by disease, accident, maladjustment, or war. These numbers have now increased to an estimated 28,000,000 persons as a result of the Second World War, our increase in population, and the rising age level of the population.

One of the principal causes of the increasing prevalence of chronic disease and its resultant disability has been the great advance in medical and surgical care which has prevented death and produced an aging population. Two thousand years ago the average length of life was 25 years; at the turn of the century, it was 49; recently compiled 1948 mortality statistics of the National Office of Vital Statistics show that the average length of life in the United States has increased to 67.2 years.

As our population becomes older, it can be expected that the incidence of chronic disease and disability will increase correspondingly; studies indicate the higher the age group, the greater the percentage of chronic disease. In the National Health Survey, 1935–1936, the following incidence rates per 1,000 persons were found of persons with a chronic disease or impairment on a given day: over 65 years of age, 515; age 45 to 64, 309; age 20 to 44, 177; age 5 to 19, 70; and under 5, 34. Rates for total and permanent disability per 1,000 population were: over 65 years of age, 75; age 45 to 64, 22; age 20 to 44, 8; age 5 to 9, 4; and under 5, 1.6.

There are a great many persons in the groups listed above for whom neither physical medicine and rehabilitation nor this book has implications. But there are many for whom they mean the bridging of the gap between the "bed and the job" or the difference between dependence and usefulness.

Age plus disability will prevent many chronically ill persons from returning to employment. Vocational placement, however, is not the only goal of rehabilitation. Self-care and the ability to do productive work while still living in a hospital, home, or institution are also worth-while objectives. They are valid medically and socially for their effect on the well-being of the person, and economically, in that personnel and operating costs of the institution or the patient's home are thereby reduced.

Lacking specific measures in the cure of many of the chronic diseases, medicine must look to rehabilitation to teach those afflicted by disability to live and to work as effectively as possible with their remaining physical abilities. Until medicine finds the answer and specific treatment to the problems of the diseases of the heart and circulation, rheumatic fever and arthritis, cerebral palsy, multiple sclerosis, poliomyelitis, and the other crippling diseases, we must utilize the techniques of physical rehabilitation, psychology, social service, vocational counseling, and the auxiliary specialties to teach the disabled to live within the limits of their disabilities but to the full extent of their capabilities.

Although we have in this nation the world's finest institutions and programs for definitive medical care of our chronically disabled and aged, with but a few exceptions there are no programs equipped to provide the patient who has a physical disability with the necessary retraining in the physical skills essential in performing the activities inherent in daily living. The physician in the past has thought too much about the physiological and clinical aspects of the patient's disability and too little about the physical retraining in skills necessary for carrying on the basic activities of daily living.

Except in a few isolated instances, the physically handicapped person must be retrained to walk and travel, to care for his daily needs, to use normal methods of transportation, to use ordinary toilet facilities, to apply and remove his own prosthetic appliances, and to communicate either orally or in writing. Too frequently, these basic skills are overlooked. The patient is given numerous medical, psychological, and vocational services in preparation for employment or self-care, but retraining in the activities of daily living is overlooked—with the result that the patient, being unable to walk and travel and care for himself, is also unable to utilize effectively the other medical, psychological, social, and vocational services he has received for richer and fuller living. Retraining in the basic activities of daily living is primary; it is simply a matter of "first things first," for daily-activity skills are the basis for all subsequent activities.

Because of the necessity for presenting the activities listed in this book in detail, they have been limited to rehabilitation activities for persons with impairments of the lower extremities. The activities described in this book are so simple that they are frequently overlooked, but the personal, vocational, and social success of the handicapped person is dependent upon them. They are the foundation of rehabilitation.

Howard A. Rusk

PREFACE

A.D.L. means activities of daily living, or, as a patient once said, "all the little things that make you miserable when you cannot do them—you know, like putting on your shoes, or eating your soup, or switching on the light, or getting from the bed to the wheel chair, or walking through a door."

They are little things, to be sure. But if one is on braces and crutches, they become strenuous exercises. They assume utmost importance, because when they are all added up, they make the difference between constantly needing help and being on one's own.

Therefore, A.D.L. play an important part in a rehabilitation program for the physically handicapped. The only way to learn these activities lies in long and strenuous *practice;* the only possible way of reaching the goal is through exercise. Exercise is used not as an end in itself, but as a means to becoming independent. Therefore, the exercise program is based on the motions inherent in the essential A.D.L. In this way, there is a close interrelation between A.D.L. and exercise. The A.D.L. may be regarded as exercises and the exercises as A.D.L.

Exercise increases strength and promotes coordination, endurance, and agility and thus enables the patient to perform the necessary motions. But there are much more far-reaching effects of exercise.

When a child wants to do something very badly—to turn a somersault or to dive—he practices and tries again and again, day after day, until finally he has mastered the skill he set out to learn. There follows a wonderful feeling of satisfaction, the stimulating feeling that he has done something with his own power, just through practice and persistence.

In a sick person, because of shock or injury, or often because of sheer weakness, this feeling of being able to achieve something, this desire to act and plan, is very low. The most important aim then of our entire rehabilitation program is to help the patient to experience again what it means to do things and to show him that he is capable of reaching a goal. The starting point for this reeducation to "doing" is exercise. The exercises must be very simple in the beginning. We have to be reasonably sure that the patient will learn to perform them in a comparatively short time. They also have to be given regularly every day and always at the same time. Another important point in the program is a carefully planned schedule for the entire day. In the beginning the rest periods will be much longer than the work periods, but gradually as the patient's strength increases, the time for work will be much more extensive than the time for rest.

Once the patient realizes that he can actually perform a given task, even if it is the simplest exercise, like bending and straightening the fingers of the hand, then he himself will try for the next more difficult step. And as the human being is a mosaic which reacts and acts as a whole, this feeling of satisfaction which results from carrying out a plan will carry over from the neuromuscular level to all other levels of human activity. The patient will become more active in his entire attitude, and gradually, under proper guidance, he will try to take part in the life around him, eventually even finding his place as a working member of his community.

The activities of daily living discussed in this book are based on the original work of one of the collaborators (George G. Deaver, M.D.), and of Mary Eleanor Brown, A.R.P.T., formerly at the Institute for the Crippled and Disabled, New York City, and of Marjorie P. Sheldon, A.R.P.T. The modifications and additions were developed at the Institute of Physical Medicine and Rehabilitation, New York University-Bellevue Medical Center, and the departments of Physical Medicine and Rehabilitation of Bellevue Hospital, Goldwater Memorial Hospital, and the University Hospital of the New York University-Bellevue Medical Center. A number of them are shown in teaching filmstrips distributed by Filmstrips, Inc., New York City.

The author is deeply indebted to her collaborators, Dr. Howard A. Rusk, Dr. George G. Deaver, and Dr. Donald A. Covalt, for their invaluable assistance. She is further indebted, and wishes to express grateful thanks to all members of the staff and students of the Institute of Physical Medicine and Rehabilitation, particularly former staff members Miss Dorothy Harris, A.R.P.T., and Captain Dorothy Peterson, A.R.P.T.; to all patients who participated in the development of the activities of daily living and who posed for the photographs, particularly Mrs. Thomas Miley and Miss Jamie Coffman; to Mrs. Emily Keyes Belt, Miss Mary Steers, and Mr. Stanley Simmons for their photography; to Mrs. Grace Blanchard, Miss Margaret McCormack, R.N., and Mr. Eugene J. Taylor for their critical reading and analysis of the manuscript; and to The National Foundation for Infantile Paralysis for its assistance in the teaching program during which much of this material was developed.

It is a privilege to be able to work with patients in the Institute of Physical Medicine and Rehabilitation, to see how ingenious and courageous they are, to see how much persistence they have once we have aroused their drive to do things and have challenged them to help themselves instead of being helped. Anyone who has had this privilege realizes that exercise may become the magic formula on the road from helplessness and mere existence to independence and life.

Edith Buchwald

New York, N.Y.
January, 1952

CONTENTS

Physical Rehabilitation for Daily Living

CHAPTER I

Functional Training*

Functional training involves the physical reconditioning of the patient through a carefully devised exercise and activity program in order to make him able to handle his body in the most efficient way so that he will be as independent as possible.

The basis for this independence lies in the performance of the activities necessary during the course of an ordinary day. The entire program is based on medical findings and other necessary examinations and will be carried through according to medical prescription and under close medical supervision.

Activities of Daily Living (A.D.L.) can be divided into three main groups:

"I. Self-care activities.
II. Ambulation, elevation, and traveling activities.
III. Hand activities."†

The motions inherent in the essential A.D.L. become the basis for an exercise program.

How are A.D.L. taught? In general we approach the problem in the following way:

1. A given A.D.L. is broken down into its simplest motions.
2. Exercises are selected to enable the patient to perform these specific motions.
   a. The motion itself may be practiced as an exercise, *e.g.*, grasping a fork—the exercise for this motion may be grasping a fork or similar objects.
   b. If for some reason, such as lack of strength or lack of coordination, it is not possible to practice the motion itself, preparatory exercises, *e.g.*, strengthening hand and finger muscles, have to be practiced first.
   c. In some cases special gadgets may have to be devised.
3. The particular A.D.L. itself is practiced as a whole in a real-life situation.

In this book we deal with patients with lower extremity involvement, but for better understanding of the problem as a whole we include hand disabilities in the general introduction.

The discussion of the specific activity "eating a meal while sitting in bed" will make the above approach clearer, and Chart I may serve as an example.

The first column shows the breakdown of the activity into its simplest motions. The second column shows examples of exercises to be practiced so that the motions can be accomplished. The third column shows examples of preparatory exercises, if the patient for some reason or other is not ready for the exercise itself.

The above analysis of the motions is in the natural sequence of the A.D.L. itself. The sequence to be practiced with the patient will depend entirely on what he is able to do. It will be best to let him start with the parts of the A.D.L. he can do and then gradually teach him the parts he cannot do. For example, he may be able to put food into his mouth only when it is put on a spoon for him, or he may be able to maintain his balance in sitting before he has learned to come to a sitting position by himself.

Since the goal is to teach him a given A.D.L., the starting point should be selected according to his condition and in such a way that he will feel that although the task is difficult it is not altogether impossible.

In the program described here the term "exercises" is used as long as motions as such are practiced, *e.g.*, sitting up or grasping eating utensils. Once the patient combines motions in a real-life situation, *e.g.*, sits up and actually eats a meal, then the term "A.D.L." is used. It must be remembered that this differentiation is artificial and serves only for the purpose of simplification.

* Adapted from Buchwald, Edith, Functional Training, *Am. Phys. Therapy Rev.*, Vol. 29, No. 11, November, 1949.

† Deaver, George G., and Mary Eleanor Brown, "Physical Demands of Daily Life," Institute for the Crippled and Disabled, New York, 1945.

CHART I—EXAMPLE OF HOW TO SELECT EXERCISES BASED ON THE BASIC MOTIONS OF A GIVEN A.D.L.
Basic Motions and Exercises to Be Considered When Teaching "Eating a Meal while Sitting in Bed"

SIMPLEST MOTIONS OF A.D.L.	EXERCISES (TEACHING THE MOTIONS)	PREPARATORY EXERCISES (IF INDICATED)
1. Changing from supine to sitting position	Sitting up 1. using hands and elbows 2. with help 3. with gadgets	Rolling over, strengthening of arms
2. Maintaining balance while sitting, with and without arm movements	Exercises for sitting balance, with back supported and unsupported	Strengthening of shoulder girdle, back muscles, abdominal muscles
3. Grasping and holding eating utensils	Grasping and holding spoon, fork, knife. Wooden spools or rubber handles may be used at first to make grasping easier	Strengthening of finger and hand muscles Eye-hand coordination (All hand exercises in connection with occupational therapy)
4. Using eating utensils, such as getting food on utensils and cutting	Going through real motions: 1. using regular food 2. using plasticine for learning how to cut	Same as above
5. Putting food into mouth	Movements practiced: 1. putting utensil in mouth without food 2. putting utensil in mouth with food	Same as above
6. Chewing and swallowing	Specific exercises in connection with speech therapy	

CHART II—MOTIONS AND PROBLEMS INVOLVED IN TEACHING "EATING A MEAL WHILE SITTING IN BED" (ACCORDING TO DISABILITY)*

I. PARAPLEGIA: involvement of both lower extremities with or without abdominal muscles (poliomyelitis, spinal cord lesions, etc.). Motions 1 and 2 have to be learned

II. HEMIPLEGIA: involvement of upper and lower extremity on the same side, with or without aphasia (cerebral hemorrhage, cerebral palsy, etc.)
- A. Probably motions 1–6 have to be learned
- B. Two-handed activities must be performed with one hand
- C. The problem of aphasia has to be considered

III. QUADRIPLEGIA: involvement of all four extremities with or without abdominal or back muscles (poliomyelitis, spinal cord lesions, etc.)
- A. Probably motions 1–5 have to be learned
- B. Special problem: hand and finger activities, use of special gadgets

IV. AMPUTATION: Loss of one or more extremities
- A. Motions 1 and 2 must be learned for double amputation above the knee, and motions 3–5 for single or double amputation of the hand or entire arm
- B. Special problem: management of artificial limb(s); if stump(s) is too short for prostheses, use of special gadgets may have to be considered

V. MISCELLANEOUS DISABILITIES resulting from arthritis, poliomyelitis, cerebral palsy, multiple sclerosis, Parkinson's disease, etc., with one or more special problems such as deformity, extreme incoordination, loss of sensation, loss of strength, severe spasticity, severe tremor, and rigidity
- A. Probably motions 1–5 will have to be learned
- B. Special problems: use of gadgets, hand-eye coordination, relaxation, etc.

* See Chart I for motions referred to.

It cannot be stressed often enough that there are no rigid rules. The principle is to test the patient for what he can do, observe him carefully, and then work out with him the methods that will be the easiest (best) for him and also show him what other patients in similar conditions have found helpful.

There are also no rigid rules in regard to different disabilities when teaching A.D.L. Consideration must be given, in general, to (*a*) the motions that in all probability a patient with a certain disability may have to learn and (*b*) the specific problems connected with his disability. Specific problems vary according to the degree of disability.

Keeping Chart I in mind, the teaching of "eating a meal while sitting in bed," to persons with different disabilities, is considered. Chart II may serve as an outline to show in general what motions may have to be learned and what problems are to be considered.

If patients are classified as follows: (*a*) bed patients, (*b*) wheel-chair patients, and (*c*) ambulatory patients, it may be seen that A.D.L. involve different problems for the different levels. The motions necessary for "eating a meal while sitting in bed" were shown on Chart I. For a wheel-chair patient, "eating a meal sitting in a wheel chair at a table" will involve

1. Getting dressed (which again includes getting washed, etc., first)
2. Getting out of bed into a wheel chair
3. Propelling the wheel chair to the table (with maintenance of balance in the wheel chair)
4. Necessary motions for eating

For an *ambulatory* patient the problem again is different. "*Eating a meal sitting at a table (using crutches, canes, etc.)*" will involve

1. Walking (which again involves getting dressed, getting out of bed)
2. Sitting down in a chair at a table
   a. At home
   b. In a cafeteria or restaurant (which involves traveling to get there)

On the basis of the above examples, it may be said that a given A.D.L. for a given group of patients (bed, wheel-chair, or ambulatory) is the sum total not only of all the motions of the specific activ-

---

CHART III—ACTIVITIES OF DAILY LIVING: GENERAL CLASSIFICATION

I. SELF-CARE
  A. Toilet activities
    1. Hygiene: washing, bathing, care of teeth, etc.
    2. Appearance: care of hair, make-up or shaving, etc.
    3. Problems of elimination: bowel and bladder training, attending to toilet needs, etc.
  B. Dressing activities
  C. Eating activities
II. AMBULATION, ELEVATION, AND TRAVELING
  A. Getting from place to place—using wheel chair
    1. Indoors
    2. Outdoors (assistance will be needed for curbs, steps, etc.)
    3. Using a transportation medium (car)
  B. Walking—with or without appliances (crutches, prostheses, etc.)
    1. Indoors
    2. Outdoors (including crossing street)
  C. Using a transportation medium (car, bus, etc.)
  D. Elevation
    1. From sitting to standing position (getting in and out of bed, chair, etc.)
    2. Climbing (curbs, stairs, etc.)
III. HAND ACTIVITIES
  A. Communication, e.g., signal light, pressing bell button, writing, using telephone, etc.
  B. Management of buttons, zippers, shoelaces, etc.
  C. Handling of furniture and gadgets, e.g., drawers, faucets, keys, etc.

Note: In cases of speech disturbance, *Speech Therapy* may be added to the above.

CHART IV—OUTLINE OF EXERCISES FOR TEACHING A.D.L.

I. EXERCISES WITHOUT APPLIANCES—basis for A.D.L. in bed and wheel chair
- A. Moving about supine in bed, or on mat
- B. Coming to a sitting position in bed, or on mat
- C. Sitting balance: exercises (in bed, in wheel chair, on mat) for maintaining balance with or without arm and–or trunk movements
- D. Push-ups in bed, in wheel chair, on mat
- E. Moving about while sitting in bed, on mat
- F. Moving from place to place using wheel chair
  - 1. Managing wheel chair
  - 2. Getting from wheel chair to bed, chairs, toilet, tub, etc., and back
- G. Moving on hands and knees on mat

II. AMBULATION EXERCISES with appliances and without appliances—basis for A.D.L. involving walking
- A. Preparation for walking
  - 1. Management of braces (putting on, taking off, caring for, locking, unlocking) in bed, in wheel chair, on mat
  - 2. Precrutch exercises in parallel bars
    - a. Balancing
    - b. Push-ups
    - c. Walking
    - d. With crutches or canes
  - 3. Crutch-balancing exercises
    - a. Against wall
    - b. Away from wall
    - c. Rhythm exercises
- B. Crutch-walking exercises
  - 1. Gaits
  - 2. In different directions and through doors
  - 3. Over obstacles
  - 4. On different floor coverings
  - 5. Walking for endurance
  - 6. Walking for speed
  - 7. Outdoors on smooth and rough surface
- C. Elevation exercises
  - 1. From sitting to standing position and reverse:
    - a. Getting up and down from wheel chair (in parallel bars, against wall, away from wall, at table)
    - b. Getting up and down from different pieces of furniture
    - c. Getting in and out of car, up and down from floor, etc.
  - 2. Climbing exercises: graduated and standard ramps, curbs, steps, bus steps

---

ity but also of everything that was learned on the preceding level.

The approach used in teaching one activity can be applied to all activities, as will be clear from the following discussion of the total functional training program. Chart III gives the main groups of the A.D.L. and all the subdivisions of these groups to be considered.

If all A.D.L. (Chart III) are analyzed according to the same principle used in analyzing "eating a meal while sitting in bed," it will be seen that there are groups of motions basic to all A.D.L. and that these motions in turn become the exercises that are shown in Chart IV.

It should be repeated at this point that the division into A.D.L. and exercises is artificial and is made solely for classification purposes.

Summary: To simplify the very complex problem, the entire functional activity program is divided as follows:

1. A.D.L. for bed patients and the necessary bed exercises.
2. A.D.L. for wheel-chair and ambulatory patients and the necessary wheel-chair and mat exercises.
3. Ambulation, elevation, and traveling activities and the necessary exercises.

Each group of exercises is selected to teach the daily activities belonging to the respective group, and unless the patient is able to perform the exercises (motions) in a given group he will not be ready to perform the A.D.L. in this group. Under most circumstances he should not be taught A.D.L. or exercises of a particular group before he has mastered the preparatory activities.

For example: (*a*) a patient should not be permitted to stand up in his braces until he has already learned how to maintain his balance in the sitting position, or (*b*) he should not be taught how to walk with crutches unless he has been taught all crutch-balancing exercises.

For further simplification we classify the patients as follows: (*a*) bed patients, (*b*) wheel-chair patients, and (*c*) ambulatory patients.

A.D.L. are important on every level. It is of course desirable to regard each level as the preparatory stage for the following level, but it is also desirable to make every patient as independent as possible at his particular stage. For example, wheel-chair patients should be able to travel in a car in order to get to their job, so that they can work even though walking cannot be taught for some reason or other. In any case the elimination of lifting the patient and the use of the wheel chair will form the basis for independence.

Outlines for a functional training program for bed, wheel-chair, and ambulatory patients are shown in Charts V, VI, and VII. Only the most basic exercises and activities are included, and it is hoped that this basis may serve as a guide in building up a rich and flexible program. It is necessary to adapt the basic program to the particular problems of specific disabilities (see Chart II).

Although a patient may have normal upper extremities, hand activities as a part of daily life must be considered; *e.g.*, in using the telephone, the problem is not *how* to use the hands, but where to

CHART V—OUTLINE OF FUNCTIONAL TRAINING PROGRAM FOR BED PATIENTS

A.D.L. IN BED

I. SELF-CARE
  A. Toilet Activities
    1. Hygiene
      a. Washing and drying: face, hands, arms, body and back, legs and feet
      b. Care of the skin
      c. Oral hygiene
    2. Appearance
      a. Care of hair and nails
      b. Shaving or make-up
    3. Toilet needs
      a. Using the bedpan
      b. Using the urinal
      c. Using toilet paper
      d. Adjusting clothing
      e. Bowel and bladder training
  B. Dressing Activities
    1. Two-piece pajamas
    2. Nightgown
    3. Special pants and pads
  C. Eating Activities. Sitting up and eating a meal
II. HAND ACTIVITIES
  A. Pressing bell button or pulling signal cord
  B. Turning light on and off
  C. Using telephone and radio

EXERCISES IN BED

1. Rolling over
2. Moving sideward—supine
3. Sitting up
4. Sitting balance
  a. Back supported
  b. Back unsupported
5. Push-ups in sitting
6. Moving forward and backward while sitting
7. Placing legs over edge of bed while sitting

Note: The numbers in the two columns have no relationship to each other.

place the telephone, so that a patient in bed, in the wheel chair, or on crutches can reach it.

It should not be forgotten that the primary goal is the teaching of A.D.L., and the exercises serve only as a means to this end. Finally it is important to remember that A.D.L. are always more than the sum of their motions and have to be practiced as a whole in a real-life situation, so that they may truly become the foundation for a maximum of independence of the patient.

Outline of Exercises and Activities

The exercises and activities are described in outline form. To make the description as brief and practical as possible, simple everyday language is used, rather than technical language.

The outline is as follows:

Title: to identify exercise or activity.

Purpose: to explain why an exercise or activity is done. If the purpose is obvious, as in "getting up and down curbs," it will be omitted.

Preparation for: to indicate specific activities for which the exercise is essential.

Preliminary exercises: to list the most essential exercises for a given movement.

Equipment: to list necessary equipment. Special equipment will be shown in brackets. Full description of a given piece of equipment will be found under "Equipment" in Chapter VII.

Starting Position: to describe the exact position from which the exercise or activity is begun. If necessary there will be a picture on the opposite page with the title "Starting Position." This will be indicated in the text with the abbreviation S.P.

Instructions: to give concise directions as to performance of the exercise or activity. Whenever necessary the text will be supplemented with a picture on the opposite page. This will be indicated in the text by a number corresponding to that of the picture.
The starting position as well as the instructions will be directed to the patient, in order to serve as a guide for the therapist in giving directions for the exercises.

Precautions: to highlight the difficult phases (with or without illustrations).

Helpful remarks: will be added if necessary (with or without illustrations).

Variations: of activity or exercises will be added if practical (with or without illustrations).

The exercises and activities are described to the patient's right or left, as shown in the pictures. The opposite directions can easily be worked out by the therapist and the patient. Whenever the procedure can be reversed completely, it will be so indicated and then the pictures can be read in reverse sequence.

Frequency and length of time are not discussed, since they will vary according to the doctor's prescription.

CHAPTER II

Bed and Mat Exercises

The purpose of the bed and mat exercises is to develop strength, mobility, and balance, to enable the patient to perform the necessary motions for self-care activities in bed and in the wheel chair, and to prepare him for crutch walking.

The exercises are outlined in order of difficulty from a maximum of support to a minimum of support. They proceed from the supine position to sitting with back supported, then unsupported, to exercises on hands and knees, so that finally the patient is ready for standing and walking.

Although the goal is complete independence for the patient, in the beginning the therapist should always be *ready* to support him if necessary. Support should be given around the waist. The patient should be taught to support himself on his arms whenever he loses his balance; the therapist, therefore, should avoid grasping his arm. This applies also to crutch walking.

Throughout the exercises "pushing on hands" is stressed, since a patient with involvement of the lower extremities will need this particular motion to move about in bed, to transfer to the wheel chair, and to walk on crutches. If the patient cannot *push*, a device may be used to provide better leverage. In the beginning many patients will *pull*, using parts of the furniture or ropes. The more their strength increases, the more the pulling will be replaced by pushing. The following outline includes 10 basic exercises. The therapist may vary and add to the exercises according to the condition of the patient.

Exercises 1 to 6 can be done in bed as well as on the mat. It is better to exercise on the mat for the following reasons: (*a*) the mat provides a more stable surface than the mattress, (*b*) psychologically it is helpful for the patient to get out of bed as early as permitted by the doctor.

Precautions: In the presence of pressure sores on the lower back or buttocks the patient is not allowed to lie on his back or to sit up, but is permitted to stand and walk. In this instance standing and walking activities may be taught before activities that involve lying on the back and sitting.

1. **Rolling over,** on bed or mat (Fig. 1).
2. **Moving sideward—supine,** on bed or mat (Fig. 2). These first two exercises are essential for changing position in bed, a very important factor in preventing pressure sores. They are also the first step in learning to move about.
3. **Sitting up.** Sitting up is the basic motion for nearly all self-care activities, in bed as well as in the wheel chair. Four different methods are shown.
   a. **Sitting up—pushing on hands,** on bed or mat (Fig. 3A). This aids in strengthening the "crutch-walking" muscles.
   b. **Sitting up—placing legs over edge of bed first** (Fig. 3B). Patients with spastic lower extremities must place their legs over the edge of the bed, in order to release their tight hamstrings, before sitting up.
   c. **Sitting up—holding on, for flaccid lower extremities,** on bed or mat (Fig. 3C). Some patients have to pull themselves into a sitting position by holding on to ropes, etc.
   d. **Sitting up—by holding on to two ropes, for spastic lower extremities,** on bed (Fig. 3D). The legs are placed over the edge of the bed before the patient pulls himself into a sitting position.
4. **Sitting balance,** on bed or mat. Once the patient has learned to sit up, he must learn to balance in the sitting position while moving his arms and trunk, with his back supported as well as unsupported.
   a. **Sitting balance—starting positions** (Fig. 4A).
   b. **Sitting balance—back supported** (Fig. 4B).
   c. **Sitting balance—back unsupported** (Fig. 4C).
5. **Push-ups in sitting,** on bed or mat (Fig. 5).
6. **Moving forward and backward while sitting,** on bed or mat (Fig. 6). These exercises are most important because the patient will use these motions in almost all A.D.L., in bed and in the wheel chair, as well as on crutches.

7. **Placing legs over edge of bed—while sitting** (Fig. 7). This exercise is helpful in learning sitting balance while handling the lower extremities.

Exercises 1 to 7 (in bed) comprise the basic movements for transfer from the bed to the wheel chair and back (see "Self-care," p. 42).

8. **Balancing on hands and knees,** on mat (Fig. 8). Balancing in the four-legged position is a step toward standing balance.
9. **Crawling,** on mat (Fig. 9).
10. **Raising arms alternately in a four-legged position,** on mat (Fig. 10). These exercises are an aid in relearning reciprocal motion patterns for walking as well as for balance.

Fig. 1. ROLLING OVER

Purpose: to move from place to place in bed in order to facilitate making bed; to change position in order to prevent pressure sores; to increase mobility.
Preparation for: sitting up; dressing and toilet activities; getting in and out of bed.
Equipment: bed or mat (side railing).

Starting Position: Lie on back, arms at sides, knees extended if possible. Do not lie too near edge.
Instructions: Roll to left.
1. Turn body to left until you lie on left side.
2. Using arms if necessary roll...
3. ...over on to abdomen.
4. Push down on right hand and roll back to left side...
5. ...returning to starting position.

Repeat complete exercise to the right.

Precautions: Therapist should be ready to catch patient but should help only if necessary. Care must be taken of pressure sores, and sharp corners on bed or night table must be avoided.
Helpful remarks:
1, 2. Rolling over will be facilitated by grasping mattress or holding on to head of bed.
Sometimes it is helpful to have therapist cross patient's legs before patient starts to roll.
6. A side railing can be attached to either or both sides of bed so that patient can practice by himself, every hour on the hour, without any help, since all danger of falling out of bed is eliminated.
Variations: Exercise can be done on mat and repeated to each side for entire length of mat.

Fig. 1. ROLLING OVER

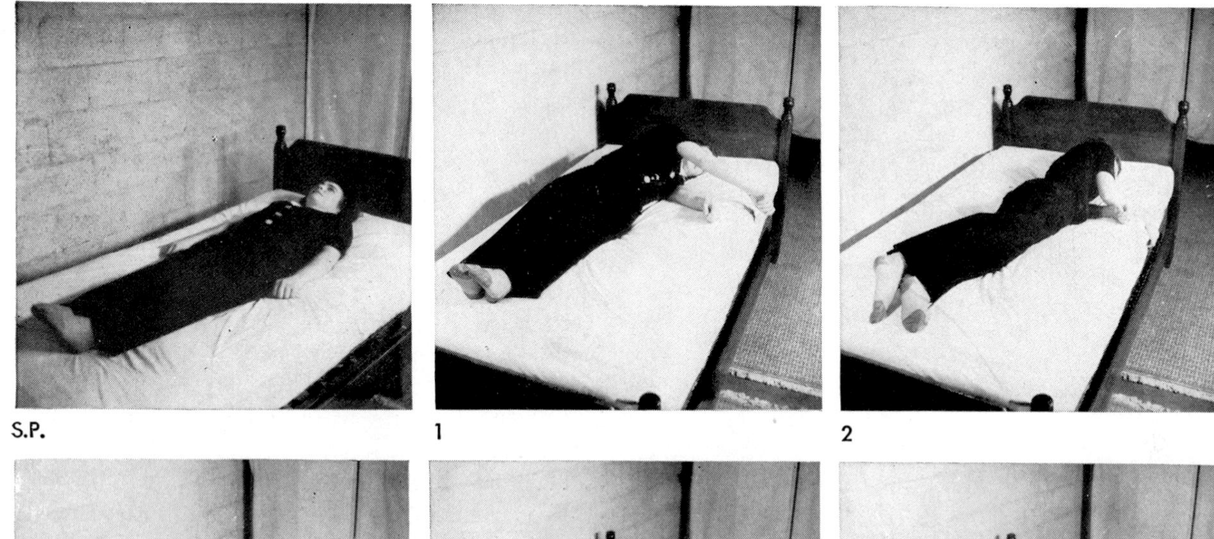

S.P. 1 2

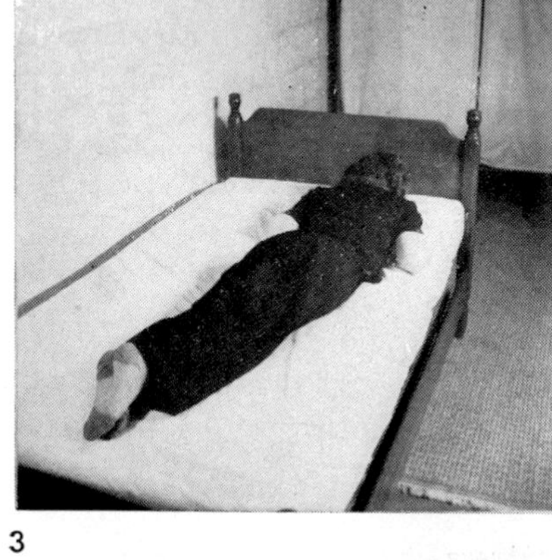

3

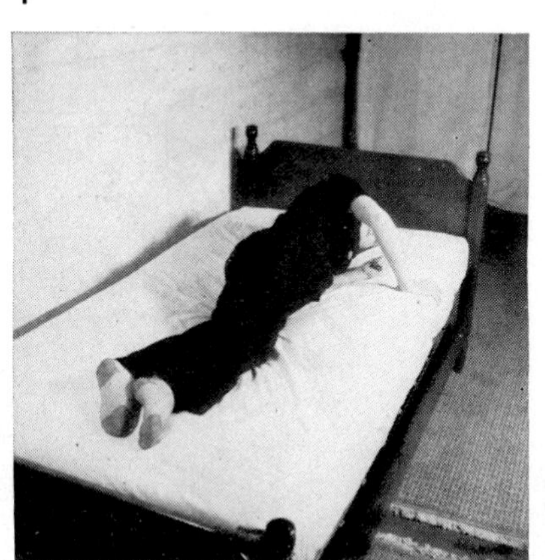

4

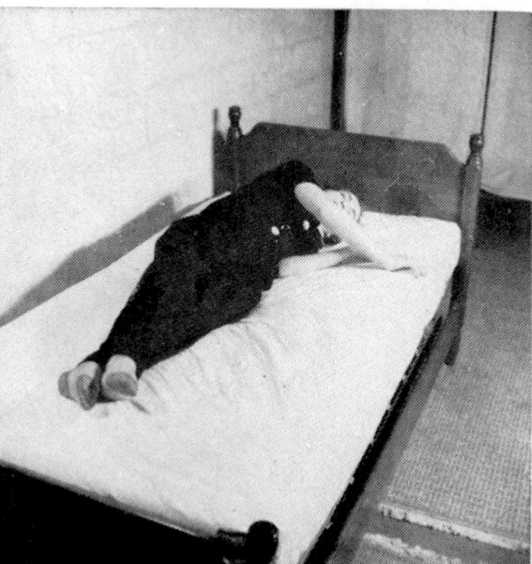

5

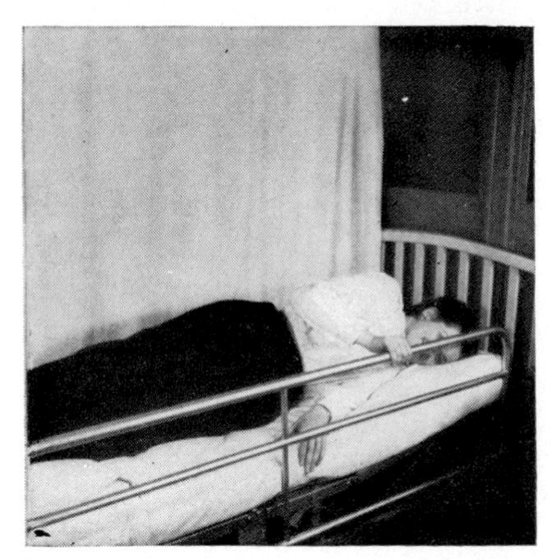

6

Fig. 2. MOVING SIDEWARD—supine

Purpose: to move from place to place in bed to facilitate making bed; to increase mobility; to handle lower extremities.
Preparation for: sitting up; sitting with legs over edge of bed; dressing and toilet activities; getting in and out of bed; handling of braces.
Preliminary exercises: rolling over.
Equipment: bed or mat.

Starting Position: Lie on back, arms at sides, knees extended if possible.
Instructions: Move toward left.
1. Move head and shoulder to left.
2. Use hands if necessary to move hips in line with...
3. ...head and shoulders.
4. Use arms and hands if necessary to move lower extremities into line with head and trunk. First left leg...
5. ...then right leg until you are straight.

Repeat complete exercise to right.

Precautions: Therapist should be ready to catch patient but should help only if necessary. Care should be taken of sharp corners on bed, wall, or night table.
Helpful remarks:
1, 2. Grasping mattress or head of bed will help to move body sideward.
4, 5. Moving legs sideward will be aided by rolling back and forth.
If only one leg is affected, the stronger one may be used to push or lift the weakened leg sideward.
A side railing may be attached to either or both sides of bed so that patient can practice by himself, every hour on the hour, without any help, since danger of falling out of bed is eliminated. (See Fig. 1·6 and repeat to each side.)
Variations: The exercise can be done on mat for entire length of mat.

Fig. 2. MOVING SIDEWARD—supine

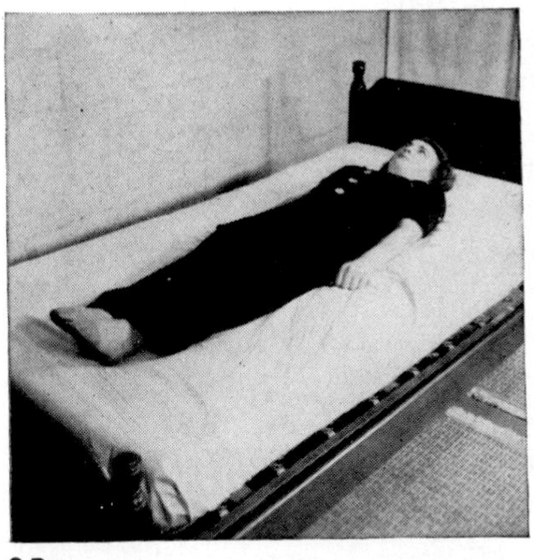

S.P.

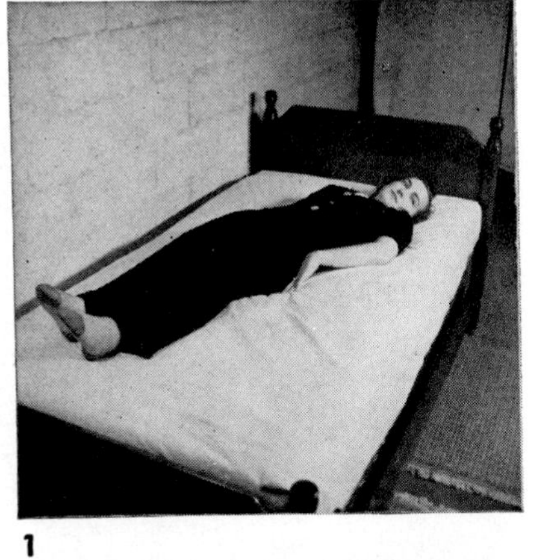

1

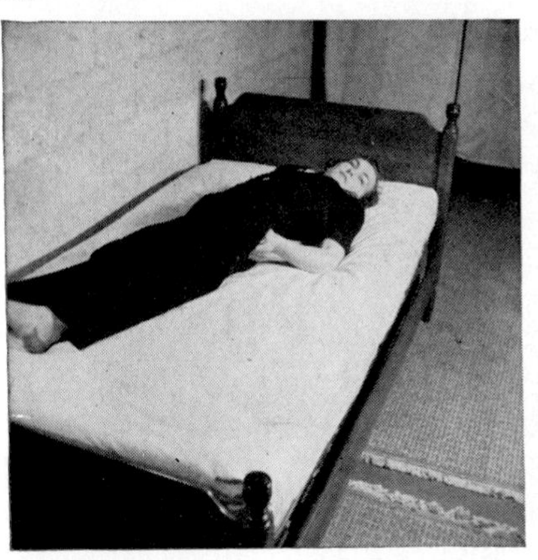

2

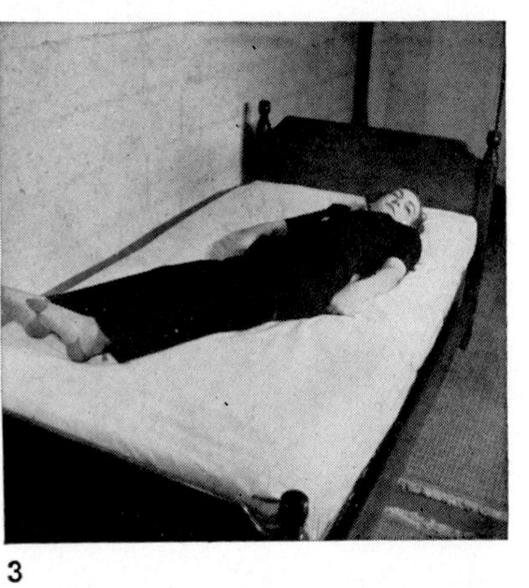

3

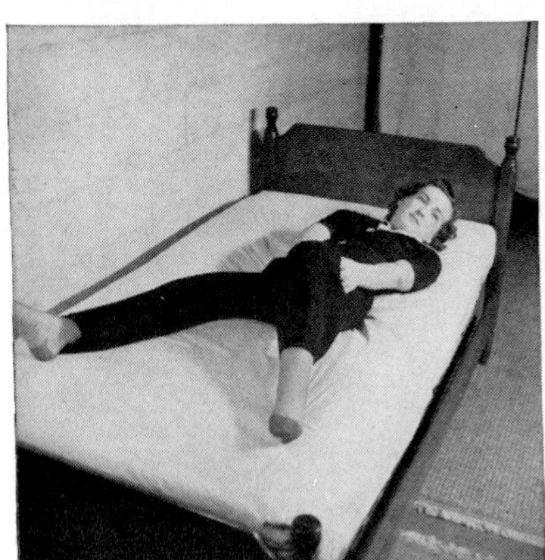

4

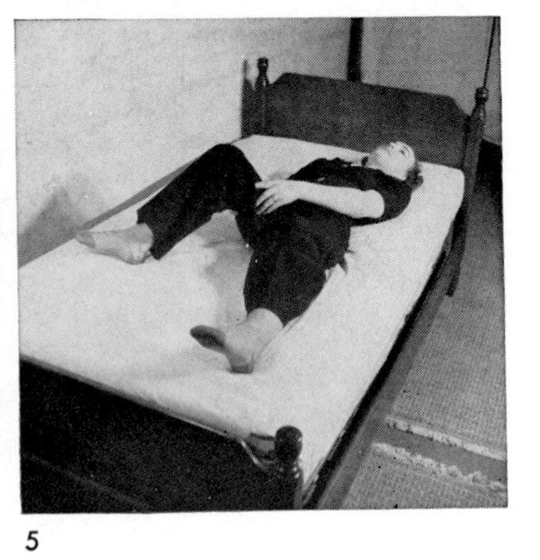

5

Fig. 3A. SITTING UP—pushing on hands

It is extremely important to emphasize "pushing" on hands at all times, since the ability to push up is essential for all A.D.L. as well as crutch walking. This method is the easiest one for patients with flaccid lower extremities.

Purpose: to sit up without help.

Preparation for: push-ups; all self-care activities in bed.

Preliminary exercises: rolling over.

Equipment: bed or mat (rope, trapeze).

Starting Position: Lie flat on back. Place palms near hips.

Instructions:

1. Lean on elbows, raise head and shoulders.
2. Slide elbows back as far as possible under shoulders and *quickly*...
3. ...push on right hand, extending right elbow.
4. Push on left hand. Extend left elbow, raising body to a sitting position.
5. Take small steps forward with hands. Right hand...
6. ...left hand, until you sit straight.

Lie down: Reverse entire procedure. Take small steps back with your hands. Round back and duck head as you bend elbows slowly in returning to starting position. (Read pictures in reverse sequence.)

Precautions: Patients who have been in bed for a prolonged period of time will get dizzy easily. Therefore, it is important to sit up for only a few minutes at first and to increase the time gradually.

Helpful remarks:

1, 2. It is important to slide elbows as far back as possible, in order to have a better mechanical advantage for pushing on hands.

2, 3, 4. Keeping head ducked forward will ensure balance and prevent falling backward.

Fig. 3A. SITTING UP—pushing on hands

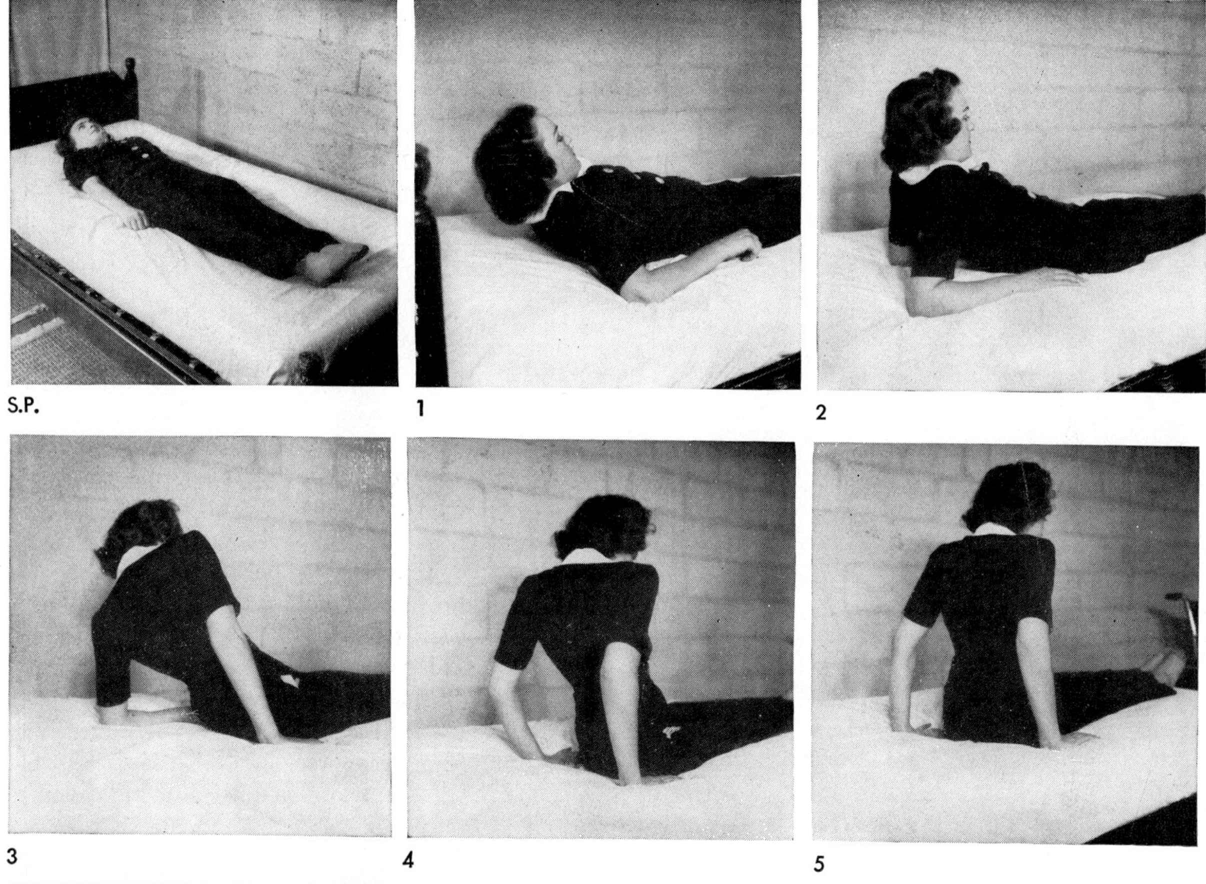

S.P. 1 2

3 4 5

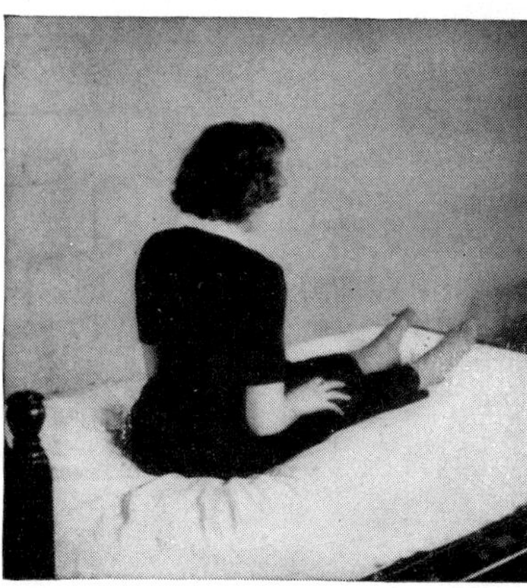

6

Fig. 3B. SITTING UP—placing legs over edge of bed first

If lower extremities are spastic, it will be easier to place legs over edge of bed first and then sit up. Bending the knees will release tight hamstrings. Sitting up by holding on and pulling up to a sitting position can be practiced in the beginning when patient cannot push on hands at all or loses his balance too easily. Gradually, as strength and balance increase, pulling is eliminated and pushing is used exclusively if possible.

Purpose: to sit up without help; to handle lower extremities.

Preparation for: push-ups; handling of braces; transfer from bed to wheel chair and back; dressing activities; toilet activities in bed and wheel chair.

Preliminary exercises: moving sideward—supine.

Equipment: bed.

Starting Position: Lie flat on back in bed.

Instructions:

1. Lean on left elbow, raising head and shoulders. Grasp left leg with both hands and push (or lift) it over...
2. ...edge of bed.
3. Repeat the same procedure with right leg and push (or lift) it over edge of bed next to left leg. Then lean on both elbows and come to a sitting position by pushing on both hands (as in Figure 3A).
4. Adjust legs and body so that you sit straight.

Lie down: Reverse entire procedure. (Read pictures in reverse sequence.)

Precautions: Therapist should stand in front of patient ready to support him when he sits up since patient may be apprehensive, especially after prolonged bed rest. As skill and confidence are gained, a chair may be placed with back rest toward bed, and patient can hold on to back rest for support (Fig. 15·4).

Helpful remarks:

4. Sometimes it will help to hold patient's knees.
5. A rope may be used in the beginning to pull up to a sitting position (Figs. 3C and 3D).

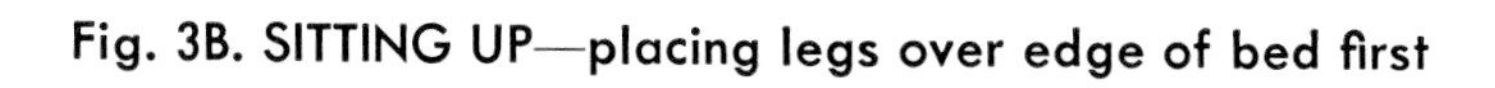

Fig. 3B. SITTING UP—placing legs over edge of bed first

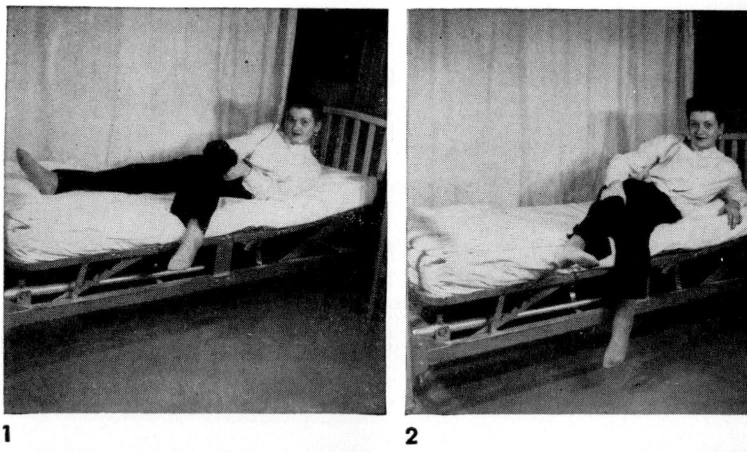

1 2

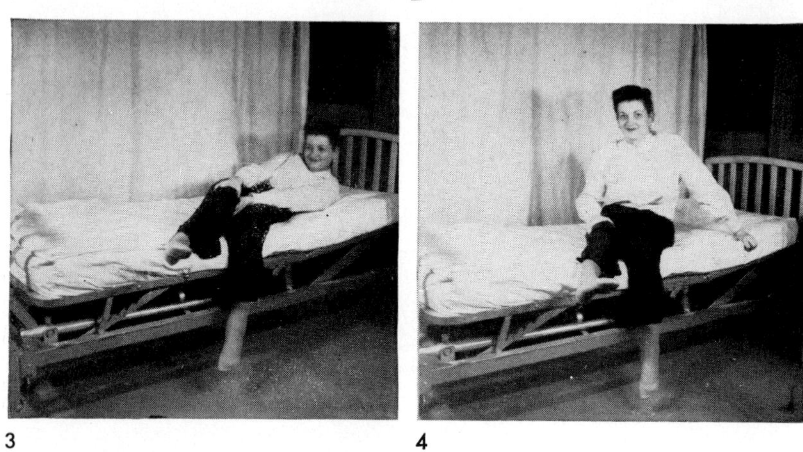

3 4

Holding on to rope attached to foot of bed (for patients who cannot push up yet)

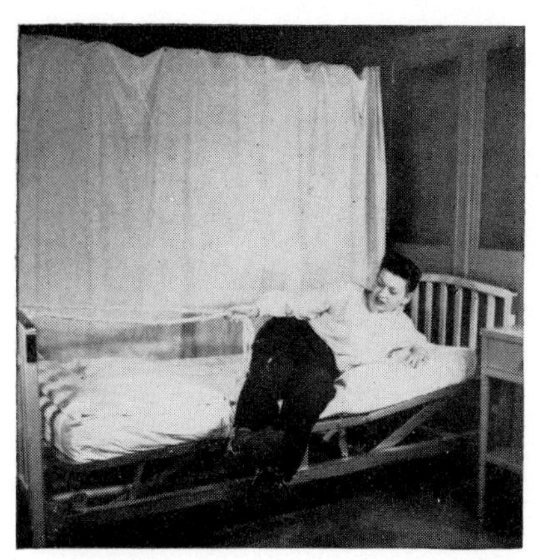

5

Fig. 3C. SITTING UP—holding on

This is for patients with flaccid lower extremities. The patient pulls himself up to a sitting position by

1. Holding on to hands of therapist, or
2. Holding on to trapeze, or

3a, b, c. Holding on to rope which is attached to foot of bed.

Pulling up on hands of therapist and lying down slowly (can also be done on mat)

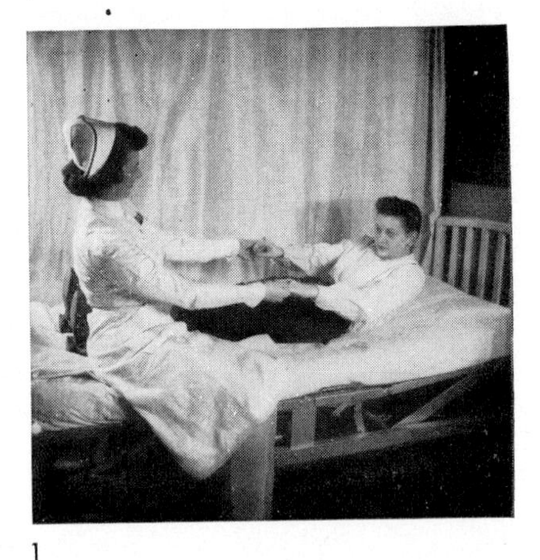

1

Pulling up on trapeze and lying down slowly

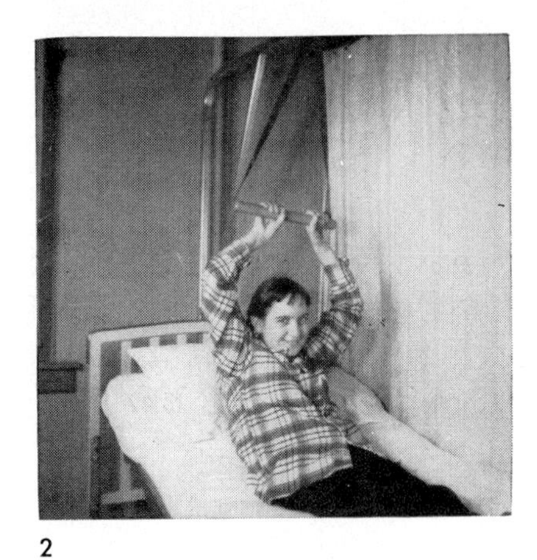

2

Pulling up on rope. (For lying down slowly, read pictures in reverse sequence.)

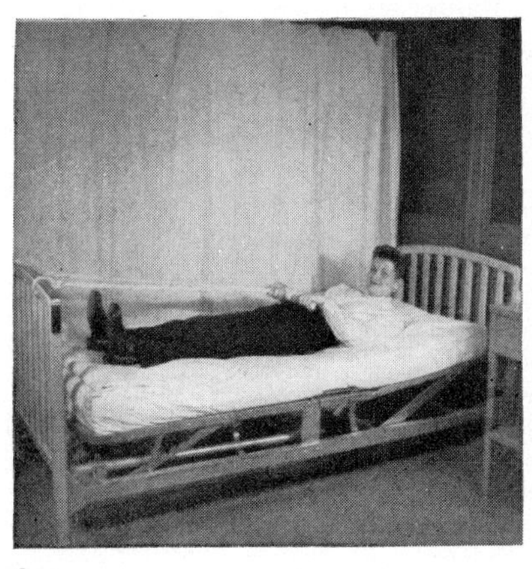

3a

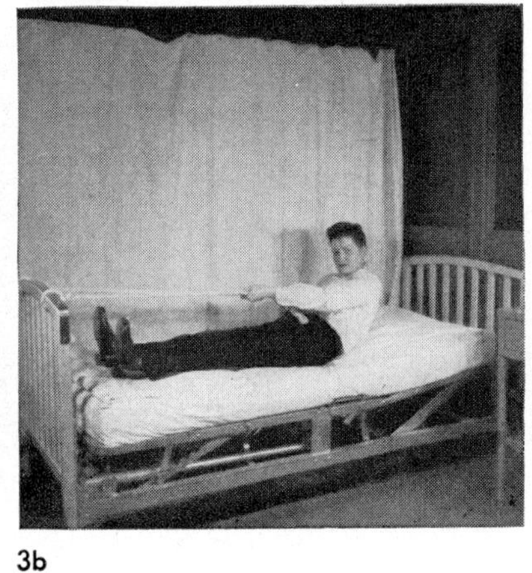

3b

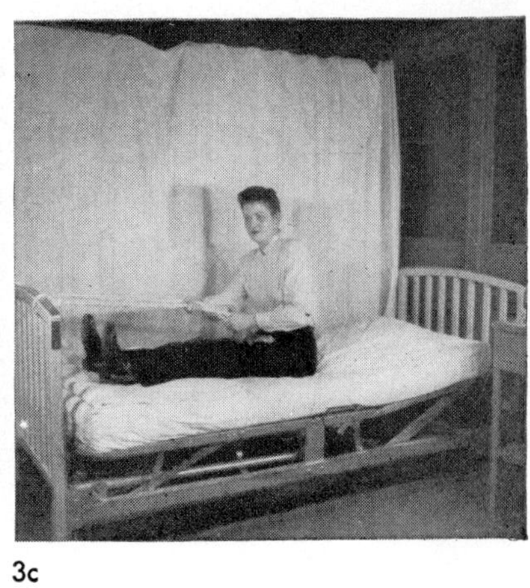

3c

Fig. 3D. SITTING UP—holding on to two ropes

(For lying down, read pictures in reverse sequence.)

This is for patients with spastic lower extremities. The second rope is especially helpful for heavy patients and for those wearing braces when moving body from edge to center of bed. Lying down should be done slowly, rounding back and ducking head. It may also help to

1. Crank up the bed (or place pillows behind back of patient) so that he does not have to push up (or pull up) from a completely flat position, but starts partially raised. As strength and skill increase, bed is cranked down gradually (or pillows eliminated).
2. Roll over before pushing up or pulling up to a sitting position.

If lower extremities are flaccid, both legs are on the bed; if they are spastic, legs are placed over edge of bed first.

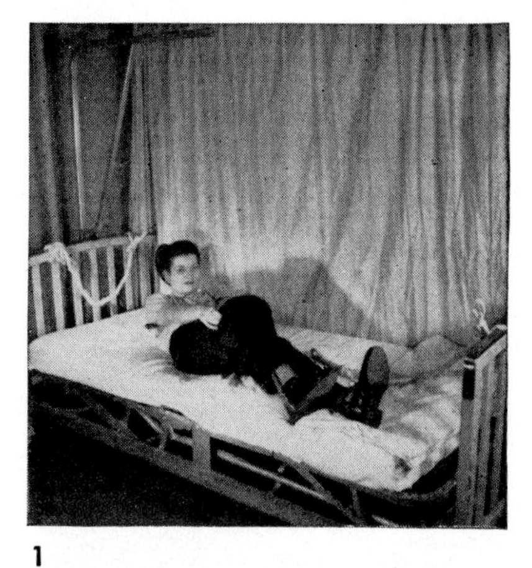

1

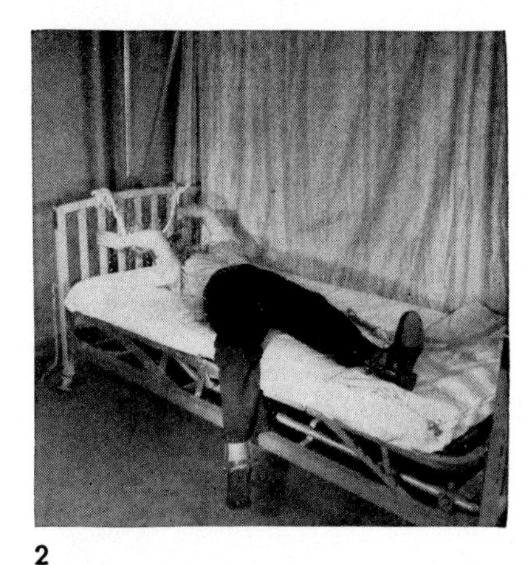

2

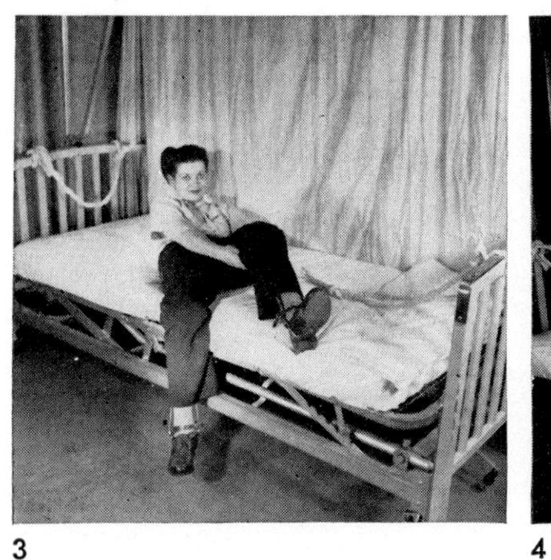

3

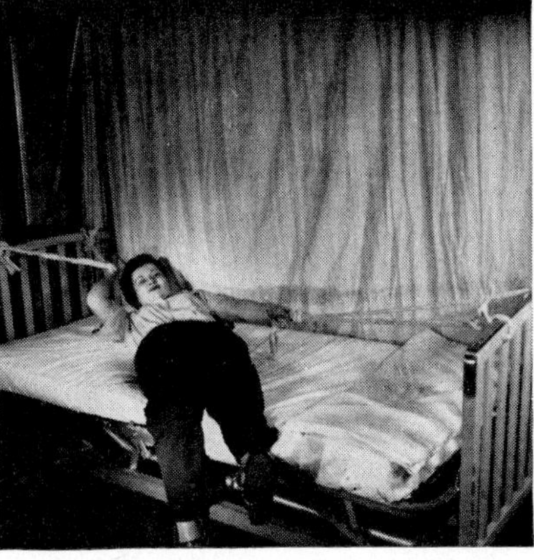

4

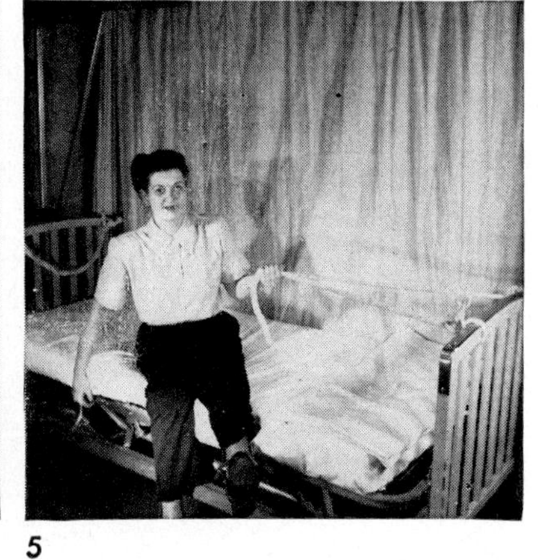

5

Fig. 4A. SITTING BALANCE—starting positions

Purpose: to maintain balance in sitting while moving arms and trunk.
Preparation for: all self-care activities in bed as well as in wheel chair.
Preliminary exercises: sitting up.
Equipment: bed or mat.

Starting Positions:* *Sitting balance with back supported* is practiced first. Back is supported from small of back up to shoulder blades by any of the following methods:
1. Bed is cranked up, or
2. In bed, pillows are placed behind patient's back with (or without) therapist holding arms of patient.
3. On mat, patient leans against the wall, or
4. Therapist kneels behind patient.

As strength and balance increase, *sitting balance with back unsupported* is practiced:
5. In bed or on mat with legs straight.
6. In bed with legs over edge of bed.

* Precaution: Therapist should be ready to support patient when exercises are started, especially for Position 6.

Fig. 4A. SITTING BALANCE—starting positions

Back supported

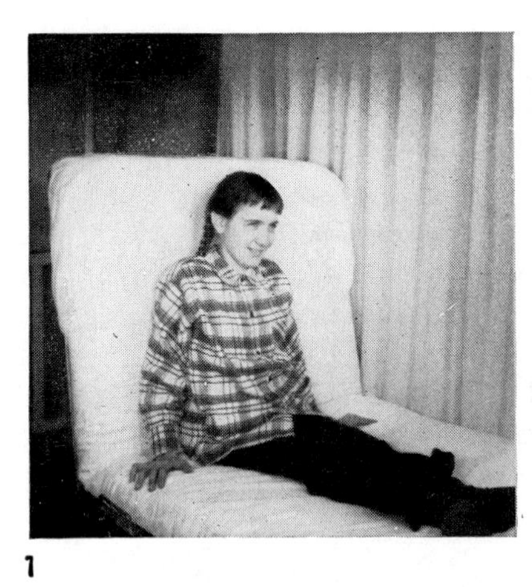

1

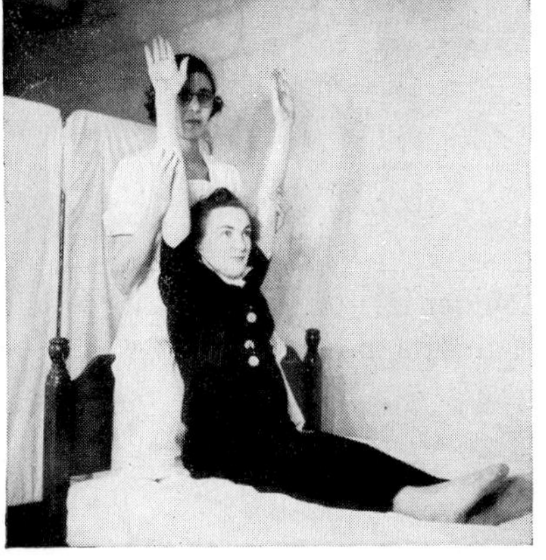

2

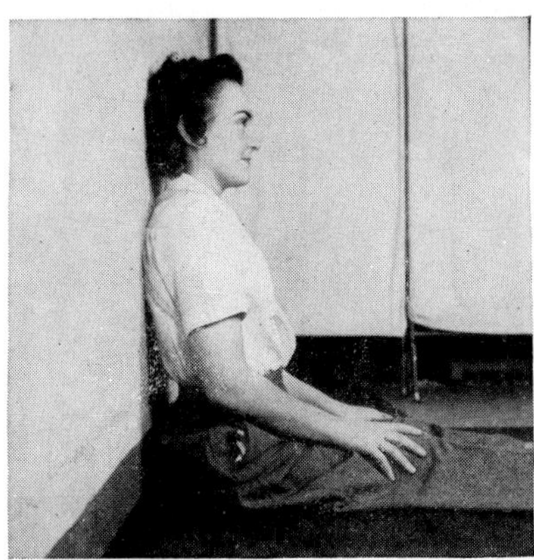

3

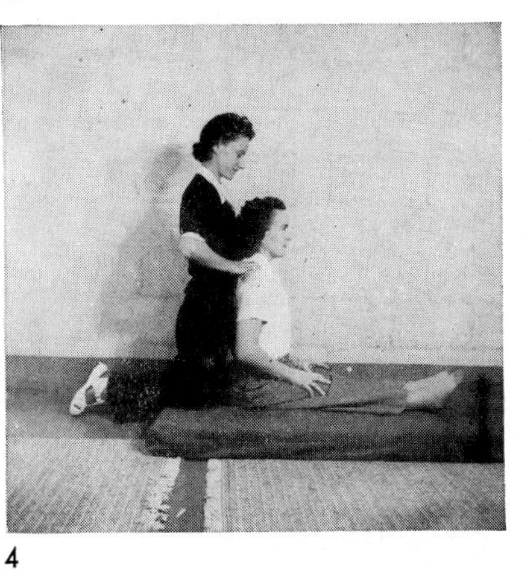

4

Back unsupported

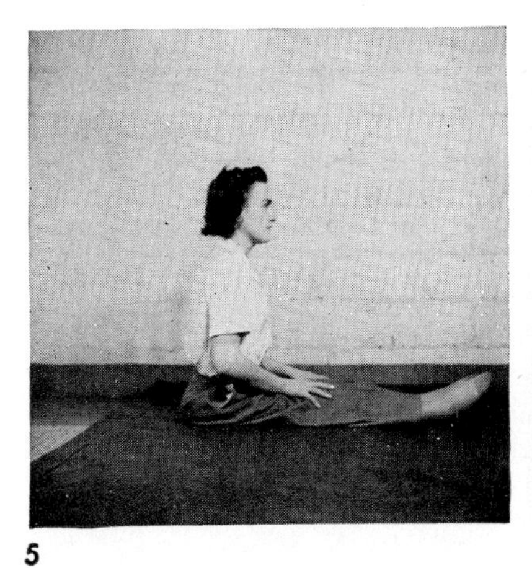

5

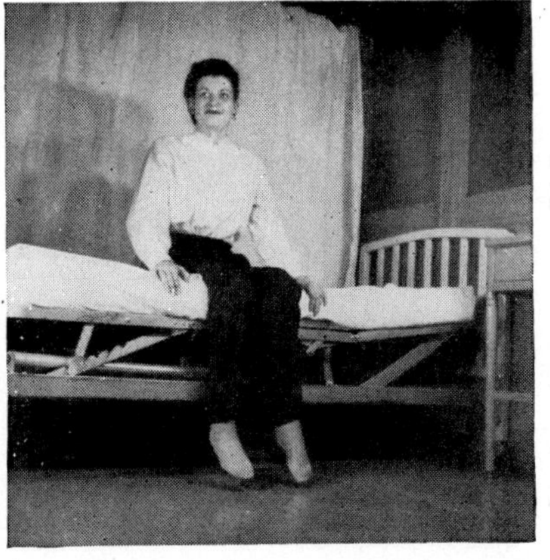

6

Figs. 4B and 4C. SITTING BALANCE—back supported and unsupported

Starting Position: Use any of positions shown in Fig. **4A.** Begin with maximum support and gradually work to minimum or no support.

Instructions: Hold each of following positions 30 seconds and then return to starting position. Do not hunch shoulders at any time.

1a, b. Place hands near hips on mat (or bed).

2a, b, 1c. Raise arms sideward to shoulder level.

3a, b, 2c. Raise arms forward to shoulder level.

4a, b, 3c. Raise arms overhead, close to ears, palms facing each other.

5a, b. Bend forward, hands sliding over thighs, until head is as close to knees as possible.

6a, b. Bend forward until fingers touch toes.

Helpful remarks:

1b, 2b, 3b. If patient has spastic lower extremities, he will not be able to keep his sitting balance with knees straight. He, therefore, has to place his legs over the edge of the bed (to release his hamstrings) and raise his arms sideward, forward, and overhead in this position.

Variations: All movements may be combined with clapping hands. As strength, balance, and confidence develop, number of clappings between movements increases. All sorts of ball games may be played in bed and on mat with back supported as well as unsupported. Catching and throwing a ball (small and big) will involve all essential arm and trunk movements. Children will enjoy this and do more "exercising" while playing.

Fig. 4B. SITTING BALANCE—back supported

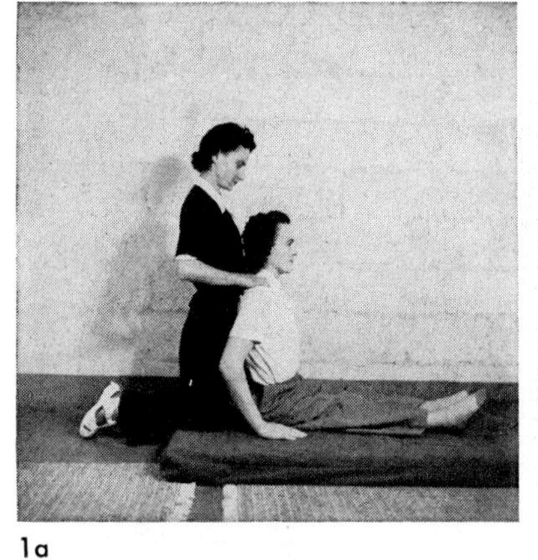

1a

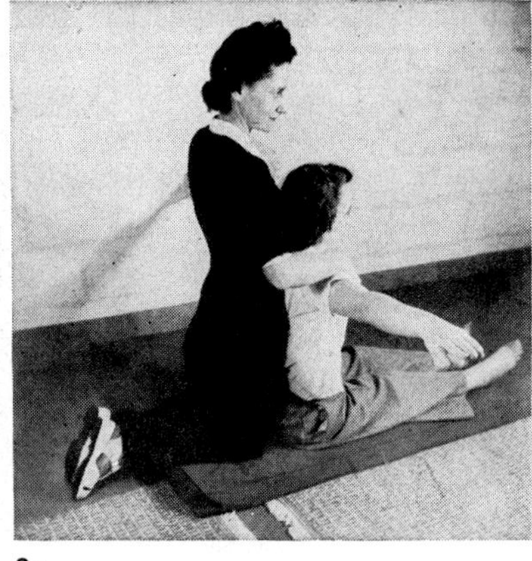

2a

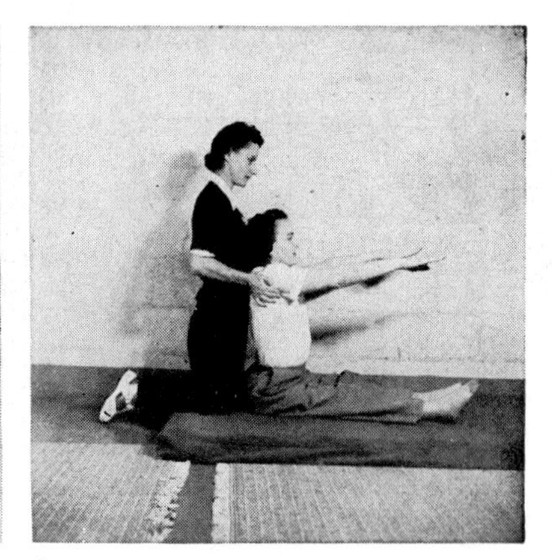

3a

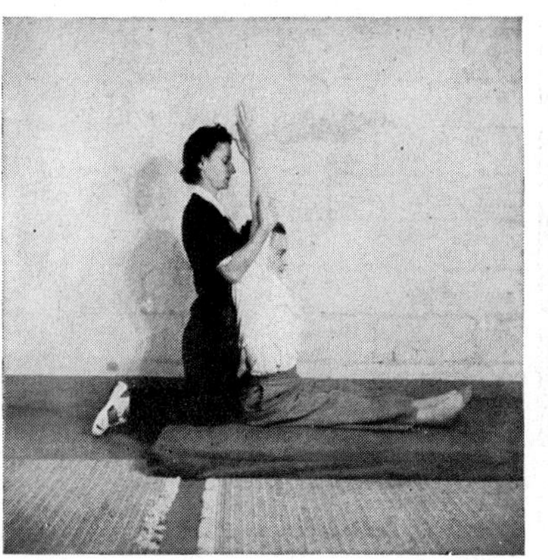

4a

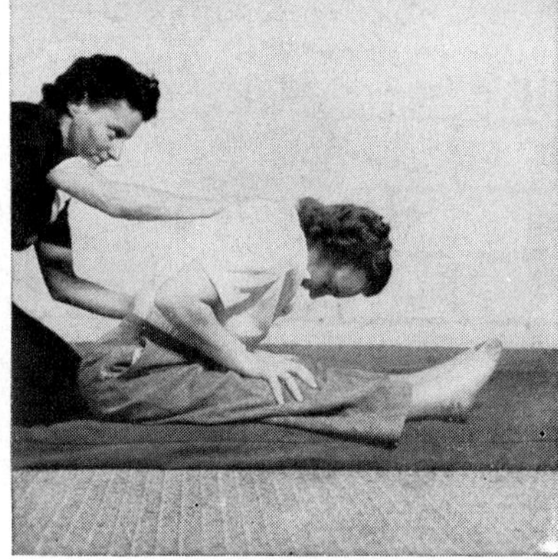

5a

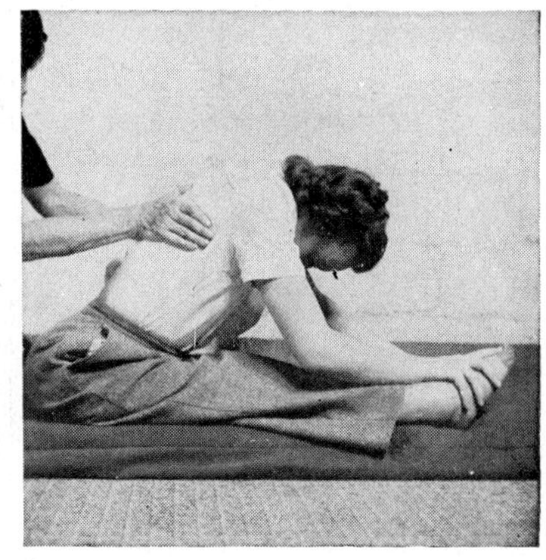

6a

Fig. 4C. SITTING BALANCE—back unsupported

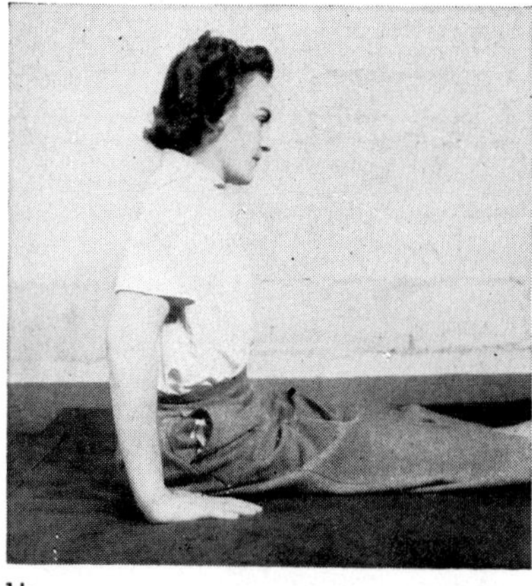

1b

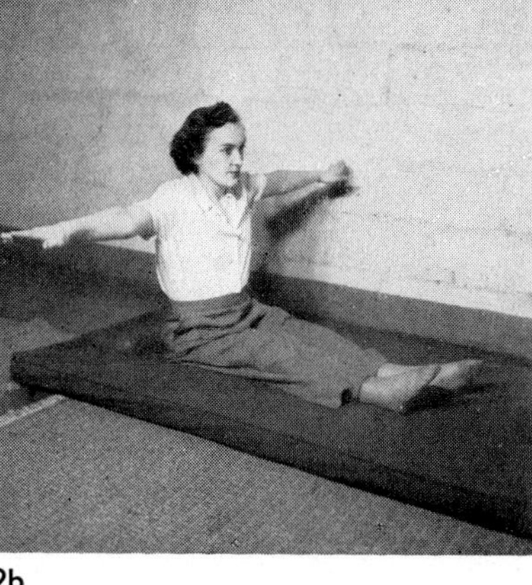

2b

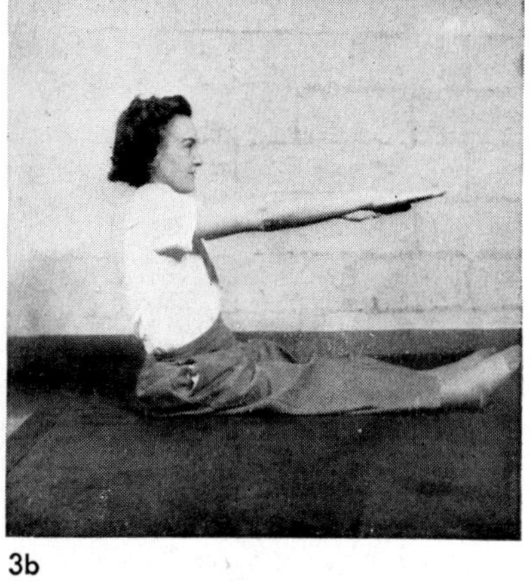

3b

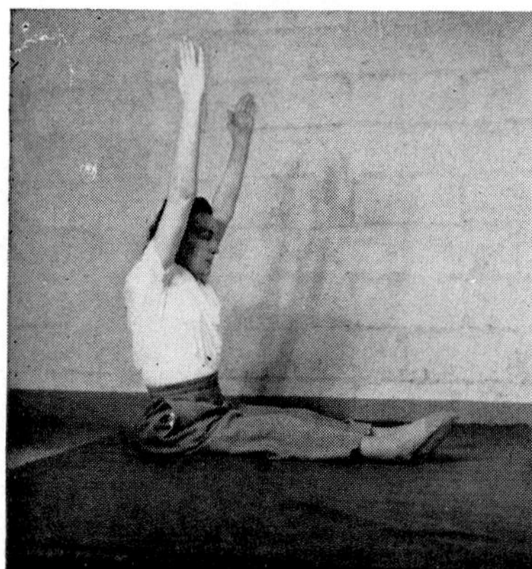

4b

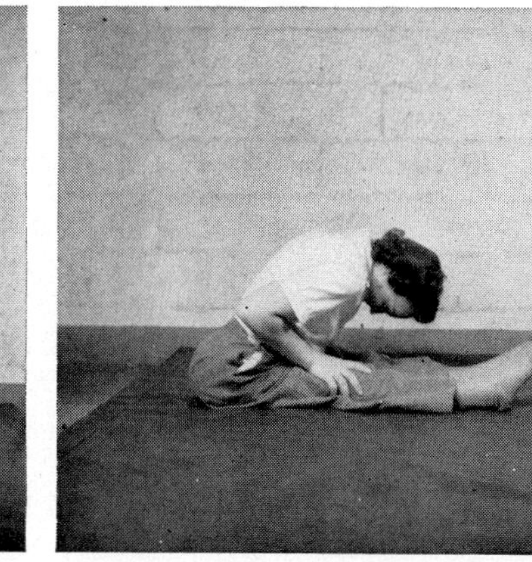

5b

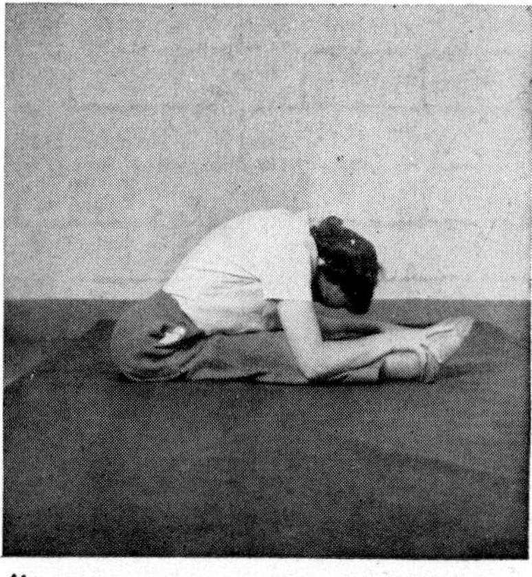

6b

in bed

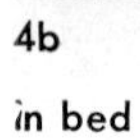

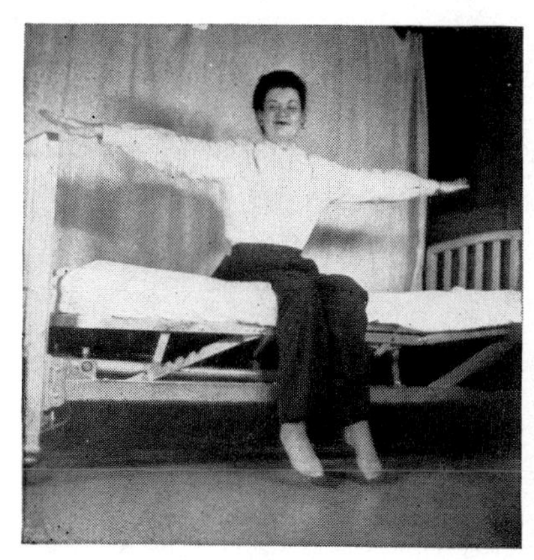

1c

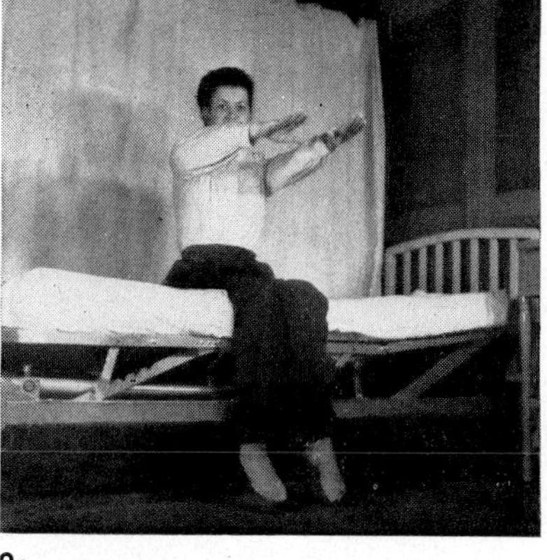

2c

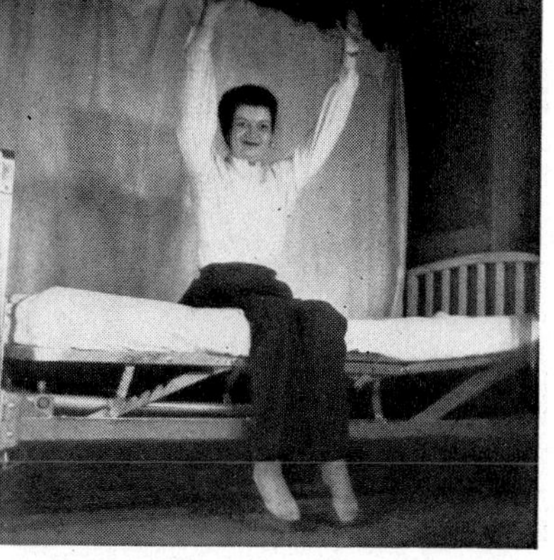

3c

Fig. 5. PUSH-UPS IN SITTING

Purpose: to strengthen arm and shoulder muscles.
Preparation for: all A.D.L. in bed as well as in wheel chair; transfer from wheel chair to bed, chairs, toilet, and car. Most important preparation for crutch walking.
Preliminary exercises: sitting balance.
Equipment: bed, mat (sandbags).

Starting Position: Sit on mat or bed, arms at sides; palms, fists, or fingers down on mat (or bed) near hips. Keep shoulders down. Extend knees if possible.

Instructions:

1. Put all weight on hands, extend elbows until body is off mat. Hold 3 seconds if possible.
2. Lower body by bending elbows slowly.

Precautions: To prevent falling backward, head is bent forward.
Helpful remarks: If there is any difficulty in balancing, hands are placed farther forward. To gain more height and to ensure balance, head is ducked.
1a, b. Small sandbags may be used for better leverage if arms are too short.
If lower extremities are spastic, it will be impossible to push up with knees straight. Therefore, legs have to be placed over edge of bed (Fig. **4A**·6) or push-ups practiced in wheel chair (Fig. **12**).
Variations: As strength develops, one can increase number of push-ups, count for "holding" push-up position, and count for bending elbows.

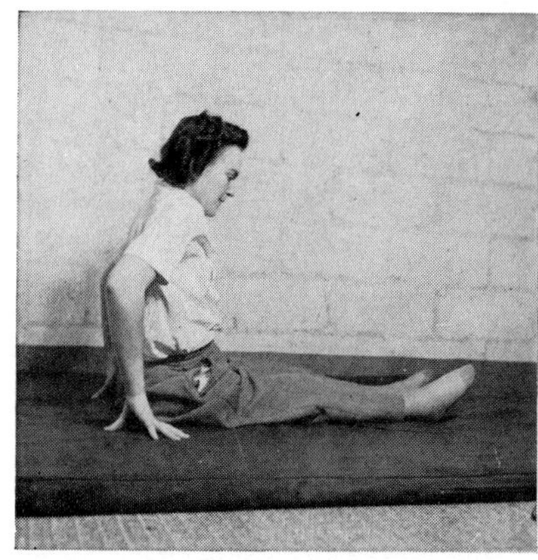

S.P.

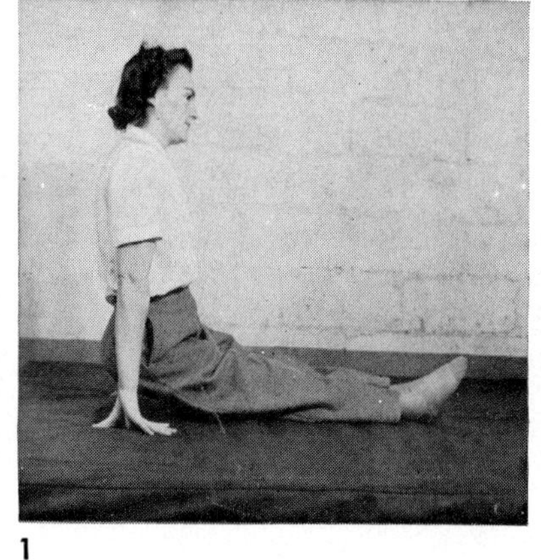

1

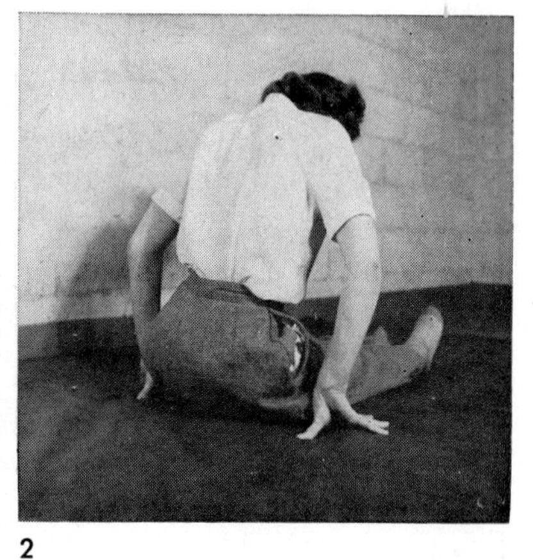

2

Using sandbags for better leverage

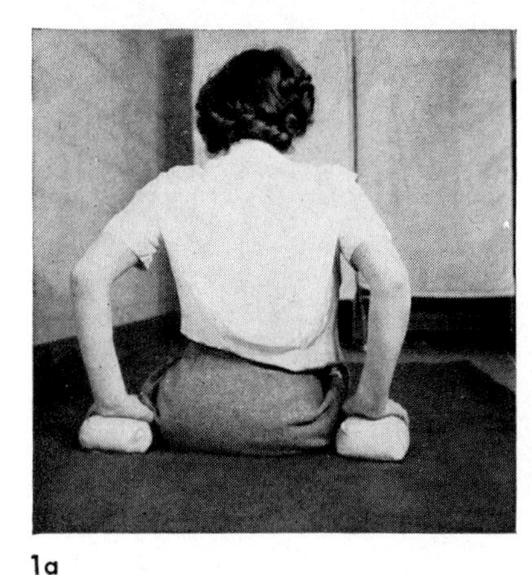

1a

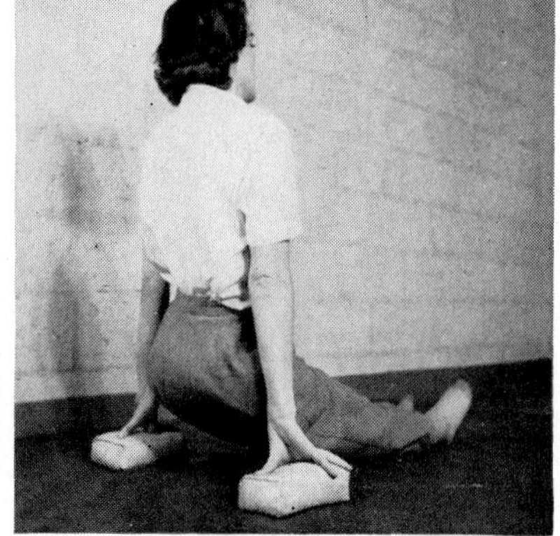

1b

Fig. 6. MOVING FORWARD AND BACKWARD WHILE SITTING

Purpose and preparation: same as for Figure **5**.
Preliminary exercises: push-ups in sitting.

Moving forward:

Starting Position: Same as for Figure **5**.
Instructions:

1. Push up on both hands until both elbows are extended, bending forward slightly and ducking head so that body is off mat.
2. Extend trunk slightly and raise head, still pushing as much as possible on hands so that a minimum of weight is on heels, and slide body forward.
3. Sit down, release hands, and...
1. ...place them in front of hips and start new sequence.

Moving backward: Reverse entire procedure. (Read pictures in reverse sequence.)

Precautions: In case of pressure areas, sufficient height must be gained to avoid irritation of sensitive areas. This may be achieved by using sandbags as above (Figs. **5**·1a, **5**·1b) or when in bed, holding on to trapeze and pulling body up instead of pushing up before moving forward or backward (Fig. **3C**·2).

Helpful remarks: For better mechanical advantage, hands are placed farther forward when moving forward, and farther backward when moving backward. Push-ups as well as moving forward and backward will be much easier on a harder surface, such as a mat, than on a mattress in bed.

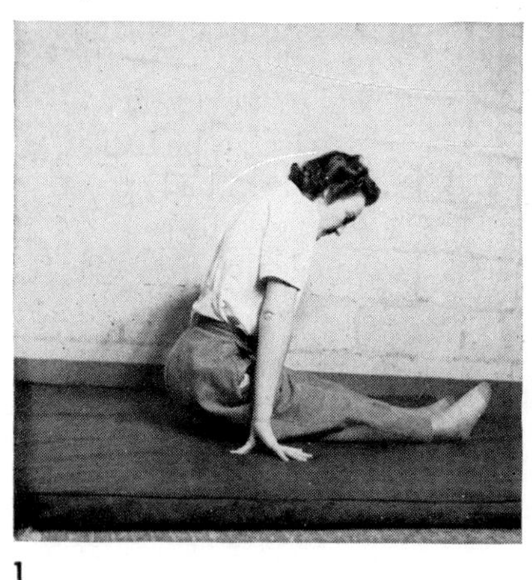
1

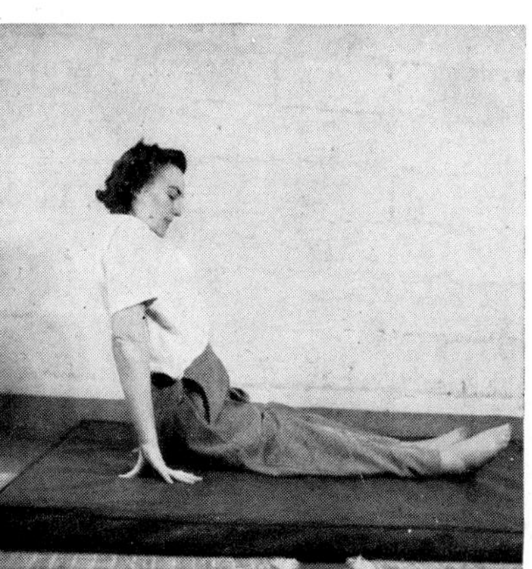
2

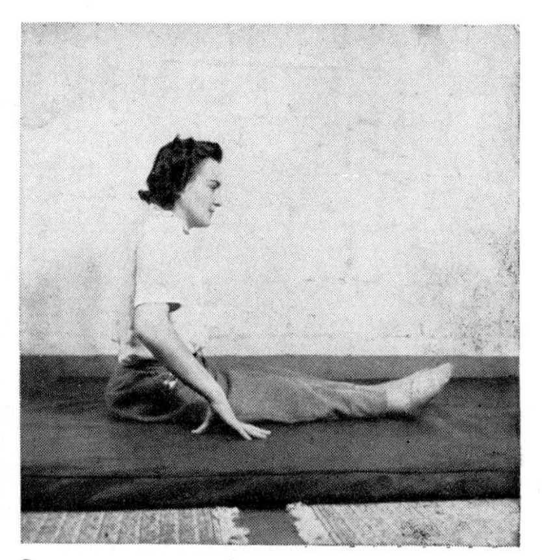
3

Fig. 7. PLACING LEGS OVER EDGE OF BED WHILE SITTING

Purpose: to maintain sitting balance while handling lower extremities.
Preparation for: transfer from bed to wheel chair and back; transfer from wheel chair to car and back; dressing and toilet activities; handling of braces.
Preliminary exercises: moving sideways supine; sitting balance; push-ups.
Equipment: bed.

Starting Position: Sit erect in bed with knees extended if possible.
Instructions: Turn to right, if bed stands with left side against wall.
1. Lift right leg with hands over edge of bed, turning body to right at the same time.
2. Lift left leg with hands...
3. ...place it near right leg. Repeat as often as necessary until both legs are well over edge of...
4. ...bed. Place both hands on bed, each hand next to hip. Push up on hands and turn body to right, until...
5. ...you sit straight on the edge of the bed.

Practice also while turning to the left. For this the bed has to be moved.

Lie down: Reverse entire procedure. (Read pictures in reverse sequence.)

Precautions: Patient is likely to be apprehensive when doing this exercise for the first time, especially if he has been in bed for a prolonged period. Therefore, therapist should stand in front of patient ready to give support around waist. A chair can be placed in front of patient with back close to bed so that patient can hold on to back rest for support (Fig. 15·4).
Helpful remarks: This exercise is more difficult than (although similar to) exercise shown in Figure 3B. In Figure 3B patient places his legs over the edge of bed first, whereas in this exercise he must be able to sit up first and maintain his balance while placing his legs over edge of bed.

Fig. 7. PLACING LEGS OVER EDGE OF BED WHILE SITTING

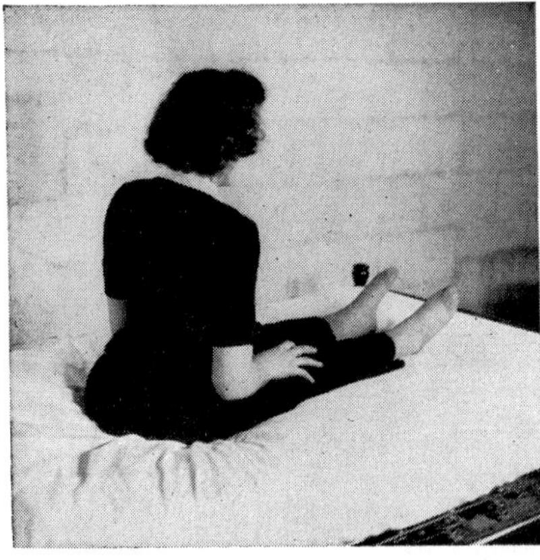

S.P.

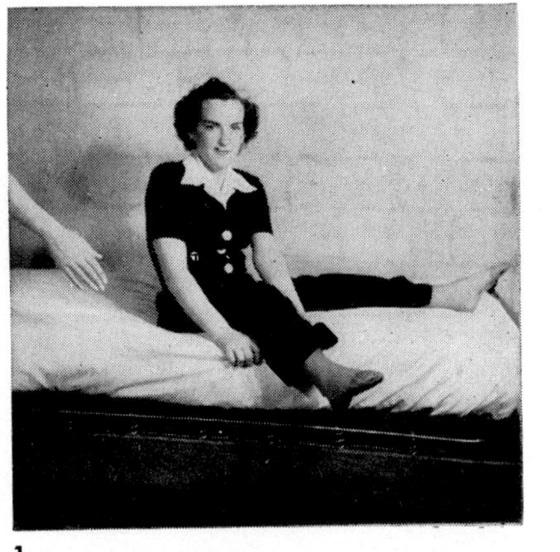

1

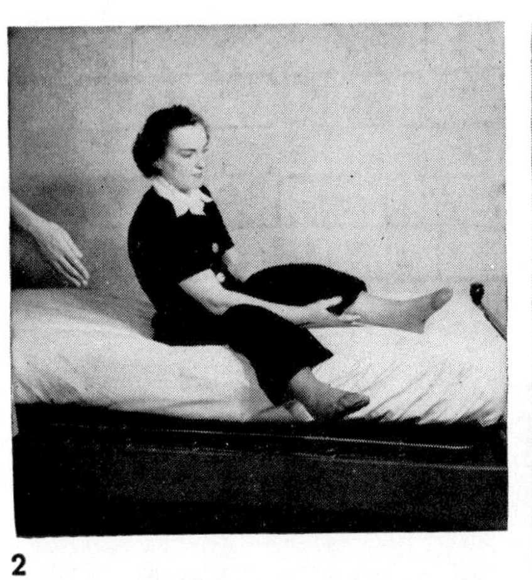

2

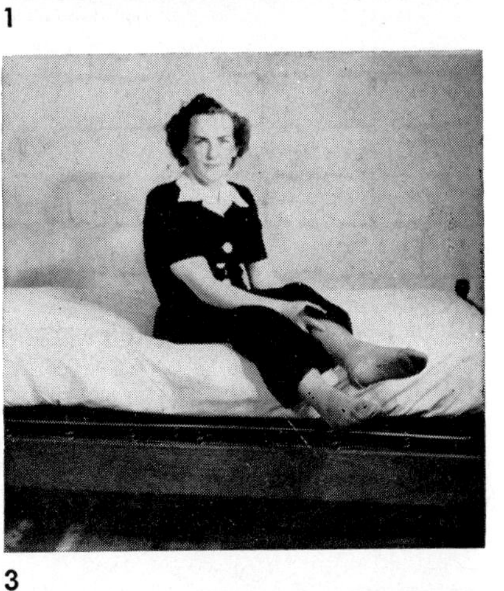

3

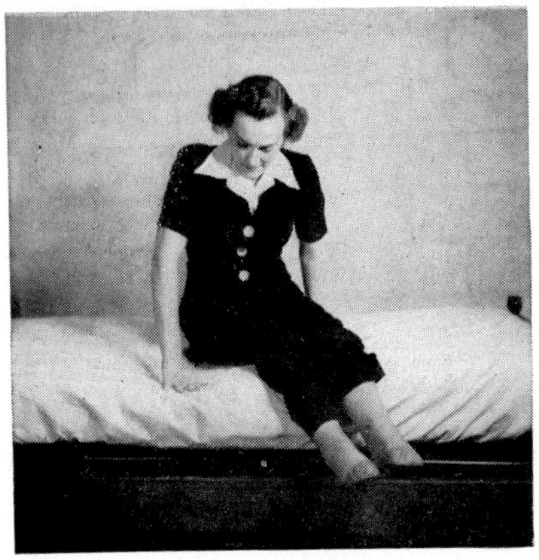

4

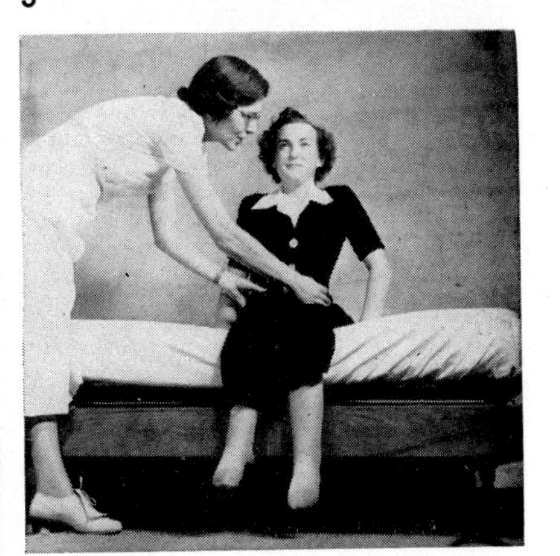

5

Fig. 8. BALANCING ON HANDS AND KNEES

Purpose: to strengthen arm and shoulder muscles; to shift and distribute weight between hands and knees.
Preparation for: crutch walking.
Preliminary exercises: rolling over; push-ups.
Equipment: mat, sandbags.

Starting Position: Lie flat on stomach. Palms beneath shoulders on mat. Knees extended and apart. Fingers pointing forward. Sandbags or pillows under feet to prevent pressure.
Instructions:
1. Put all weight on hands raising head and shoulders and...
2. ...extend elbows.
3. Shift weight to one hand while taking small step with other hand toward knees. Start with left hand...
4. ...then right hand. Put all weight on both hands and push down hard, ducking head and thereby raising pelvis and bending knees. Start to take weight on knees.
5. Repeat steps, left hand...
6. ...right hand, until you are well balanced on hands and knees.
7. Pull in abdomen and straighten spine, look up. Hold for 3 seconds.
Return slowly to starting position, reversing entire procedure. (Read pictures in reverse sequence.)

Precautions: To prevent fractures this exercise should not be done unless physician has found no evidence of osteoporosis in the x-rays of patient.
8. Patient will have a tendency to fall sideward. Therapist should guide patient's body by holding his pelvis around hips. Support should not be given by holding lower extremities down, since the downward pressure may cause fractures.
Helpful remarks: In coming to a four-legged position, patient gradually shifts his weight in the following way:
1, 2, 3. All weight is on hands.
4. Beginning of transfer of weight to knees.
7, 8. Weight distribution between hands and knees.
Entire movement is controlled by continuous pushing on hands. When returning to prone position, the movement is controlled by shifting more and more weight to hands and by bending elbows slowly when finally lying down.

Fig. 8. BALANCING ON HANDS AND KNEES

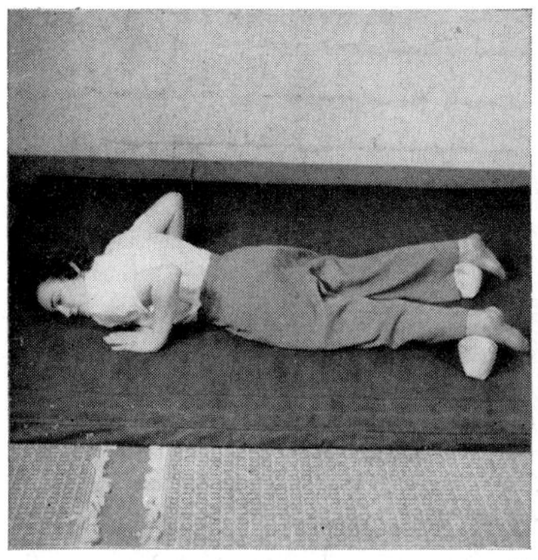

S.P.

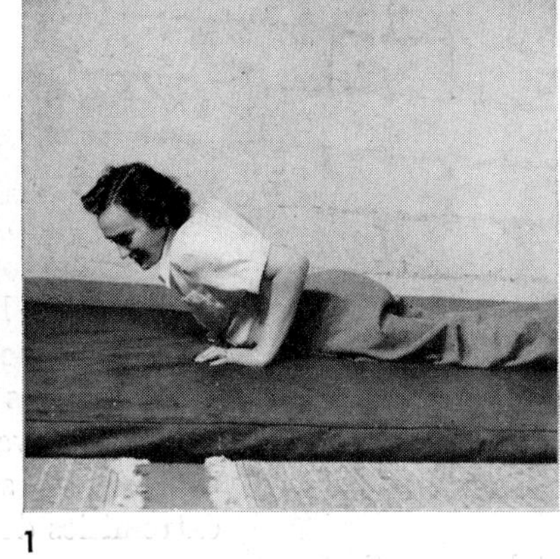

1

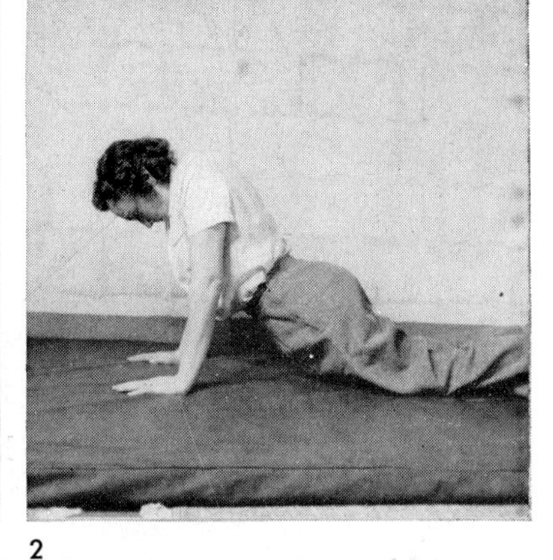

2

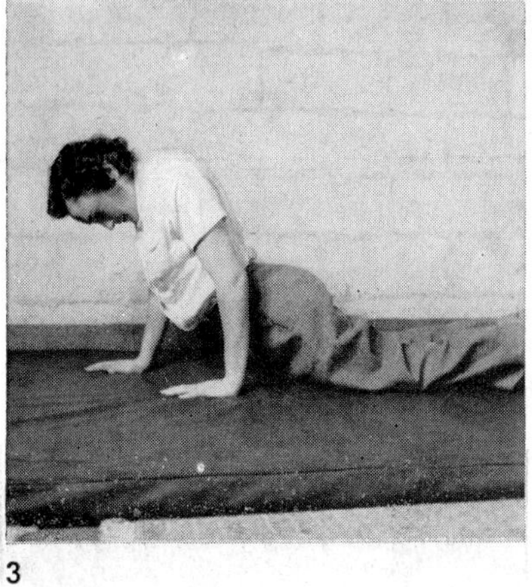

3

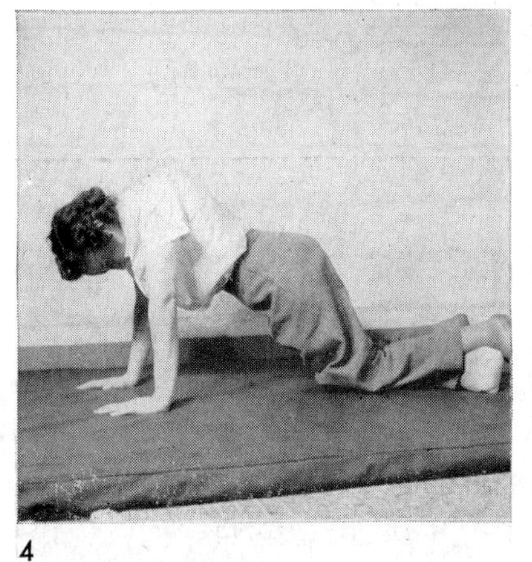

4

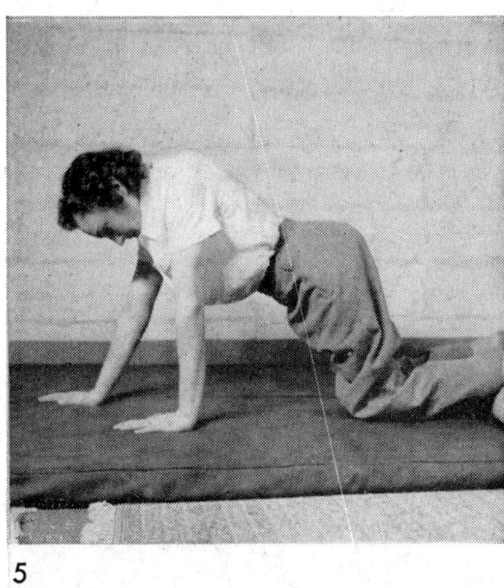

5

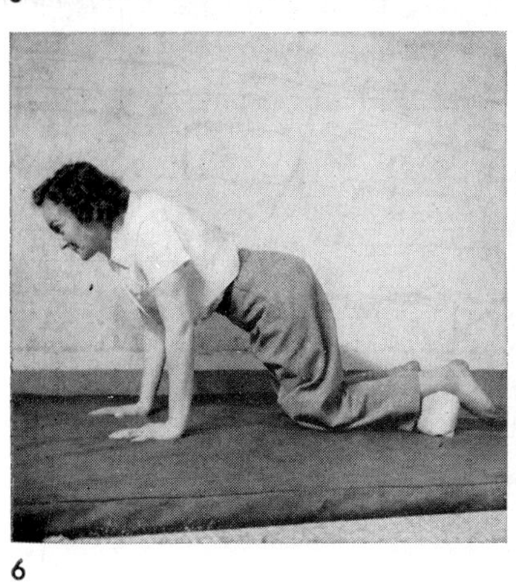

6

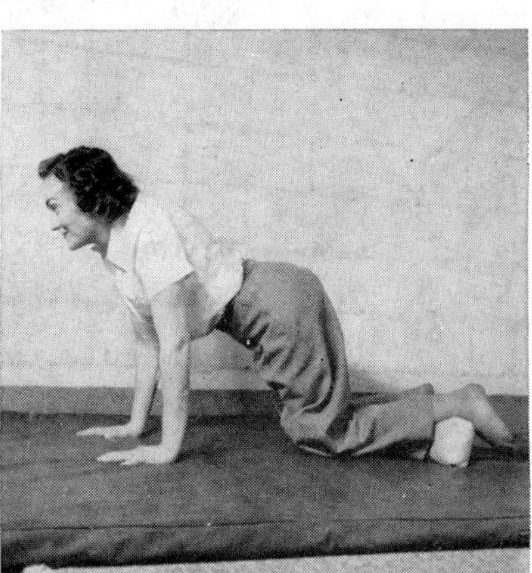

7

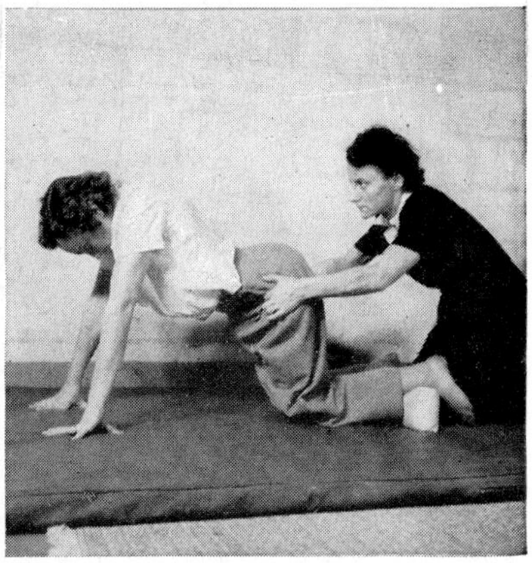

8

Fig. 9. CRAWLING

Purpose: to strengthen arm, shoulder, and thigh muscles; to maintain balance while moving forward in a four-legged position.

Preparation for: crutch walking, especially for four-point and two-point gait.

Preliminary exercises: balancing on hands and knees.

Equipment: mat.

Starting Position: Assume four-legged position (see Fig. 8).

Instructions:

1. Balance on both knees and left hand, raise right hand and take a small step forward; shift weight to it.
2. Balance on both hands and right knee so that left knee can be raised, bring it forward and take a small step shifting weight on it.
3. Repeat with left hand...
4. ... and right knee.

Precautions: This exercise should not be done unless physician has found no evidence of osteoporosis in x-rays of patient.

Helpful remarks: If patient is not able to move one knee forward at a time, he still can try to move forward in a four-legged position by dragging both knees forward simultaneously.

Patient will have a tendency to fall sideward. Therapist should guide patient's body by holding his pelvis around hips and also push pelvis slightly forward if necessary (Fig. 8·8). At no time should support be given by holding lower extremities down.

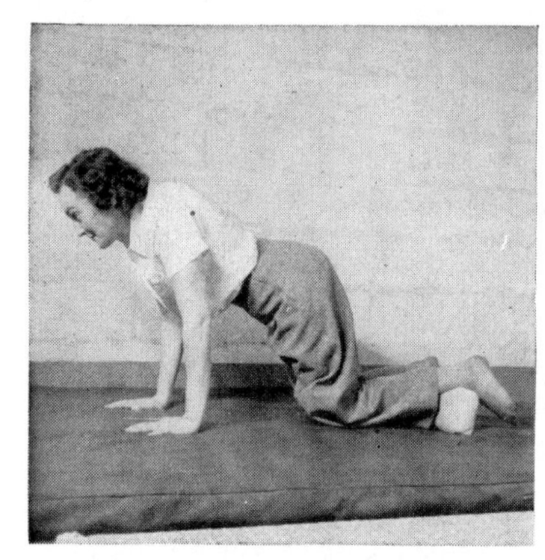

S.P.

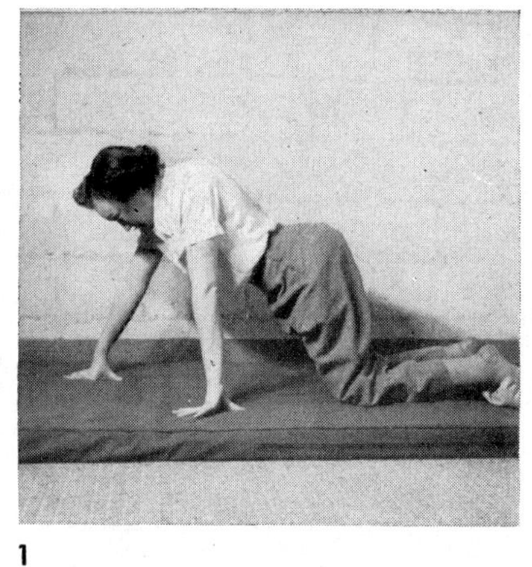

1

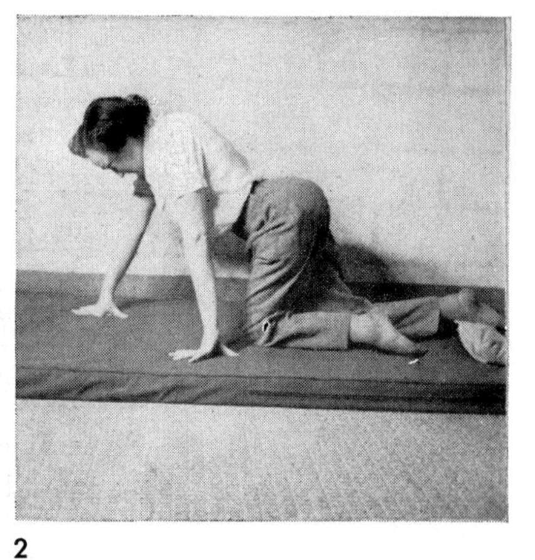

2

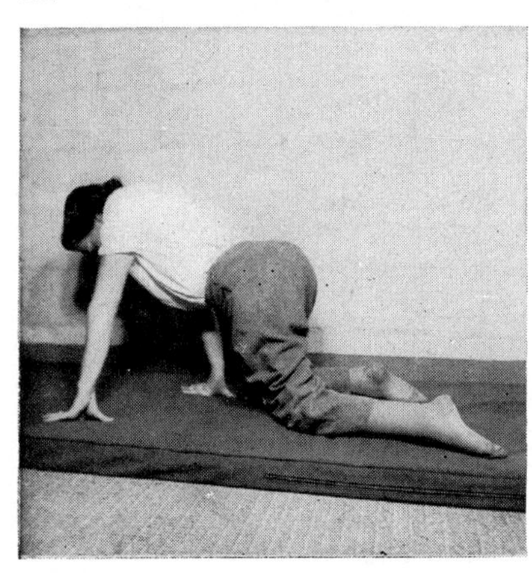

3

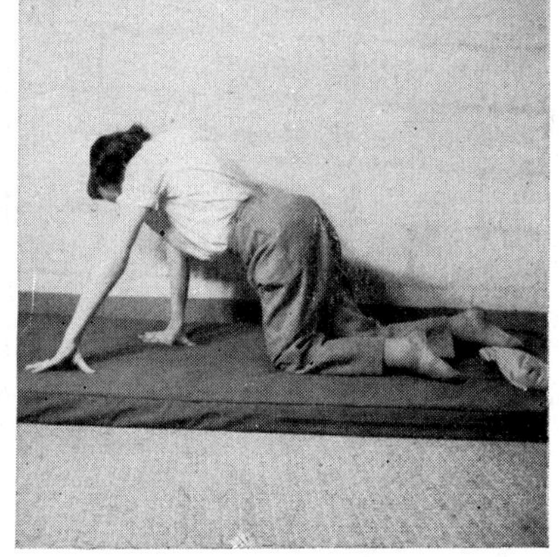

4

Fig. 10. RAISING ARMS ALTERNATELY—in a four-legged position

Purpose: to balance on two knees and one hand while raising other hand.
Preparation for: crutch balancing and crutch walking.
Preliminary exercises: balancing on hands and knees.

Starting Position: Assume four-legged position (see Fig. 8).
Instructions:
1. Distribute weight between both knees and on left hand so that right hand can be raised to shoulder level. Hold.
2. Replace hand on mat. Repeat with left arm, shifting weight to both knees and right arm.

Precautions: Same as in Figure 9.

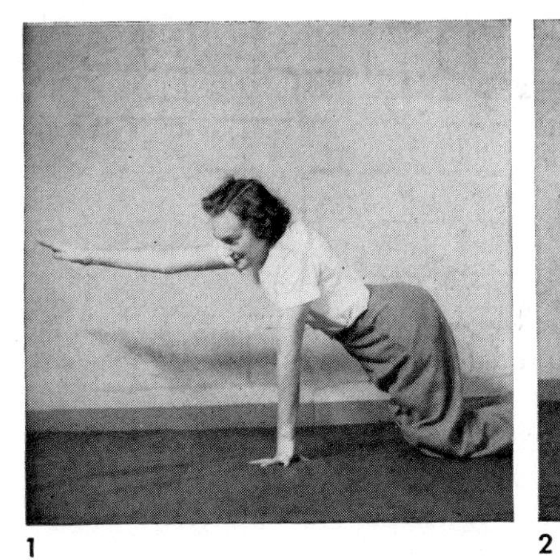
1

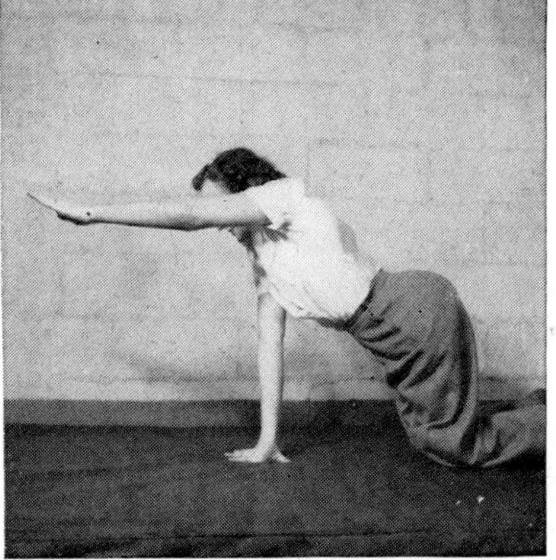
2

CHAPTER III

Wheel-chair Exercises

Once the patient has learned to move about in bed and has acquired the necessary sitting balance, he learns to transfer from the bed into the wheel chair and back (see Chap. IV, p. 46). The following wheel-chair exercises will prepare him for the wheel-chair activities as well as teach him how to get down onto the mat without being lifted.

1. **Sitting balance** (Fig. 11). The patient learns to move his arms and trunk while sitting in the wheel chair. This is a preparation for independent control of the wheel chair.
2. **Push-ups** (Fig. 12). This exercise will strengthen the "crutch-walking" muscles and also is a necessary motion when transferring from and to the wheel chair.
3. **Crossing legs** (Fig. 13). The patient learns to handle his lower extremities while sitting in the wheel chair.
4. **From wheel chair to mat (floor) and back.**
   a. **Using benches** (Fig. 14A).
   b. **Directly** (Fig. 14B).
   This exercise is a combination of Bed Exercises 1 to 7 as well as all wheel-chair exercises and teaches the patient also how to overcome differences in height.

FIG. 11. SITTING BALANCE IN WHEEL CHAIR

Purpose: to maintain sitting balance with or without arm and trunk movements.

Preparation for: dressing activities especially putting on braces, slacks, shoes, stockings; handling footrests; control of wheel chair.

Preliminary exercises: sitting balance in bed.

Starting Position: Sit in wheel chair, feet on footrests. Brakes locked.

Instructions: Hold each of following positions 30 seconds and return to starting position.

1. Raise arms forward to shoulder level (palms down).
2. Raise arms sideward to shoulder level (palms down).
3. Raise arms sideward to shoulder level, bend to right and then to left.
4. Raise arms over head.
5. Grasp hands of therapist and sit as straight as possible with shoulders away from back rest. Pull shoulder blades together and depress shoulders. Try the same without holding on.
6. Grasp hands of therapist, keeping head between arms and bend forward by rounding back. Return to starting position by pulling stomach in first and then raising head. Do not bend the elbows. Try doing the same without holding on.
7. Grasp right wheel-chair arm with right hand, bend forward and touch left foot with left hand, straighten up or...
8. ...touch left foot with left hand, right foot with right hand and straighten up.

Precautions: In the beginning patient may be apprehensive and fearful of falling out of chair. Therapist should stand in front ready for support—if necessary.

Helpful remarks:

1-6. Keeping shoulders down and attempting to pull shoulder blades together will ensure better balance.

5, 6. Patient can also hold on to gym bar, stall bar, parallel bar, or, when at home, to bed or any other *stable* piece of furniture.

Variations: Time of holding each position before returning to starting position can be gradually increased.

All eight movements may be combined into one exercise. This may be done with or without clapping of hands.

All sorts of ball games can be played which will involve above movements. When playing ball, it will be helpful in the beginning if patient is strapped into wheel chair to prevent falling out.

Fig. 11. SITTING BALANCE IN WHEEL CHAIR

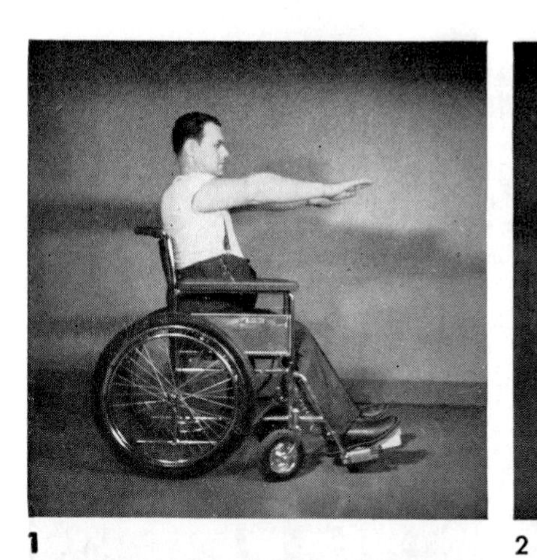
1

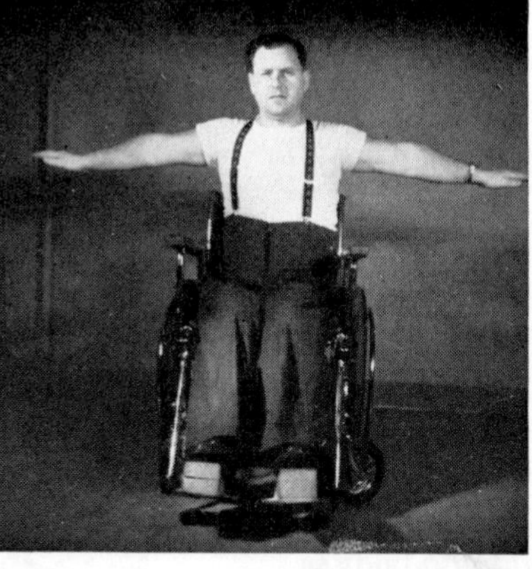
2

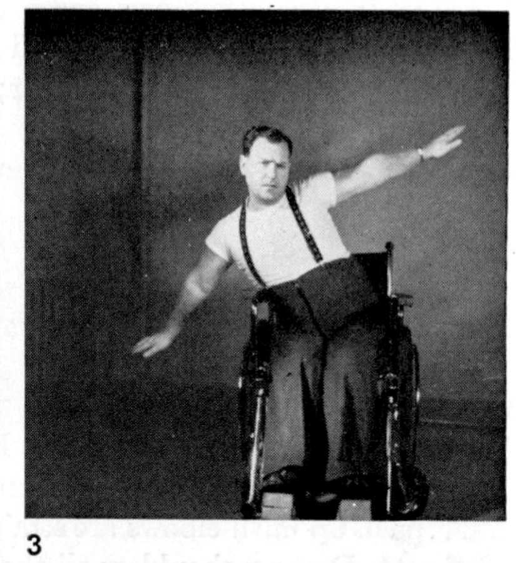
3

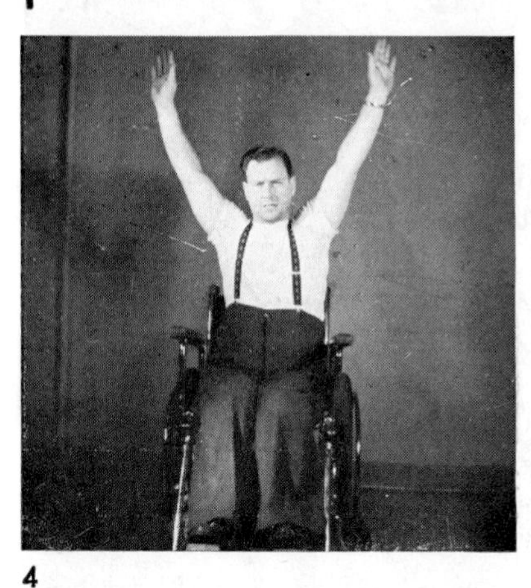
4

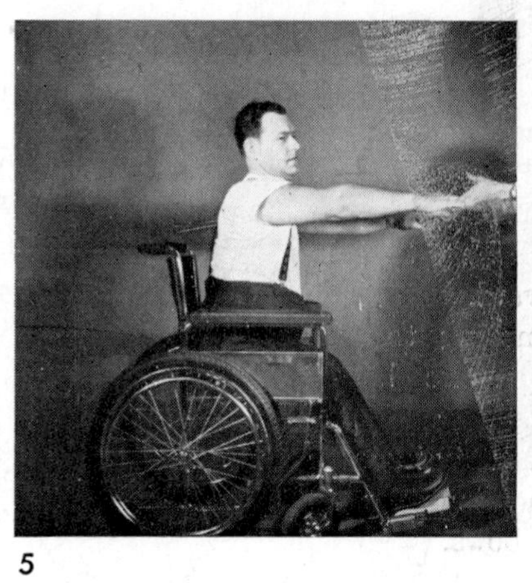
5

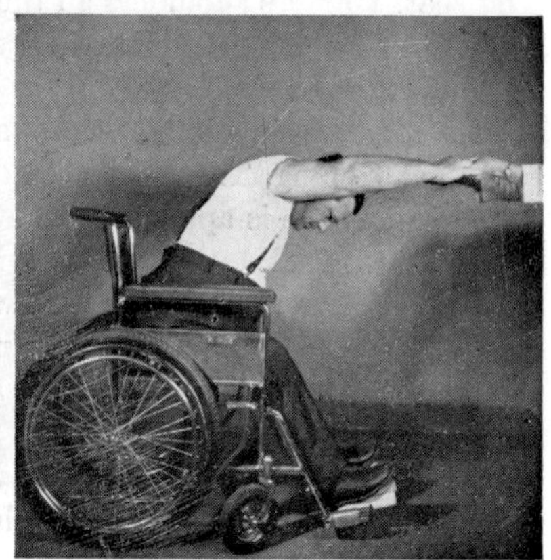
6

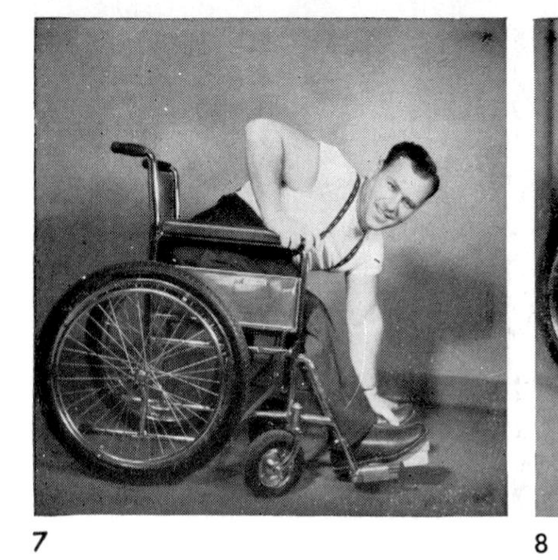
7

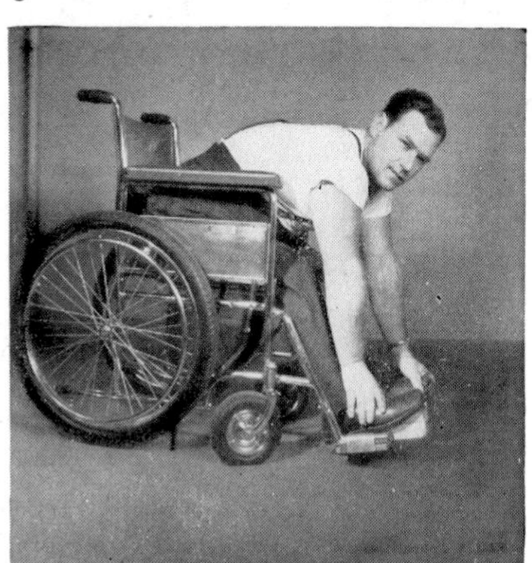
8

Fig. 14A. FROM WHEEL CHAIR TO MAT (FLOOR) AND BACK—using six benches

Purpose: to develop skill, strength, and balance to be able to get down on mat or floor without being lifted.

Preparation for: from wheel chair to bathtub, to toilet seat and back.

Preliminary exercises: sitting balance in wheel chair; push-ups in wheel chair.

Equipment: six benches of graduated height; big floor mat.

From wheel chair to mat:

Starting Position: Six benches are placed in front of wheel chair so that a ramp is formed from chair to mat. Sit in wheel chair (footrests are down).

Instructions:

1. Roll wheel chair to highest bench. Lock brakes. Lift each leg with both hands on to first bench. (Be sure there is enough space, so that toes are not bruised when lifting legs.)

2. Unlock brakes. Roll wheel chair as close as possible, let footrests slide under first bench. Lock brakes.

3. Grasp armrests, push on both hands and lift...

4. ...body off and slide on to...

5. ...first bench. Release hands and place them on bench.

6. Push on both hands, lift body off and slide down on next bench.

7. Repeat as often as necessary until...

8. ...you are on mat.

From mat to wheel chair: Reverse entire procedure. (Read pictures in reverse sequence.)

8. Sit on mat, with back against lowest bench and place hands on it. Push on both hands and lift body up to...

7. ...lowest bench. Release hands and place them behind you on next bench. Push on both hands, lift body up to next bench. Repeat...

6. ...from bench...

5. ...to bench, until...

4. ...you can grasp armrests and lift yourself back into...

3. ...wheel chair.

2. Unlock brakes...

1. ...roll chair back until only heels rest on first bench. Lift each leg with both hands from bench and place on footrests.

Precautions:

4. Therapist should be ready to support patient around waist. It also is often necessary to guide patient's feet to prevent bruising.

S.P. If there is any danger of pressure sores, a small mat should be placed on benches or benches should be upholstered.

Helpful remarks: It will aid in maintenance of balance to extend the trunk when pushing on hands and to bend the head forward and bend elbows *slowly* when sitting down.

Variations: As patient's strength and balance improve, he may try same exercise with only five benches, then with four, three, etc., until he is able to get up from and down to mat (floor) without using any (see Fig. **14B**).

Fig. 14A. FROM WHEEL CHAIR TO MAT (FLOOR) AND BACK—using six benches

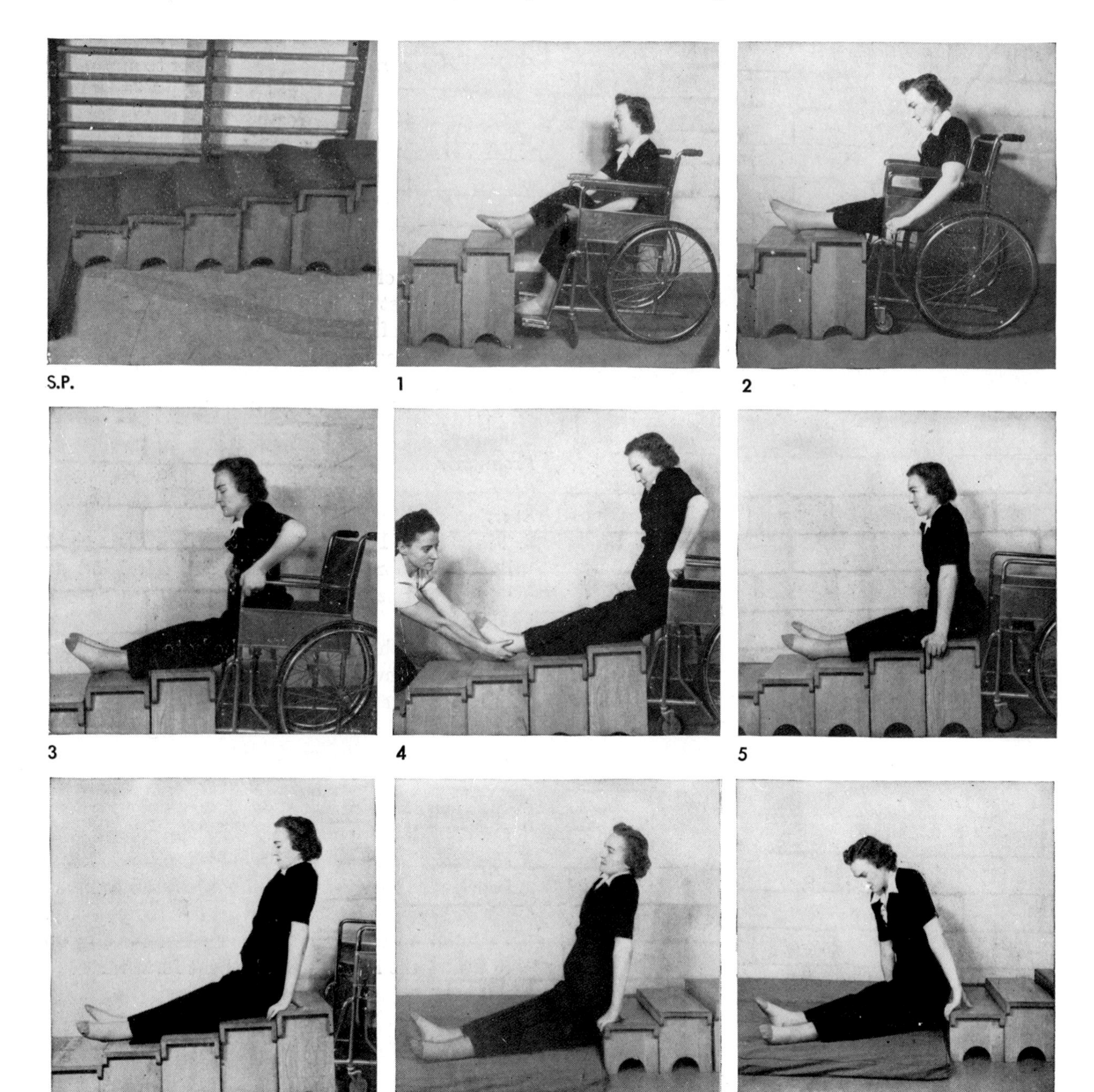

S.P. 1 2

3 4 5

6 7 8

CHAPTER IV

Self-care

Self-care consists of toilet, dressing, and eating activities, which should be taught in a situation as nearly lifelike as possible. One has to consider not only the necessary motions but many other phases of a given activity. Some of these phases may be under the direction of the physical therapy department (*e.g.*, teaching certain movements), some under the direction of the nursing department (*e.g.*, bowel and bladder training), some under the direction of the occupational therapy department (*e.g.*, adjustment of furniture). The delegation of the responsibilities will vary in different institutions. However, in order to obtain the best results, the three departments of physical therapy, nursing, and occupational therapy must work as closely together as possible.

The problems of each aspect of self-care will differ as they apply to bed, wheel-chair, and ambulatory patients. Independence, within the limits of his respective level, *viz.*, the bed, the wheel chair, the crutches, is the goal for each patient. If possible he will progress from one level to the next. Although the ideal is self-care on crutches, from a practical point of view there will always be certain activities that the ambulatory patient will perform in the wheel chair; *e.g.*, bathing will be taken care of from the wheel chair before putting on the braces.

This chapter deals with self-care for bed patients (below), self-care for wheel-chair and ambulatory patients (p. 45), hand activities as they are necessary in communication (as telephoning, reading, writing, etc., p. 78), and travel in the wheel chair (p. 79). The last two groups are included for the sake of convenience, although they are not part of the self-care activities.

Every aspect of toilet, dressing, eating, and hand activities is discussed in the following way. The main group is subdivided if necessary, the general problems are stated, and finally an outline of all essential activities with helpful suggestions is given. Pictures and detailed descriptions are included where necessary.

In many of the pictures a therapist is assisting a patient. The reason for this is to show the correct method of giving support. However, it should be clearly understood that support is to be given only when absolutely necessary.

It has to be remembered that in teaching self-care activities there are no rigid rules. The basic procedures shown and the suggestions given should only serve as a guide, since there are as many different methods as there are patients, and one has to experiment in finding the best (safest) way for each particular patient.

Self-care for Bed Patients

The basis for all bed activities are the bed exercises, which teach the patient all the necessary motions, *e.g.*, rolling over, sitting up, etc. (see Chap. I).

As long as the patient is confined to bed, it is obvious that everything necessary for his self-care must be brought to him. Careful planning of what he will need and the right selection and placement of furniture are important, if he is to become as independent as possible.

The following suggestions may serve as a guide in planning for a bed patient.

FURNITURE ADJUSTMENTS

The mattress should be firm with a board between the mattress and the spring. For patients with severe pressure sores, a foam-rubber mattress placed on top of the firm mattress is suggested.

A night table with a spacious drawer should be within easy reach. It may be helpful to have two night tables, one on each side of the bed, so that everything that is needed is accessible to the patient.

A good reading lamp should be conveniently

placed so that the patient can turn the light on and off without assistance.

The telephone and a signal light also should be near.

A bedside table is needed for eating, washing, and hand activities. The table should be sturdy, preferably with slide-on coasters, and should be the type that can be tilted for reading and writing. Small trays are satisfactory only for light meals.

POSTURE

In all bed activities good sitting posture is essential. The patient's back should be well supported by cranking up the bed (or with pillows), so that both hands will be free for the given activity, *e.g.*, *eating* (Fig. 15·1), *washing* (Fig. 15·2); and *attending to toilet needs* (Figs. 15·3 and 15·4).

In addition to good sitting posture, correct lying position must be considered. In general, when the patient is on his back (supine) a footboard is used to elevate the bedclothes, so that there is no pressure on his toes. To prevent foot drop a simple night brace (see "Braces" in Chap. VII) has proved most satisfactory.

To prevent foot drop when the patient is lying on his stomach (prone), the foot should be dorsiflexed to 90 deg. at the ankle with the toes over the edge of the mattress.

For postoperative cases or in the presence of severe pressure sores, special bed positioning according to medical prescription is essential.

Fig. 15. SELF-CARE FOR BED PATIENTS

Eating

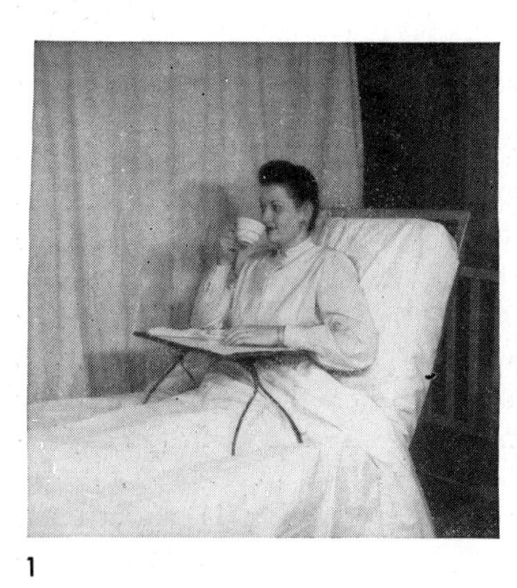

1

Washing

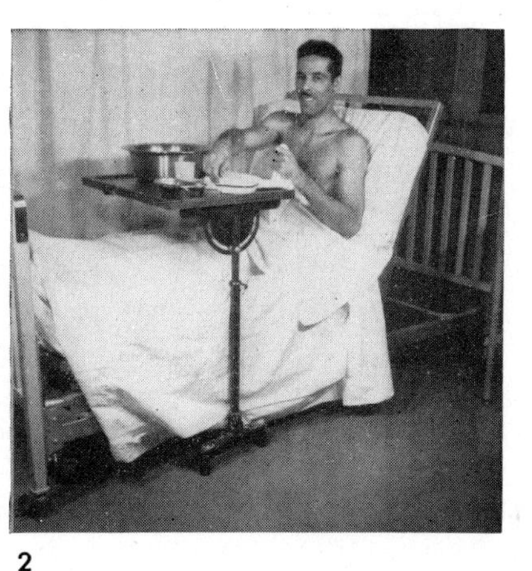

2

Toilet needs

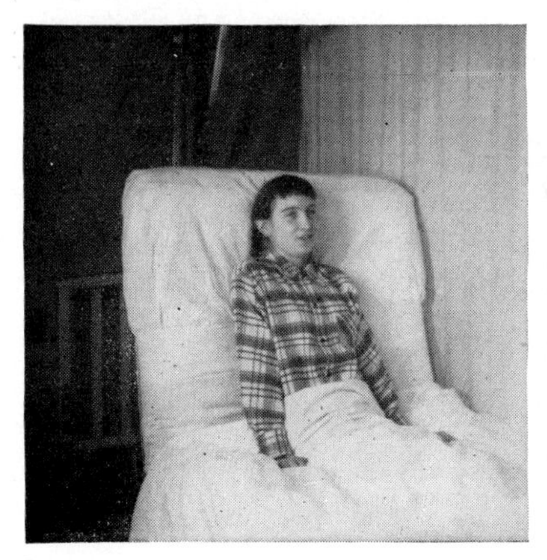

3

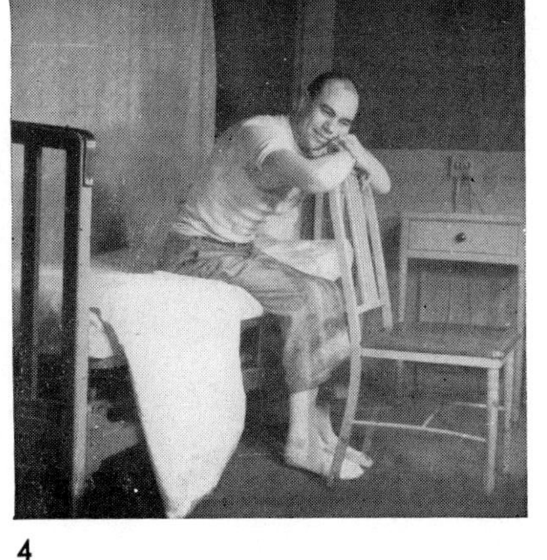

4

TOILET NEEDS*

Careful consideration must be given to toilet needs since so many patients with neurological disturbances have bowel and bladder problems.

It has been found that, when using the bedpan or urinal, sitting is the most effective position for the satisfactory emptying of the bladder as well as the bowels. Good posture and conditions which will promote relaxation are essential. The bed may be cranked up, so that the patient's back is well supported (or the back supported with pillows) (Fig. 15·3). An even better position is to sit with the legs over the edge of the bed. In order to ensure maximum security and relaxation, a chair is placed with the back rest facing the front of the bed, so that the patient can lean on it (Fig. 15·4).

In order to keep the bed dry at night, male patients with bladder problems have found the following procedure helpful. The patient sleeps on his abdomen with a shower cap placed under his genitalia. The shower cap, which should be plastic, beret type, and seamless, is prepared in the following manner:

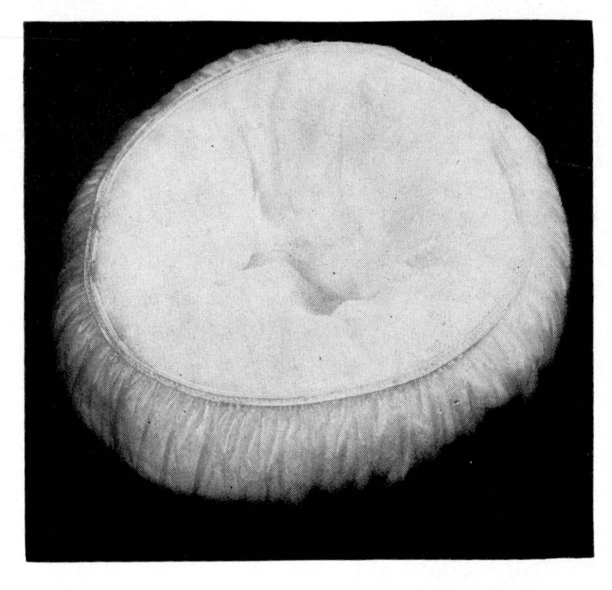

Cellucotton 1 yard square and about $\frac{1}{2}$ in. thick is rolled and tucked tightly inside the shower cap around its entire circumference. Thereby the elevated edge will form a circle which will prevent overflow. In the hollow center a thin layer of Cellucotton is placed and covered with a fine piece of gauze. This will prevent the Cellucotton clinging to the skin of the penis which is placed in the hollow center.

Whenever necessary the wet Cellucotton can be discarded and replaced. The cap will be ready for use again after being washed with soap and water.

Patients with bowel and bladder problems should be on a strict time schedule as to their liquid intake as well as output. At the present time, the bowel and bladder training program in use at this Institute is working fairly satisfactory, especially with female patients.

In general, the patients drink two glasses of liquid every two hours, from 6:00 A.M. to 6:00 P.M. They attempt to void immediately following the drinking. Once a day, at a definite time, they attempt to empty their bowels.

The whole routine, the amount of liquid taken as well as the time of elimination, must be planned for each individual patient. Since there are many variables, each patient must go through a trial-and-error period until he establishes his own particular habit patterns.

The one conclusion we have been able to draw so far is that regularity is one of the most important factors. However the whole bowel and bladder training program is considered to be in the experimental stage.

No bowel or bladder training is undertaken without a careful genitourinary study. Reexamination is essential at regular intervals.

* For further information on this subject see MORRISSEY, ALICE B., Procedures for Bladder and Bowel Rehabilitation, in "Rehabilitation Nursing," G. P. Putnam's Sons, New York. (In press.)

Self-care for Wheel-chair and Ambulatory Patients

Self-care for patients who are no longer confined to bed will involve getting from the bed into the wheel chair and propelling the wheel chair to the place where the activity has to be performed. Patients who are ambulatory will have to be able to get to the place on crutches. In both cases these activities involve the problems of going through doors, handling furniture, lights, etc., and therefore careful planning of the type and placement of furniture is essential. Bed, wheel-chair, and mat exercises (see Chaps. I and II) teach the patient all the motions necessary for his self-care, as well as his travel activities. The ambulatory patient who will use his crutches for most activities and his wheel chair only when it is practical must have mastered ambulation and elevation on crutches (see Chaps. IV and V).

The transfer from and to the wheel chair is the basis for all wheel-chair activities. When using the wheel chair the problem is to bridge the gap between the wheel chair and a given piece of furniture and to overcome possible differences in height. Any or all of the following factors are to be considered: (*a*) placement of the wheel chair, (*b*) adjustment of wheel chair (*e.g.*, removable armrests, swinging footrests, etc.), (*c*) adjustment and/or different placement of furniture (*e.g.*, cutting legs of bed), (*d*) special devices (*e.g.*, board). Often these devices can be improvised.

The following activities will illustrate the point.

1. **From bed to wheel chair and back** (six methods are shown).
   a. **Wheel chair facing bed** (Fig. **16A**). The wheel chair faces the bed and the patient backs into it. This is usually the easiest method for beginners.
   b. **Using board (wheel chair with nonremovable armrests)** (Fig. **16B**). If the armrests are not removable and the patient cannot bridge the gap, a board is used to slide over.
   c. **Using board (wheel chair with removable armrests)** (Fig. **16C**). The same method can also be used if the armrests are removable.
   d. **Using chair** (Fig. **16D**). If patients are fearful, a chair instead of a board is used to bridge the gap. This can also be done with removable armrests.
   e. **Wheel chair at angle (nonremovable armrests)** (Fig. **16E**). When the patient has very strong arms and armrests are attached, the wheel chair is placed at an angle.
   f. **Wheel chair alongside bed (removable armrests)** (Fig. **16F**). When the armrests are removable, the wheel chair can be placed alongside and very close to the bed.

   In the above methods, the transfer will be facilitated if the bed is of equal height with the wheel-chair seat. Sometimes the shortening of the legs of the bed will make the difference between lifting and not lifting the patient. A smooth sheet and a plastic wheel-chair seat cover will make for easy sliding. The placement of the wheel chair and the modifications of the wheel chair and/or the bed will have to be planned for each individual patient.
2. **From wheel chair to chair and back** (Fig. **17**). This is the next step in using the wheel chair and should be considered as the preparation for transfer to the toilet seat.
3. **Control of wheel chair** (Fig. **18**). The patient should be taught as early as possible to handle the wheel chair independently.
4. **Through door in wheel chair** (Fig. **19**). There are two methods shown, forward as well as backward. The selection will depend on the type of door.
   a. **Forward** (Fig. **19A**).
   b. **Backward** (Fig. **19B**).

Fig. 16A. FROM BED TO WHEEL CHAIR AND BACK —wheel chair facing bed

This method is easiest for beginners, especially for those with flaccid lower extremities. Later it may also be used when patient starts to wear braces.

Preliminary exercises: sitting up; sitting balance; moving forward and backward while sitting; push-ups.

Equipment: bed, wheel chair (small sandbags).

From bed to wheel chair:

Starting Position: Sit erect in bed facing foot of bed. Wheel chair stands facing bed, as close to it as possible. Footrests are down so that they can slide under bed. Brakes are locked.

Instructions:

1. Place hands near hips on bed. Push on hands and turn body toward wall.
2. Move left leg with both hands toward left edge of bed.
3. Move right leg with both hands next to left leg.
4. Repeat as often as necessary and turn back to chair. Slide backward pushing on both hands until...
5. ...one armrest can be grasped and then...
6. ...the other. Push up on both hands lifting body off bed and slide...
7. ...back into chair.
8. Unlock brakes and move chair back slowly until only heels rest on bed.
9. Lock brakes. Lift right leg with both hands off bed and place on footrest. Repeat with other leg.

From wheel chair to bed: Reverse entire procedure. (Read pictures in reverse sequence.)

Starting Position:

9. Sit in wheel chair facing bed. Be near enough to headboard so that when you get into bed (Fig. 16A-4) you can lie down without having to move up or down in bed. Brakes are locked. Leave enough space between chair and bed so that you can easily lift each leg up onto bed without bruising toes on edge of bed.

Instructions:

8. Unlock brakes. Move chair as near as...

7. ...possible. Footrests are down so that they can slide under bed. Lock brakes.

6. Grasp armrests. Push up on hands lifting body off seat and...

5. ...slide forward into bed. Place right hand on bed...

4. ...then left hand and pushing up again on both hands slide forward as much as necessary.

3. Adjust legs with...

2. ...hands and...

S.P. ...turn body.

Precautions: Brakes must be *locked* while moving in and out of chair.

9. Legs must not be lifted up or off bed unless there is sufficient space to prevent injury of toes and lower legs by jamming against bed.

Until sufficient skill and confidence are gained, therapist holds chair and is ready to support patient around waist.

Helpful remarks:

4, 5. A small sandbag may be placed under hands to facilitate push-up (Fig. 5).

If the wheel chair is much lower than bed, pillows should be placed in wheel chair to make up difference in height.

Fig. 16A. FROM BED TO WHEEL CHAIR AND BACK—wheel chair facing bed

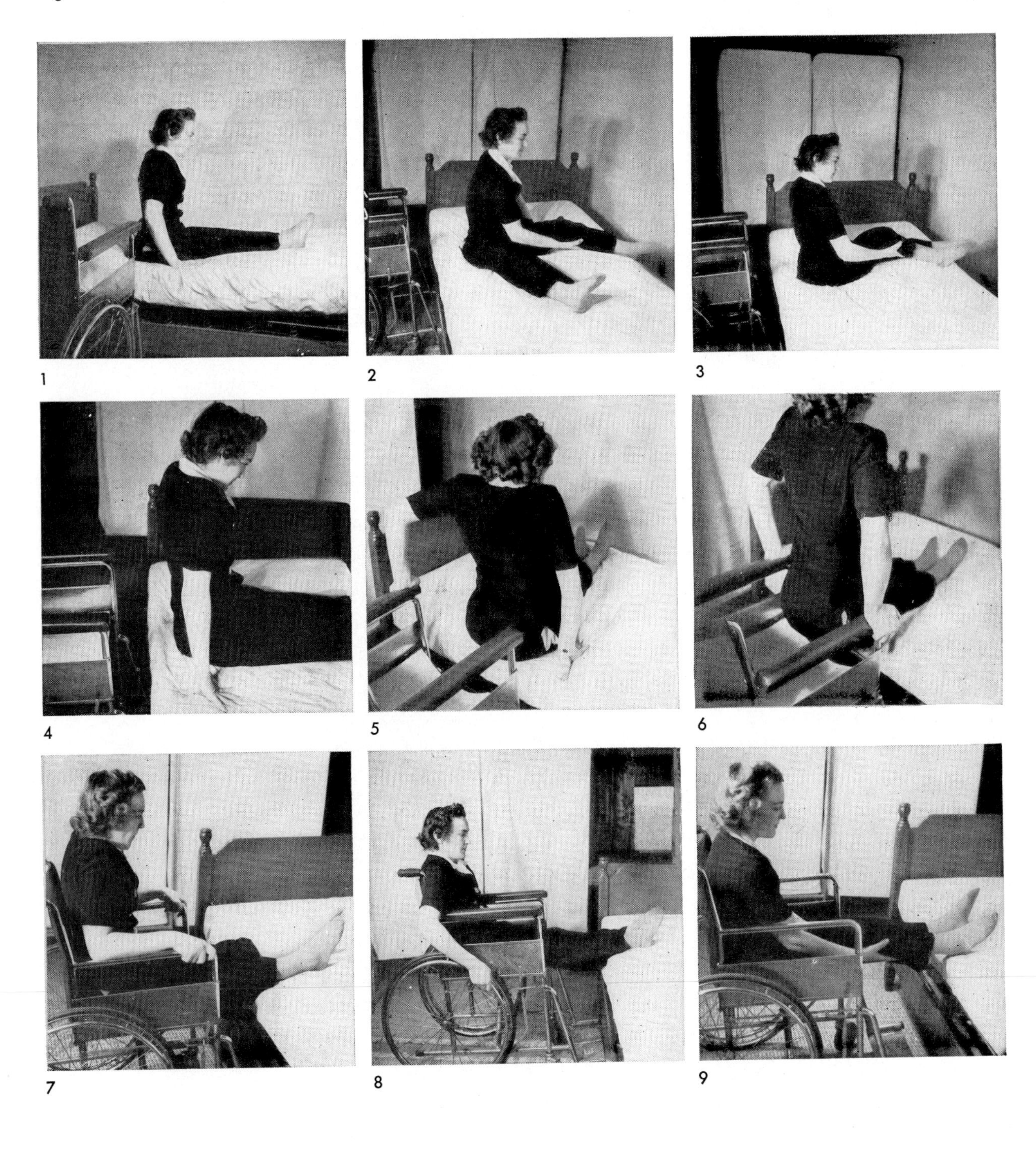

Fig. 16B. FROM BED TO WHEEL CHAIR AND BACK —using board (wheel chair with nonremovable armrests)

If patients are not strong enough to push up as in previous method, or to lift themselves across from bed to wheel chair as in next methods, a board is used to bridge gap between chair and bed. This board is also used if wheel chair cannot be brought close enough to bed because of construction of either chair or bed.
Equipment: bed, wheel chair, board.

From bed to wheel chair:

Starting Position: Sit erect in bed, facing foot of bed.

Instructions:
1. While therapist puts one end of board on bed, place both hands in front of hips on bed, push on hands and lift body until sitting on board. (If you cannot push up, roll over and let therapist place board under your buttocks and then sit up on board. No picture shown.)
2. Therapist places free end of board on wheel chair, moves chair as close as possible to bed, and locks brakes. Footrests are down so that they can slide under bed.
Slide across board into wheel chair. Let therapist remove board sideways (see also Fig. **27B**).
Adjust legs and footrests.

From wheel chair to bed: Reverse entire procedure. (Read pictures in reverse sequence.)

Fig. 16C. FROM BED TO WHEEL CHAIR AND BACK —using board (wheel chair with removable armrests)

From bed to wheel chair:

Starting Position: Sit erect in bed facing foot of bed. Therapist removes one armrest and places chair along side of bed and locks brakes.
Instructions:
1a, 2a. Same as Figure **16B.**

From wheel chair to bed: Reverse entire procedure. (Read pictures in reverse sequence.)

Precautions: To prevent tipping of board, therapist may have to hold board down on wheel-chair seat. Board also has to be placed well over half of seat when getting into chair and well under buttocks when getting into bed.
Helpful remarks:
1, 1a. It is much easier first to place one end of board under patient when he gets into as well as out of bed and then to move chair close to bed.
If there is any tendency to pressure sores, board should be upholstered. Using the board is a good preparation for getting from wheel chair to car and back.

Fig. 16D. FROM BED TO WHEEL CHAIR AND BACK —using chair

This method is helpful for patients who cannot push up sufficiently and/or easily lose their balance because of great spasticity of their lower extremities; back rest of chair supplies additional support and gives confidence and, therefore, will also be of advantage for older as well as very anxious patients.
Preliminary exercises: same as in Figure **16A,** also sitting with legs over edge of bed.
Equipment: bed, wheel chair, chair.

From bed to wheel chair:

Starting Position: Therapist places chair along side bed and places wheel chair at right angle to chair.

Instructions:
1b. Sit with legs over edge of bed. Place left hand near left hip on bed and right hand on edge of chair seat. Push up on both hands and...
2b. ...slide to chair. Place left hand behind you on chair seat and grasp right armrest with right hand so that you slide (or lift yourself) onto wheel chair. Unlock brakes, move wheel chair away from chair, place legs on footrests. (For more details see Fig. **17.**)

From wheel chair to bed: Reverse entire procedure. (Read pictures in reverse sequence.)

Precautions: If patient is very heavy, therapist must hold chair and wheel chair and also be ready to give support around waist.

Fig. 16B. FROM BED TO WHEEL CHAIR AND BACK—using board (wheel chair with nonremovable armrests)

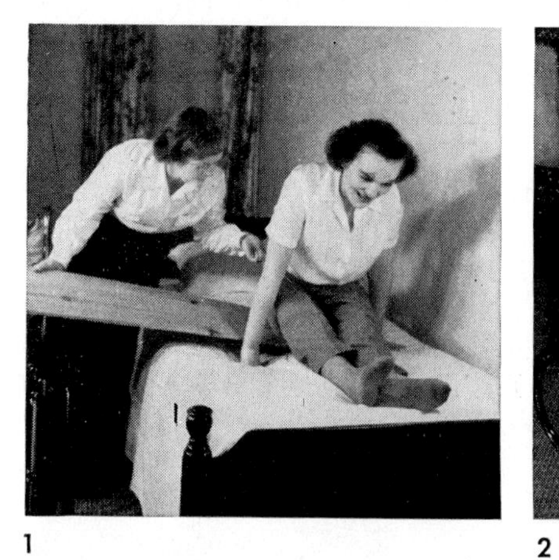

1

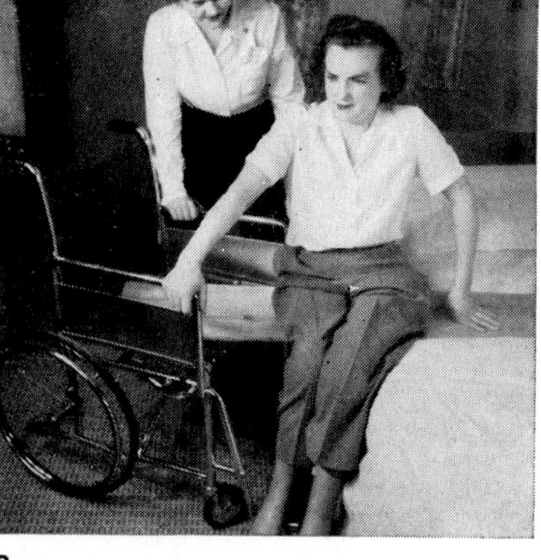

2

Fig. 16C. FROM BED TO WHEEL CHAIR AND BACK—using board (wheel chair with removable armrests)

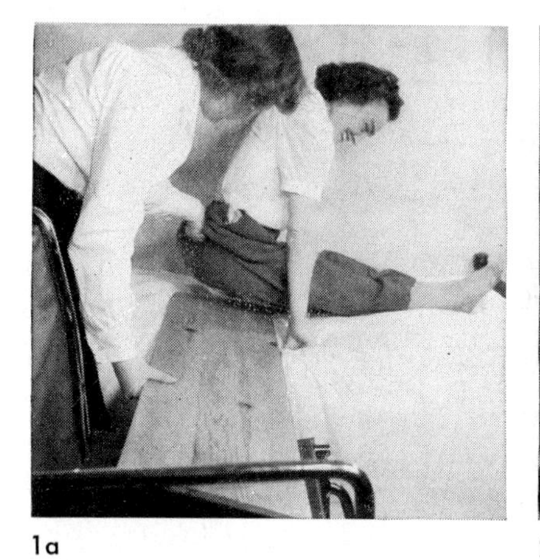

1a

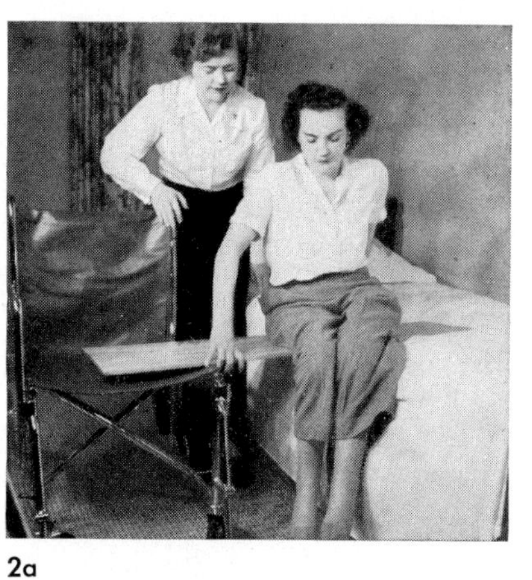

2a

Fig. 16D. FROM BED TO WHEEL CHAIR AND BACK—using chair

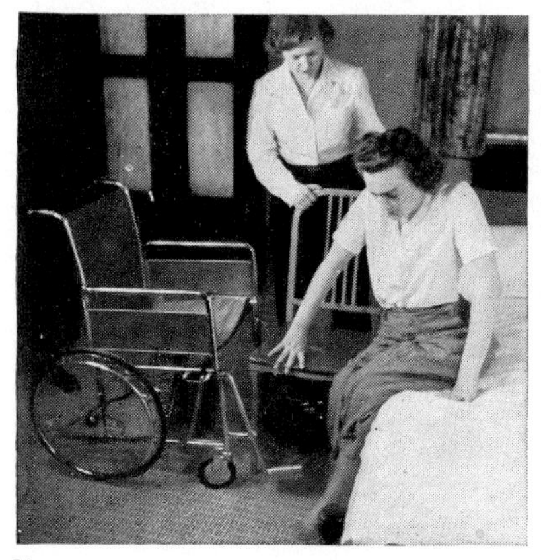

1b

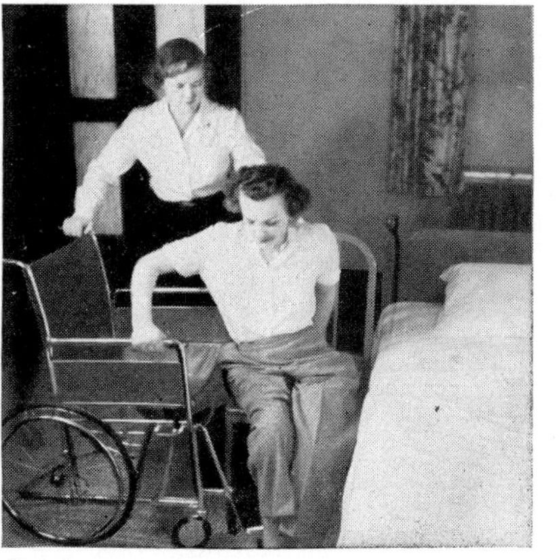

2b

Fig. 16E. FROM BED TO WHEEL CHAIR AND BACK —wheel chair at angle (nonremovable armrests)

This method is the most common one. It can be used by patients with or without braces.

Preliminary exercises: same as in Figure **16A;** also sitting with legs over edge of bed.

Equipment: bed, wheel chair.

From bed to wheel chair:

Starting Position: Wheel chair is placed at slight angle along right side of bed and facing forward. Footrests are down and brakes locked.

Instructions:

1. Sit with legs over edge of bed. Place left hand behind left hip on bed and right hand on right armrest. Turn body slightly to right.

2. Push on both hands, raise body and lift yourself across and down...

3. ...into chair. Place feet on footrests.

From wheel chair to bed: Reverse entire procedure. (Read pictures in reverse sequence.)

Starting Position:

3. Sit in wheel chair along right side of bed facing forward and at a slight angle.

Instructions:

2. Place right hand on armrest and left hand on bed near left hip. Push on both hands, raise body, and lift yourself across...

1. ...and on to bed. Slide back on bed as far as necessary. Lift legs up with hands.

Fig. 16F. FROM BED TO WHEEL CHAIR AND BACK—wheel chair alongside bed (removable armrests)

From bed to wheel chair:

Starting Position: Remove armrest, and place chair alongside and as close as possible to bed. Lock brakes.

Instructions:

1a. Place right hand next to right hip on bed and left hand on left armrest. Push on both hands, slide (or lift) sideways on to chair. Attach armrest. Place feet on footrests.

From wheel chair to bed: Reverse entire procedure. (Read pictures in reverse sequence.)

Starting Position:

2a. Sit in wheel chair along side of bed as close as possible.

Instructions:

1a. Remove right armrest, place it on bed. Place right hand near right hip on bed and grasp left armrest with left hand. Push on both hands and slide (or lift yourself) on to bed.

Precautions: To prevent tipping no weight should be on footrests. If possible, both feet, or at least one foot, should be on floor.

There is more weight on arm that is on bed. In the beginning therapist stands by ready to give support around waist.

Helpful remarks: When getting from wheel chair to bed, chair should be moved at right distance from headboard, so that when patient slides into bed he can lie down without having to move up or down in bed. This is especially true for very heavy patients.

1. Instead of placing armrest on bed, it may also be hung on handle of back of wheel chair.

Fig. 16E. FROM BED TO WHEEL CHAIR AND BACK—wheel chair at angle (nonremovable armrests)

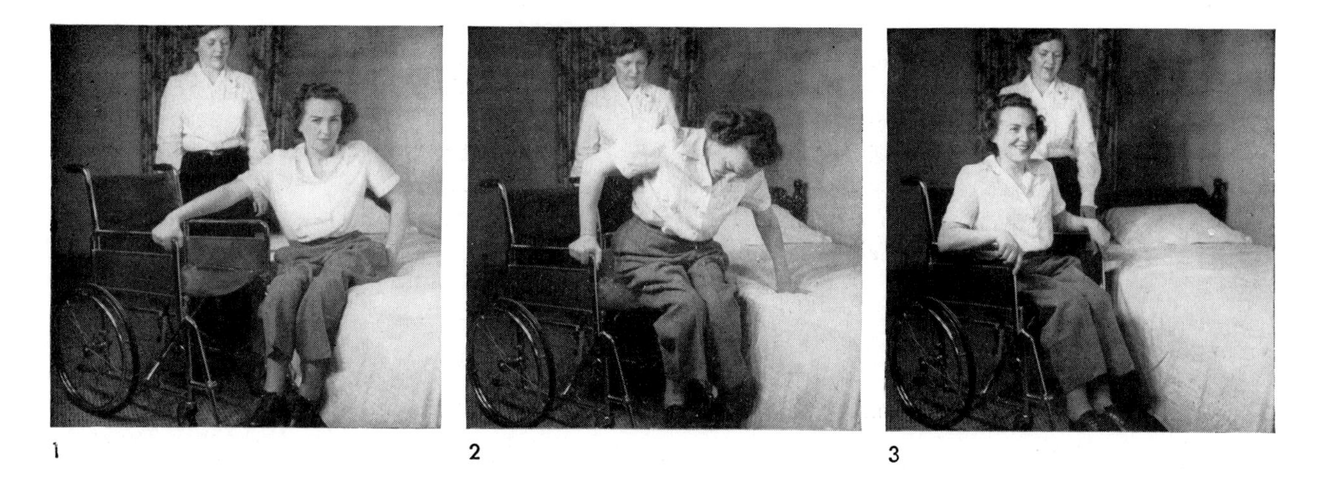

1 2 3

Fig. 16F. FROM BED TO WHEEL CHAIR AND BACK—wheel chair alongside bed (removable armrests)

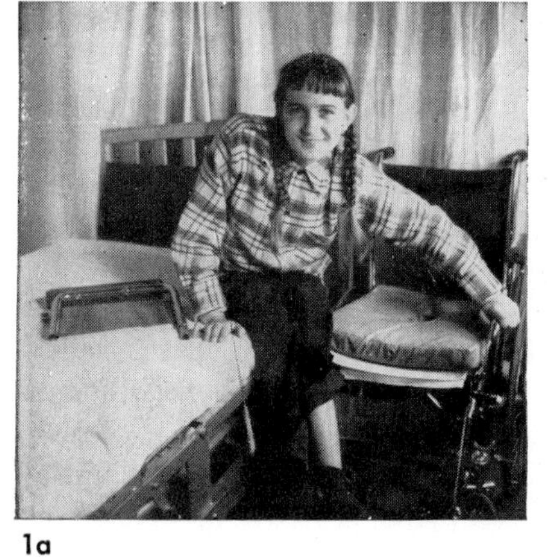

1a

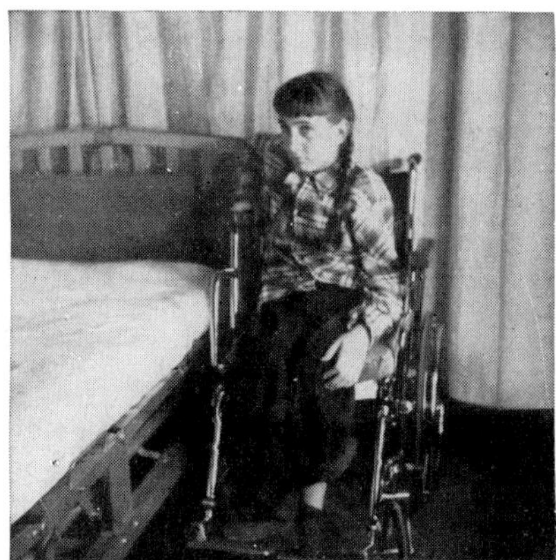

2a

Fig. 18. CONTROL OF WHEEL CHAIR

In order to make it possible for patient to control wheel chair independently, wheel chair has to be adjusted to his individual needs (see "Wheel Chairs" in Chap. VII). It is also important that wheel chair always be in perfect working order. In crowded city apartments, where the problem of space is very complicated, often a different furniture arrangement will be necessary.

Purpose: independent handling of the wheel chair.

Preparation for: getting around in the wheel chair.

Preliminary exercises: sitting balance in the wheel chair.

Instructions:

1. Lock brakes—to keep chair stationary—or...
2. ...place sandbags behind wheels, if a chair without brakes is used.
3. Raise and lower footrests.
4. Practice propelling chair in all directions as well as turning around.
5. *Wheel chair over carpet:* Sit well back in chair. Grasp hand rims at very top and give a *quick* thrust forward, so that chair is tilted into back wheels and front wheels are raised high enough to get over carpet.
   It will be helpful to secure carpets and rugs in the apartment to the floor, so that they do not wrinkle and get in the way of wheels.

Helpful remarks: When a patient is entering or leaving a wheel chair which has the small wheels in front, he should be careful to see that these wheels are always rotated forward to their fullest extent (Fig. **18**·4). With these wheels rotated forward, a greater base is had and there is less likelihood of chair tipping and throwing patient off balance.

Fig. 18. CONTROL OF WHEEL CHAIR

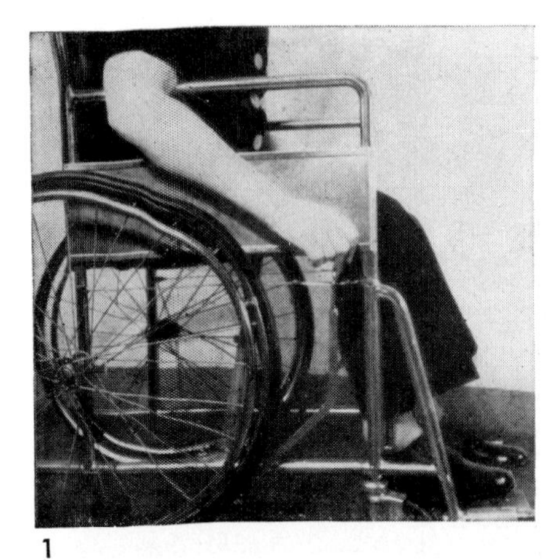

1

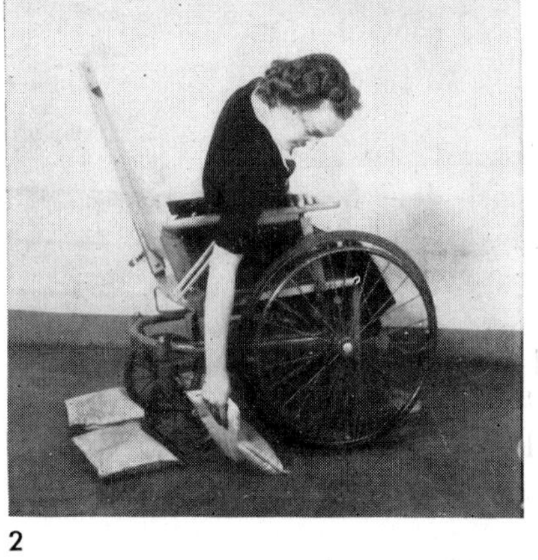

2

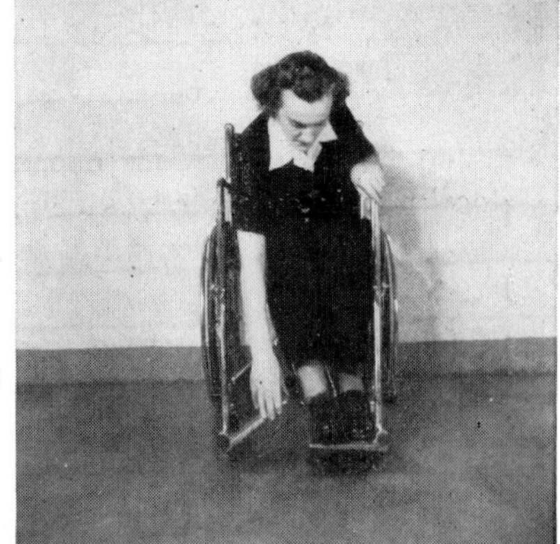

3

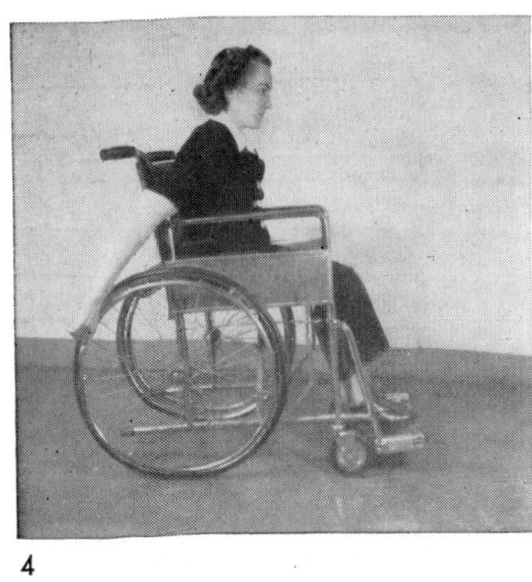

4

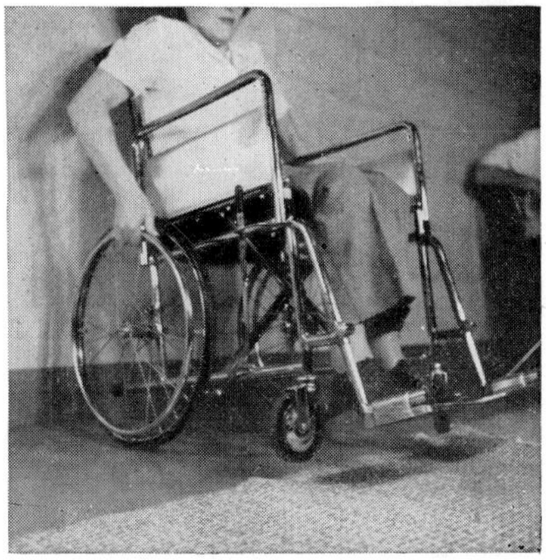

5

Toilet Activities

Toilet activities are divided into hygiene, appearance, and toilet needs. In the bathroom, transfer from the wheel chair and accessibility of all essential equipment are the major problems. If a given situation does not allow for independent handling, wheel-chair adjustments or special devices may be necessary. The following outline of the essential toilet activities with helpful suggestions will illustrate this point.

I. Hygiene
   A. Washing:* *Removable armrests* and an *old-fashioned sink* will ensure easy reach when washing hands and face (Figs. 20·1, 20·2, 20·3). Towel racks should be of wheel-chair height. Hands and face can also be washed when the patient is standing on crutches (Fig. 47B·6). *A long-handled brush* is helpful for washing the lower extremities and the back. Hanging soap on a string around the neck will prevent dropping it.
   B. Oral hygiene: A special shelf of wheel-chair height for toothbrush, tooth paste, and glass will make for convenience.
   C. Shower and bath: (See also washing, above, and Note, below.) The patient takes the shower sitting down on a small bench which is placed against the shower wall. If the patient cannot transfer directly from the wheel chair to the bench, because of the layout of the bathroom, a second bench (or as many as necessary) is used. It is easier for the patient to slide from the wheel chair to the shower bench, than to get into a tub. Also, less help is needed to clean up the shower than the tub.
      1. **In and out of shower—using two benches** (Fig. 21A).
      2. **In and out of shower—using one bench** (Fig. 21B).
      3. **In and out of bathtub** (Figs. 21C, D, E).

II. Appearance. The care of the hair and nails, make-up and shaving will be taken care of in the wheel chair, and therefore the mirrors of dressing table or bathroom should be adjusted to a convenient height. A dressing table permitting close approach of the wheel chair is suggested. For men, shaving utensils, comb, brushes, etc., should be on a shelf at wheel-chair height. If a dressing table or a shelf cannot be used, a wheel-chair lapboard may be used (Fig. 20·4).
   The care of nails, especially the toenails, should not be forgotten. Patients with sensory disturbances should check their toenails weekly. Ingrowing, rough, or overlong toenails will bruise the skin. The toenails should be cut straight across and not too short, so that the underlying tissues are not injured. It is advisable that patients, especially those who are spastic, do not trim their toenails themselves.

III. Toilet needs. If a patient has bowel and bladder problems, it has been found that the sitting position on the toilet will aid greatly in the satisfactory emptying of the bowels as well as the bladder. Therefore transfer from the wheel chair to the toilet should be taught as soon as possible. Four methods are described.
   A. **From wheel chair to toilet seat and back** (Fig. 22A). The patient transfers directly.
   B. **From wheel chair to toilet seat using small bench** (Fig. 22B). A small bench is used to bridge the gap between the wheel chair and the toilet.
   C. **Special toilet bench** (Fig. 22B·6). This is used to bridge the gap *and* overcome the difference in height.
   D. **Zipper in back rest of wheel chair** (Fig. 22A·6). This permits the patient to slide backward on to the toilet.

Once the patient has mastered ambulation and elevation, he is taught to get on and off the toilet while wearing braces and crutches.

See also dressing activities: special pants and urinal (p. 70).

* Special Note: Patients with sensory disturbances must take extremely good care of their skin. Thorough drying is essential. Daily light lubrication with skin cream will help to keep the skin smooth. The skin must be also regularly checked for red spots or breaks which may precede pressure sores. *A long-handled mirror* will aid in inspecting all areas of the skin where pressure might be suspected, *e.g.,* heels, buttocks, hips, small of back, and elbows. If any skin changes are found, pressure must be removed and treatment carried through according to a doctor's prescription.

Fig. 20. WHEEL-CHAIR ADJUSTMENTS

Hard reach—armrests attached

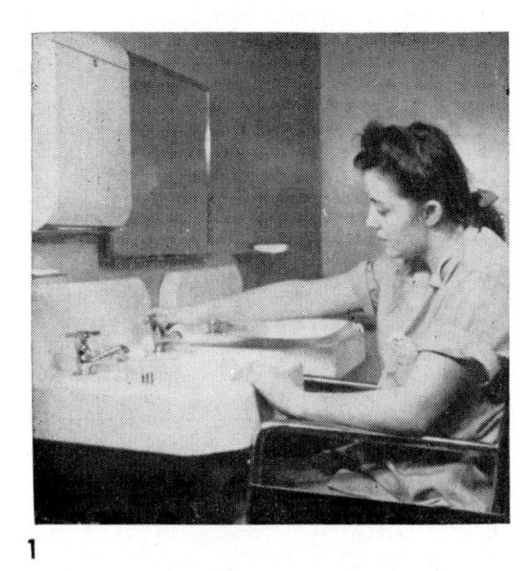

1

Easy reach—armrests removed

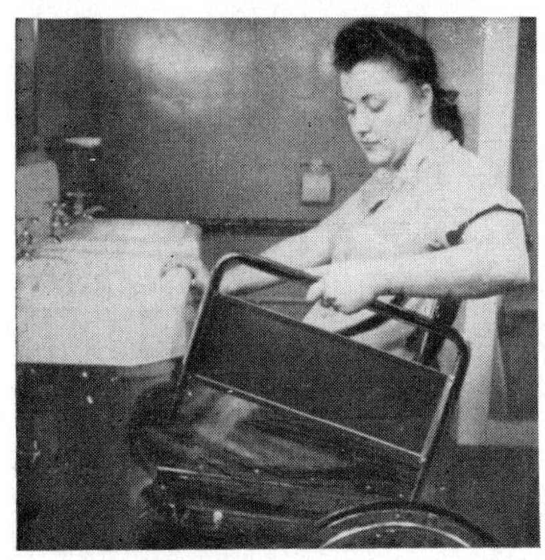

2

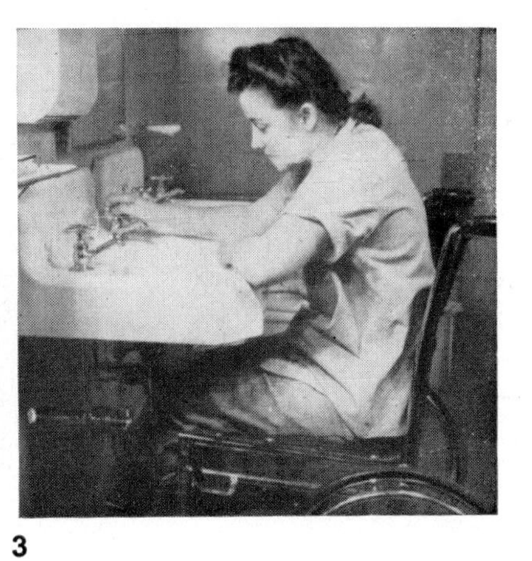

3

Lapboard (substitute for table)

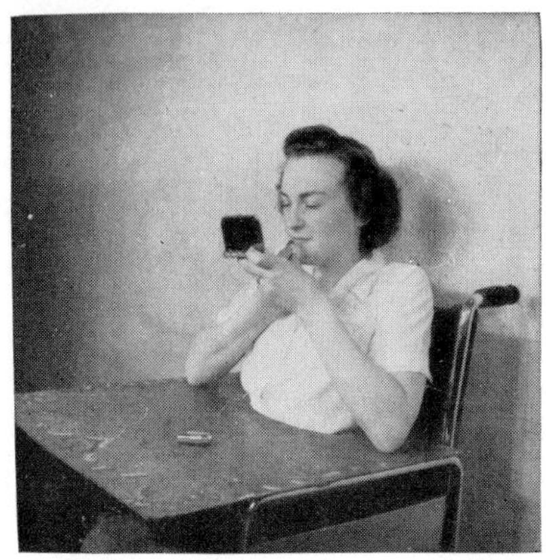

4

Fig. 21A. IN AND OUT OF SHOWER—using two benches

Preliminary exercises: transfer from wheel chair to chair; sitting balance in the wheel chair.
Equipment: two small benches.

Into shower:

Instructions:

1. A small bench is placed against shower wall. (For direct transfer from wheel chair to bench, see Figs. 21B·1a–3a.)
2. Adjoining first bench a second bench is placed outside shower. Second bench is slightly lower than wheel chair which. . .
3. . . . is placed as near as possible to it. Patient then can slide from wheel chair over outside bench on to inside bench, until he sits with back well supported against shower wall.

Back to wheel chair:
Reverse entire procedure. (Read pictures in reverse sequence.)

Helpful remarks: For easy sliding the two bench tops should be on the same level. Since shower floor is usually higher than bathroom floor, legs of inside bench should be shorter to accommodate difference in heights (or longer if shower floor is lower).

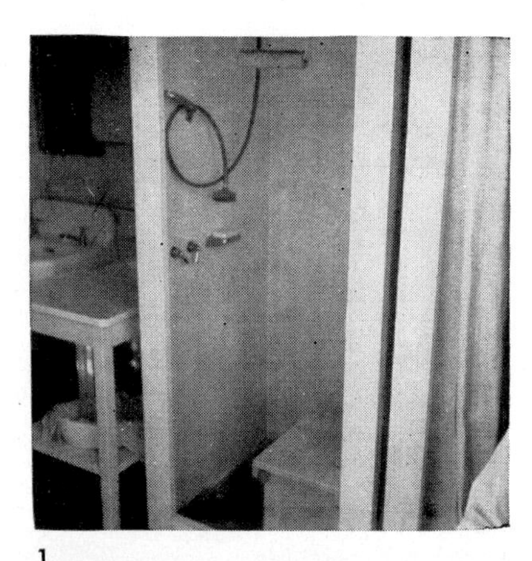

1

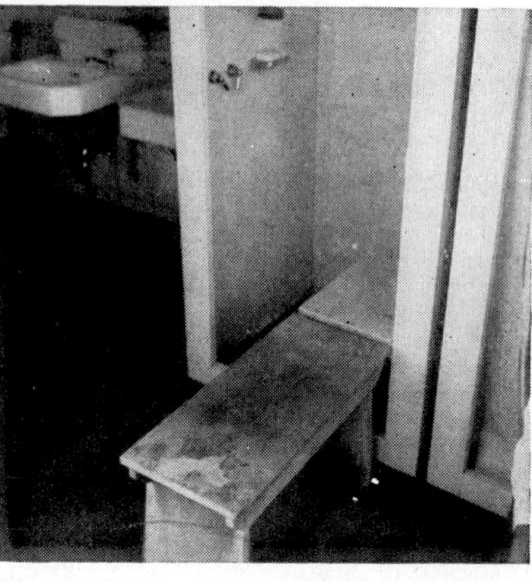

2

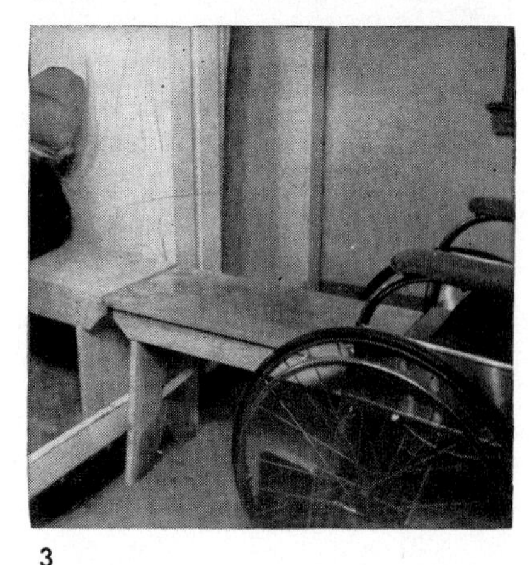

3

Fig. 21B. IN AND OUT OF SHOWER—using one bench

Equipment: See Figure 21A·1 and description.

Into shower:

Instructions:

1a. Roll wheel chair as near as possible to bench. Place right hand on bench and left hand on shower wall and slide as far forward as possible to edge of seat.

2a. Turn body and grasp left armrest with left hand and bar inside shower with right hand. Pull up with right hand while pushing down on left hand and lift body across to bench inside.

3a. Adjust legs and turn body until back is well supported against the wall, so that both hands are free when taking shower.

Back to wheel chair: Reverse entire procedure. (Read pictures in reverse sequence.)

Precautions: If there are any sensory disturbances, extreme caution has to be exercised in regard to temperature of water. A hand hose is connected with shower nozzle so that patient can easily regulate water temperature himself (Fig. 21A·1). To prevent sliding, a rubber mat with suction cups should be placed on bathroom floor. A foam-rubber pillow should be placed on inside bench.

Helpful remarks: Instead of small bench an old kitchen chair can be used inside shower. To prevent slipping, suction crutch tips should be placed on legs of chair.

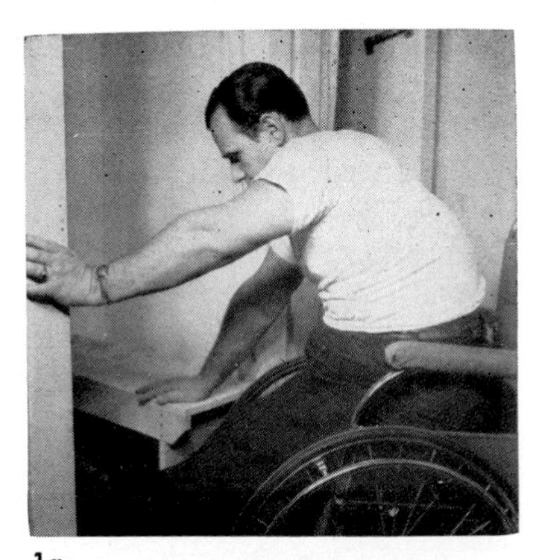

1a

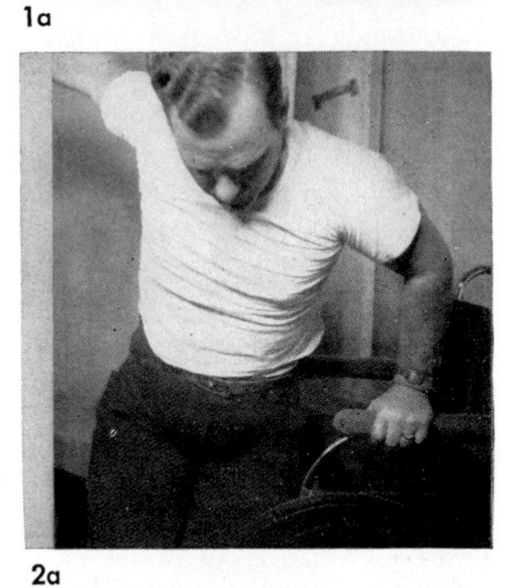

2a

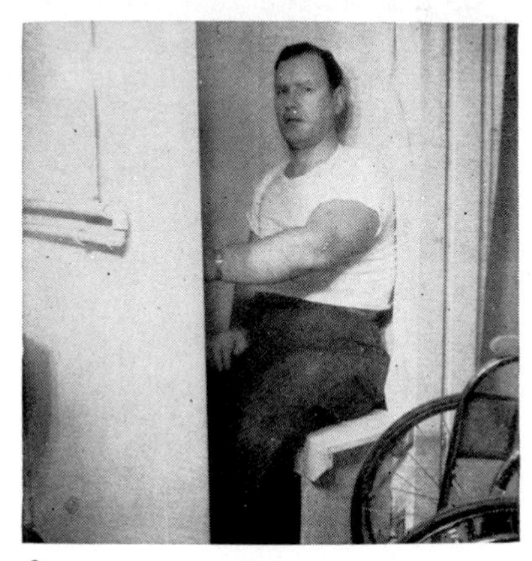

3a

Fig. 21C. IN AND OUT OF BATHTUB

Preliminary exercises: from bed to wheel chair; from wheel chair to chair, to toilet, to mat.

Into bathtub:

Starting Position: Sit in wheel chair, approach bathtub from side near free end of tub. Lock brakes. Be sure to leave enough space between wheel chair and tub, so that legs can be lifted (Fig. **21C**·1) without bruising them.

Instructions:

1. Lift left leg with both hands over edge of tub.
2. Lift right leg with both hands over edge of tub and...
3. ...place it next to left leg.
4. Unlock brakes. Place wheel chair as close as possible to tub, so that your legs hang over the edge of tub. Lock brakes and slide as far forward on wheel-chair seat as possible.
5. Place right hand on far edge of tub and left hand on left armrest.
6. Shift right hand to opposite edge of tub, while therapist grasps you around waist. Keep left hand on left armrest or place it...
7. ...on edge of tub next to you. Push hard on both hands and lower body slowly into tub. *Slow* bending of elbows will control movement.

Out of bathtub: Reverse entire procedure. (Read pictures in reverse sequence.)

Precautions: To prevent sliding, a rubber mat with suction cups should be placed on bottom of tub.

6. While patient lowers his body into tub it is important (*a*) to support him around waist, (*b*) to avoid a sudden stretch in shoulder joint by bending elbows as slow as possible, (*c*) to guide patient's legs if he is very tall, and also if he is spastic.

(The same precautions have to be taken when getting out of tub.) If there are any sensory disturbances, extreme caution has to be observed as to water temperature.

Helpful remarks: A small stool can be placed in tub, so there is less height to be overcome when getting in and out of tub. To prevent slipping, suction crutch tips should be placed on legs of stool and stool should stand on a rubber bath mat which also has suction cups. If tub is filled with water, it is easier to get in and out, but great caution must be observed.

It is essential to place wheel chair as close to tub as possible, to facilitate getting in and out of tub. Placement of wheel chair will depend on the layout of bathroom and kind of tub used.

If tub is flush against the wall, it will be helpful to attach a horizontal bar to wall, so that patient can grasp it and push on it when getting in and out (Figs. **21D**·1–4).

If wheel chair cannot be brought near enough to tub and/or if armrests are not removable, a small bench will bridge gap between wheel chair and tub (Figs. **21E**·1–3).

Fig. 21C. IN AND OUT OF BATHTUB

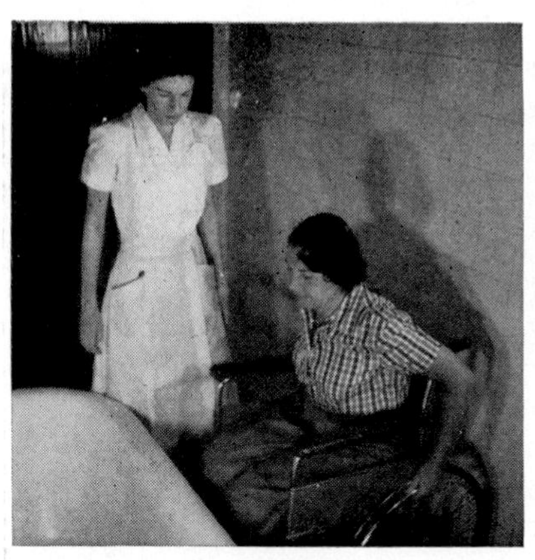

S.P.

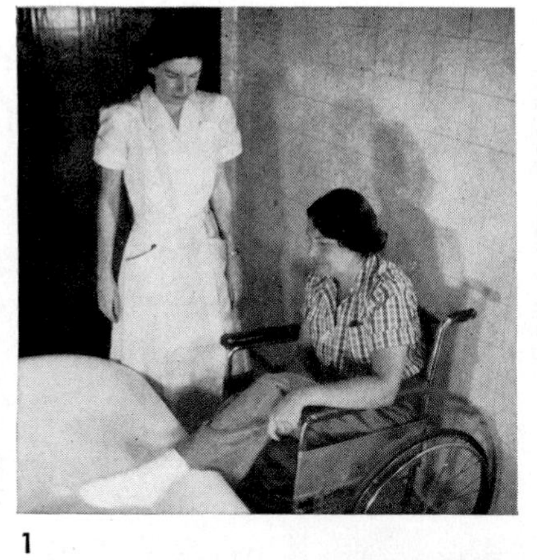

1

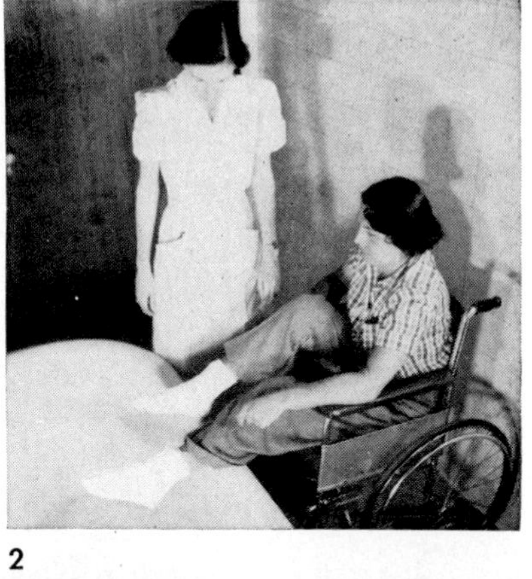

2

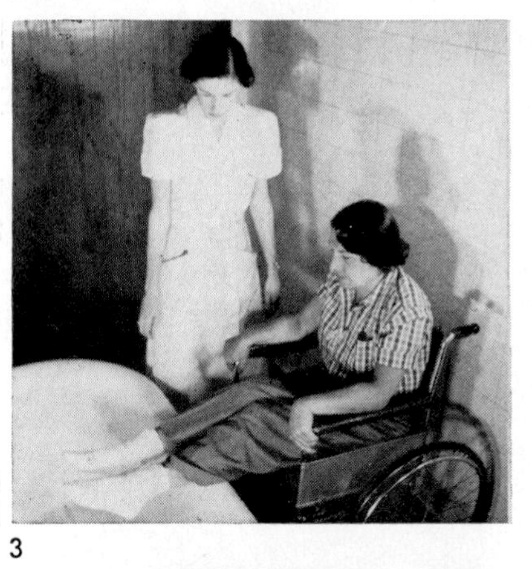

3

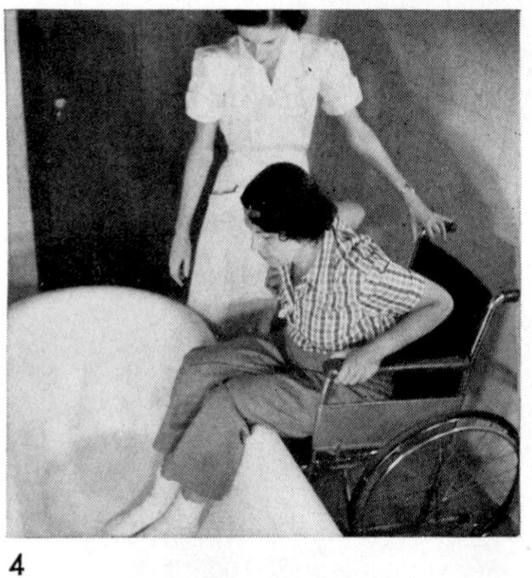

4

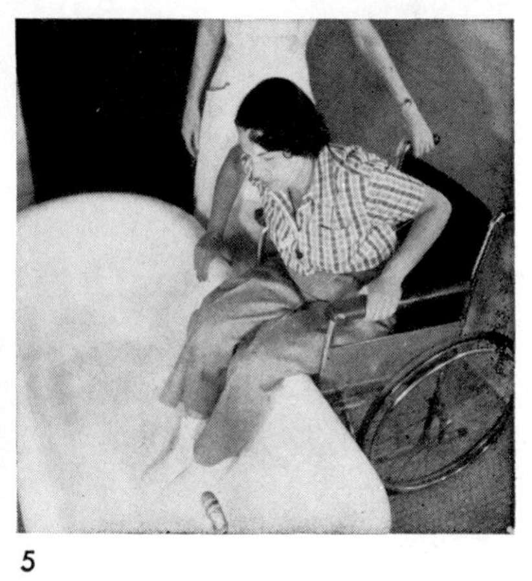

5

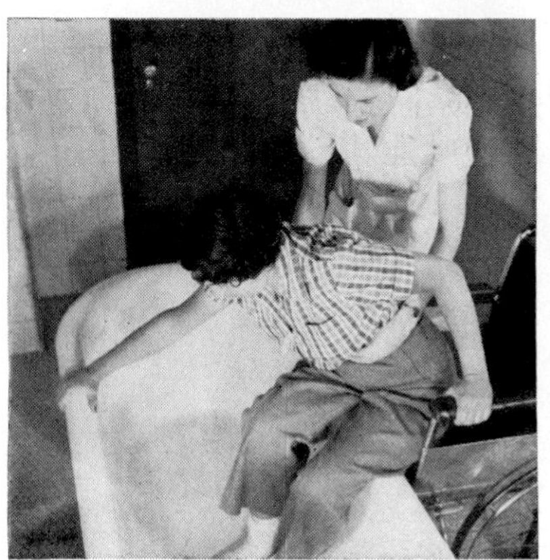

6

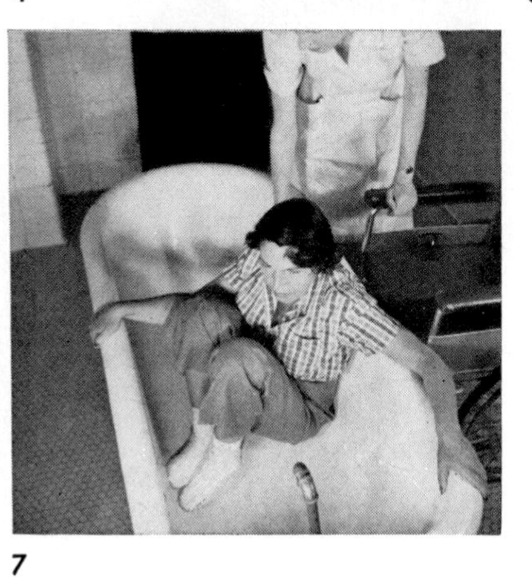

7

Fig. 21D. IN AND OUT OF BATHTUB

With bar attached to wall, so that patient can grasp it and push on it. (For out of tub, read pictures in reverse sequence.)

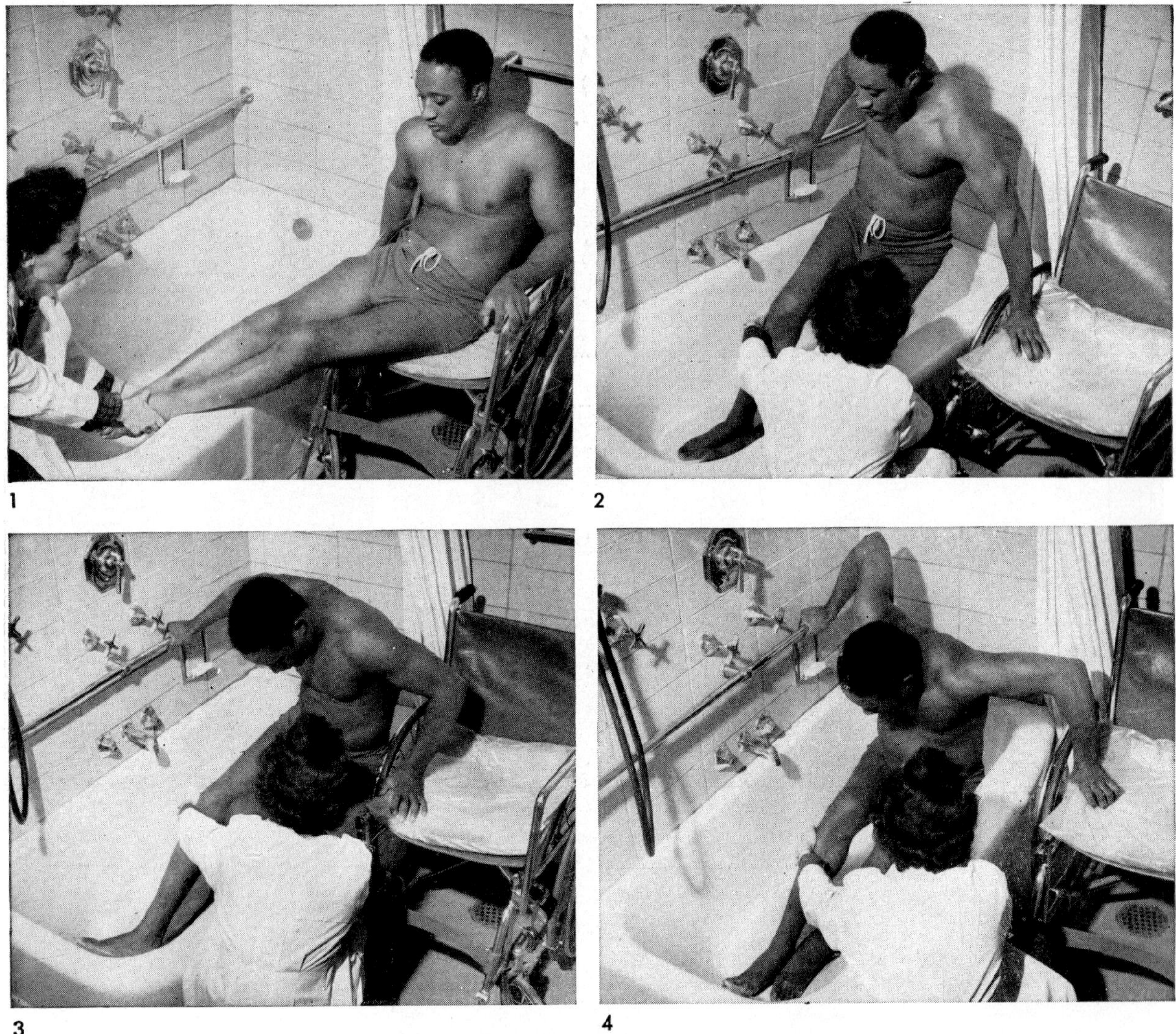

1 2 3 4

Fig. 21E. IN AND OUT OF BATHTUB

With small bench to bridge gap between wheel chair and bathtub. (For out of tub, read pictures in reverse sequence.)

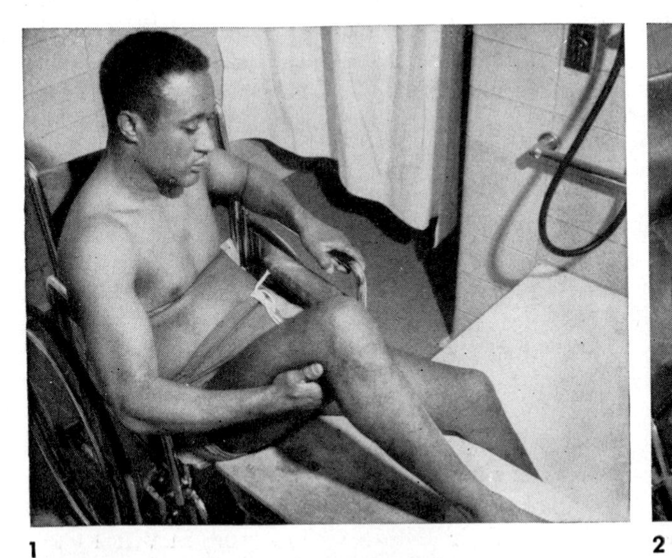

1

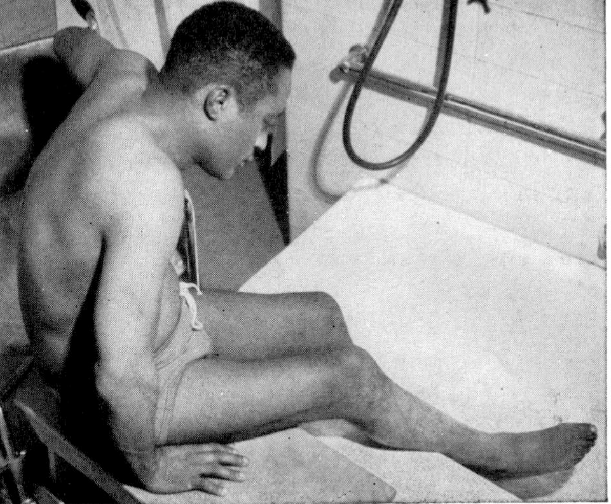

2

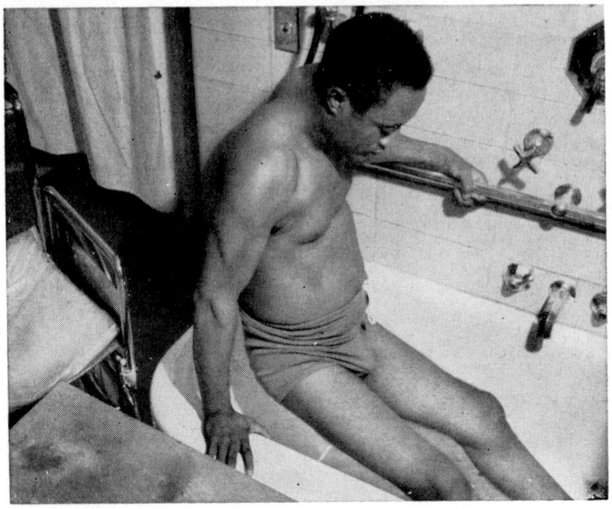

3

Fig. 22A. FROM WHEEL CHAIR TO TOILET SEAT AND BACK—directly

The transfer from wheel chair to toilet seat is basically the same as transfer from wheel chair to chair. The following method is the most commonly used. Placement of wheel chair will vary with layout of different bathrooms (see variations below).

Preliminary exercises: sitting balance; push-ups; from wheel chair to chair.

From wheel chair to toilet seat:

Starting Position: Sit in wheel chair. Roll as close as possible to toilet seat, approaching same from the side. Footrests are down. (May also be up—will depend on shape of toilet bowl.)

Instructions:

1. Place both legs with hands toward right of wheel chair. Slide to edge of chair, grasping both armrests.
2. Place left hand on toilet seat (or pipe or toilet tank), still grasping right armrest with right hand. Push on both hands...
3. ...and lift and shift body on to toilet seat, turning at the same time until...
4. ...you sit straight.

From toilet seat to wheel chair: Reverse entire procedure. (Read pictures in reverse sequence.)

Precautions:

5. If lower extremities are very spastic, therapist guides them to prevent bruising of toes and feet.

For additional support and to ensure balance when sliding on to toilet seat and back or when sitting on it, the following can be done:

a. Patient holds on to wheel chair and/or iron bar alongside wall.

b. A chair is placed in front of patient with backrest facing him so that back can be grasped for support (Fig. **15**·4).

c. Wheel chair is placed in front of patient with armrests facing him so that armrests can be grasped. Many patients find this position helpful when using toilet paper.

d. If toilet has a tank it can be used as a back rest.

If there is any tendency to pressure sores, a foam-rubber ring should be placed on toilet seat.

Helpful remarks: Most patients find it easier to adjust their clothes while sitting in wheel chair before and after using toilet.

Variations in placement of wheel chair:

a. Wheel chair is placed alongside toilet, if armrests are removable, so that patient slides or lifts himself sideways on to toilet (Fig. **16F**).

b. Wheel chair is rolled as close as possible facing toilet so that patient slides forward on to same, in a straddling position and backward into wheel chair.

c. Wheel chair is backed up to toilet if there is a zipper in back rest (Fig. **22A**·6).

For more variations see pages 68–69.

Fig. 22A. FROM WHEEL CHAIR TO TOILET SEAT AND BACK—directly

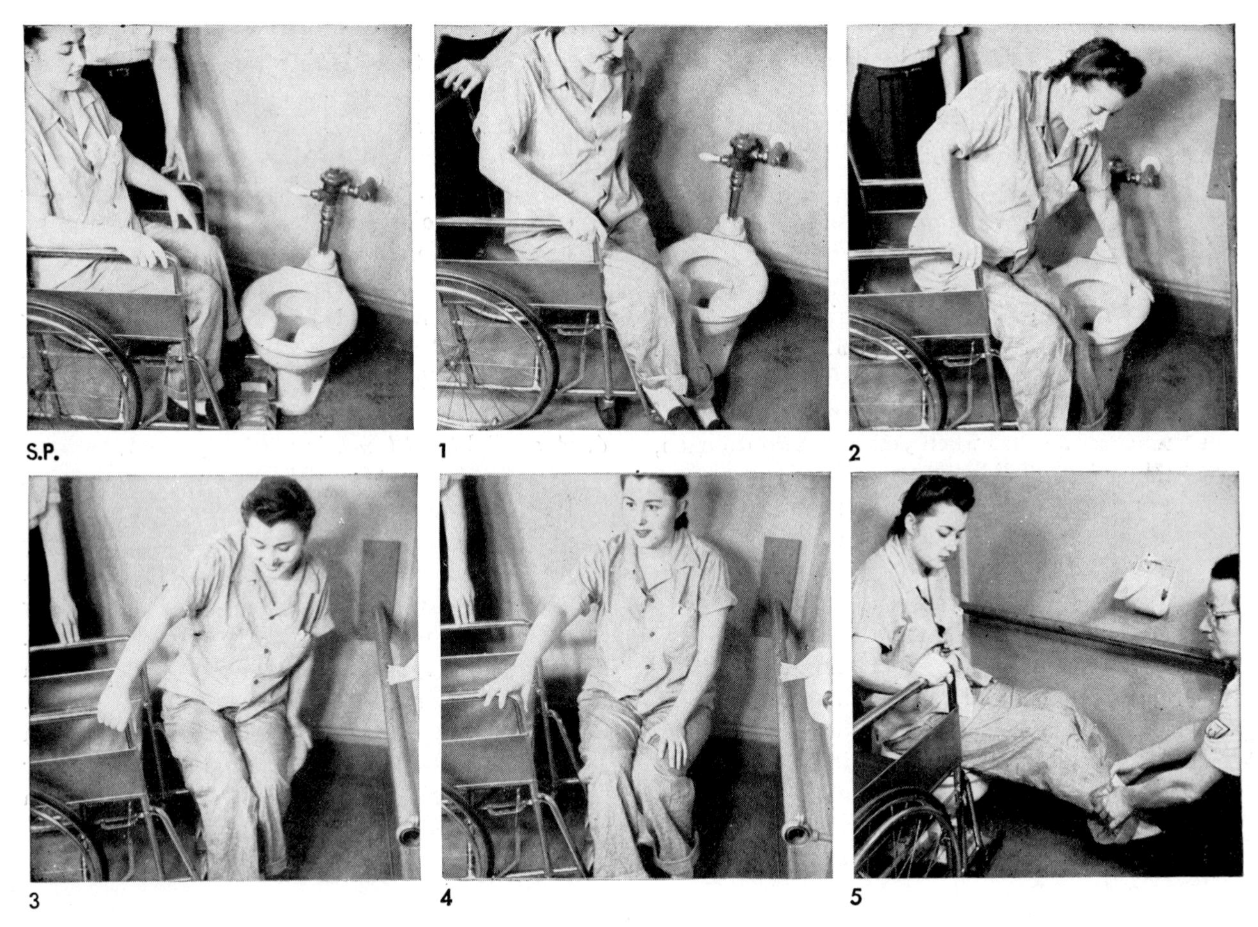

S.P. 1 2

3 4 5

Zipper in back rest

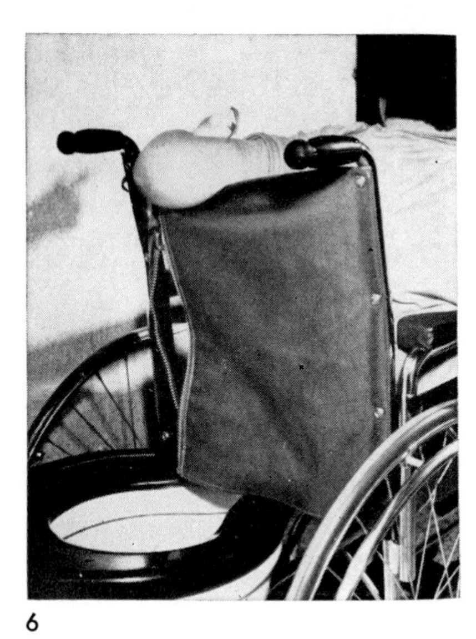

6

Fig. 22B. FROM WHEEL CHAIR TO TOILET SEAT AND BACK—using small bench

A small bench is used to bridge gap between wheel chair and toilet, if patient cannot lift himself across directly or if wheel chair for any reason cannot be brought near enough to toilet.
Equipment: small bench.

From wheel chair to toilet seat:

Starting Position: Sit in wheel chair with footrests up and face narrow side of bench. Brakes are off.
Instructions:

1. With both hands place both legs to right side of wheel chair so that when you roll toward bench, wheel chair will slide...
2. ...over edge of bench. Roll as near as you can. Put footrests down, if they are in the way of your feet.
3. By rolling wheel chair push bench as close to toilet as possible, as shown in picture.
4. Lock brakes. Slide to edge of wheel-chair seat—turning body forward, so that knees can bend.
5. Place left hand on bench—holding on to right armrest with other hand—and slide sideways on to bench. Place left hand on toilet seat—still holding on to armrest with other hand (or place it on bench). Push on both hands and slide (lift body if necessary) on to toilet seat.

From toilet seat to wheel chair: Reverse entire procedure. (Read pictures in reverse sequence.)

Precautions: If there is any tendency to pressure sores, bench should be upholstered.
Helpful remarks:

3. If space permits, the bench can be kept in position all day, ready for the patient to use it. The exact angle of placing the bench will depend on the layout and space in the bathroom. If bathroom door is too narrow to move wheel chair through, as many benches or chairs as necessary can be used to bridge distance between wheel chair and toilet (see Fig. 17).

6. *A special toilet bench* is used if patient, because of lack of strength or balance or because toilet bowl is much lower than wheel-chair seat, cannot push on hands sufficiently to overcome difference in height between wheel chair and toilet seat. The bench is $\frac{1}{8}$ to $\frac{1}{2}$ in. lower than wheel-chair seat, so that patient has only to slide on to bench. Length and width and the cutout will depend on construction as well as placement of toilet bowl. If there is any tendency to pressure sores, bench can be upholstered with one layer of foam rubber which is covered with plastic. Otherwise, bench should be painted with washable paint.

Fig. 22B. FROM WHEEL CHAIR TO TOILET SEAT AND BACK—using small bench

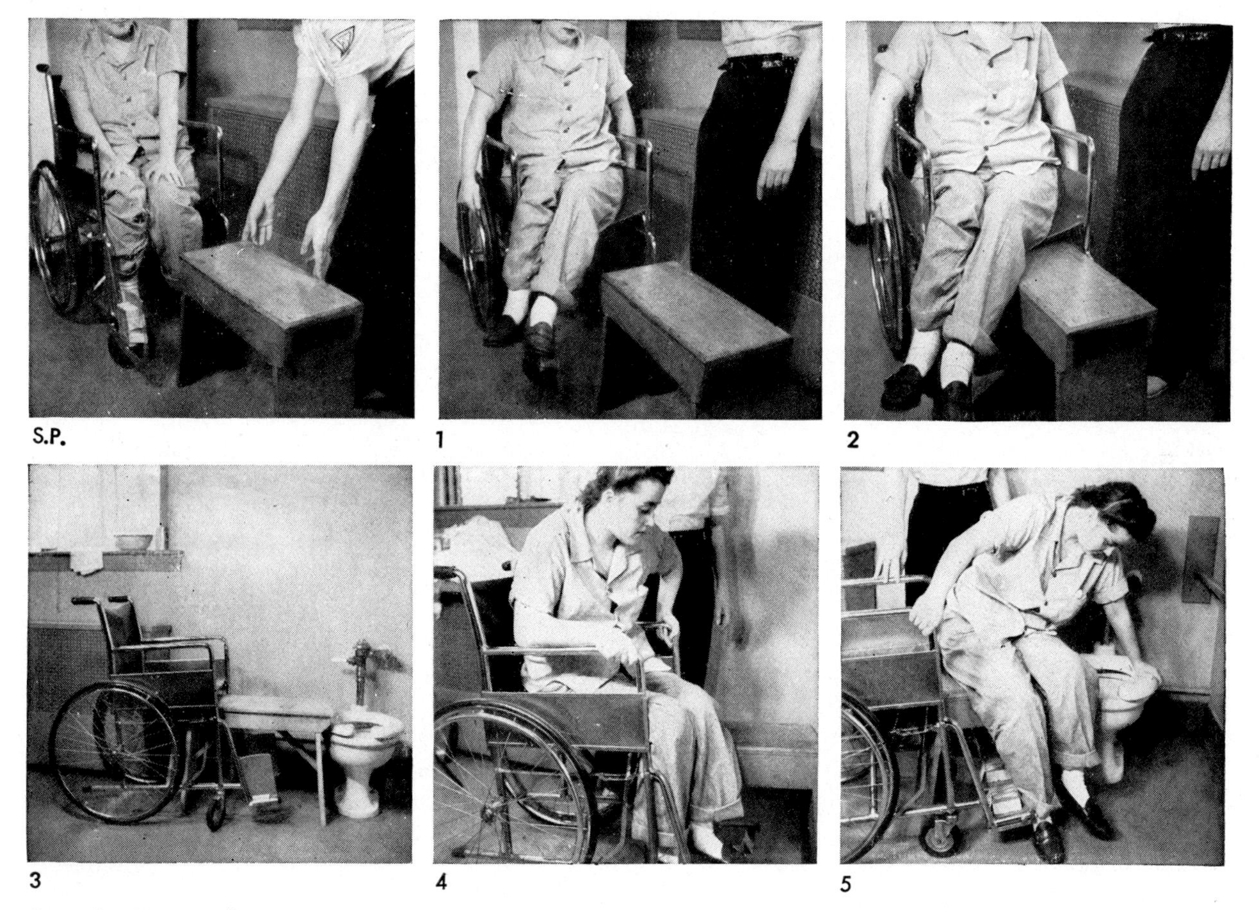

S.P. 1 2

3 4 5

Special toilet bench (used to accommodate difference in height between wheel chair and toilet seat)

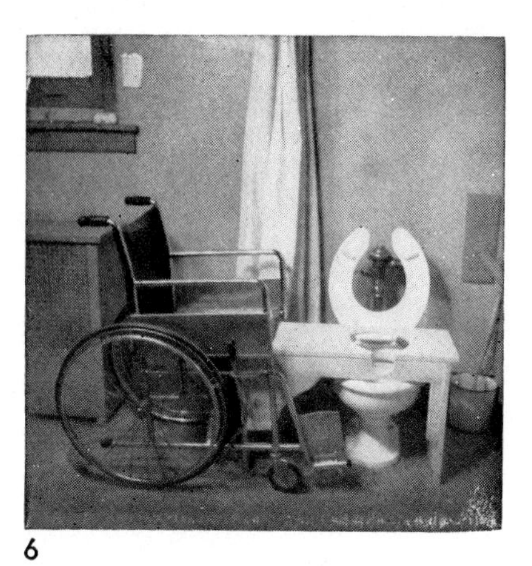

6

Dressing Activities

All clothing apparel is divided into four groups: underwear and nightwear, outer clothes and overclothes, footwear, and accessories. The main problems to be considered in dressing activities are (*a*) accessibility of apparel to patient in the wheel chair as well as on crutches, (*b*) material and style of clothes, (*c*) easy methods for dressing and undressing.

Suggestions for accessibility: Top drawers rather than lower drawers of dressers should be used. Closet rods, shoebags, shelves for shoes and accessories should all be of wheel-chair height.

Suggestions for material and style of clothes: The material should be durable and preferably wrinkle-resistant. It should also be smooth, *e.g.*, rayon or wool gabardine, to facilitate transfer from and to wheel chair. The style should be of a type that will fit easily over braces and stand the wear and tear of walking with crutches.

Following is an outline of the essential items of wearing apparel. For each item special suggestions are made which may be helpful in selecting the most practical type of clothing. Articles of men's clothing will be listed first under each item.

Underwear and nightwear:

1. Pajama tops: button-in-front
2. Pajama pants: see slacks below
3. Dressing gown: wrap-around style
4. Slippers: moccasin-type, so that they will stay on foot. The patient should not be barefoot at any time, to prevent bruising of toes.
5. Undershirt: presents no problem
6. Bra: may be helpful if fastens in front
7. Girdle: maternity-type girdle, which opens all the way down, so that the patient can roll into it
8. Garter belt: advisable if stockings are not held in place by braces. Round garters should not be worn, since they cut off the circulation.
9. Urinal: Male patients with bladder problems usually wear rubber urinals. They should be instructed by the nurse as to application, cleaning of the urinal, and care of the skin.
10. Pads and special pants: Female patients with bladder problems wear *absorbent pads* (Cellucotton or cotton) which are held in place with a thin elastic band (sanitary-napkin belt).
    Special short pants are worn in addition to prevent leakage around the pads. Rubberized nylon is the preferred material; however, if this is not available, the pants can be made of nylon and then lined with a waterproof material such as plastic or vinylite. The pants are designed as follows (see illustration, page 71): There are elastic bands around the waistline and the thighs to ensure snug fitting. To facilitate putting on and taking off the pants, there are snaps all the way down in front. There are snaps also across (at the height where the pads are fastened) so that, when the patient is attending to toilet needs, the pants can be opened without removing the braces. This opening also makes it easier to change the pads. Since the opening and closing of zippers frequently injure the skin, it is advisable not to use them. The described design will ensure longer wear of the pants.
11. Slips: Halfslips will provide extra width over the hips to fit over braces.

Outer clothes, overclothes and braces:

1. Shirts: present no problem.
2. Blouses: should button in front, have action back and sleeves with wide armholes (raglan sleeves are not satisfactory, since they tear easily).
3. Pants and slacks: For methods of putting on see Figs. **24A** and **24B.**
4. Slacks for women: Buttons or zippers in front will make for easier fastening. Zippers in the side seams of the slacks are practical for patients who wear long leg braces without a pelvic band, so that the braces can be put on as well as removed without removing the slacks. Maternity slacks are adjustable around the waist; therefore the same pair can be worn with or without braces. There are also ordinary slacks on the market that have adjustable zippers around the waist.
5. Braces: for methods of putting on and removing see Fig. **25.** Also see "Braces" in Chapter VII.
6. Skirts: should be wide with fullness around the waist and hips (*e.g.*, dirndl skirt).
7. Dresses: should have action back, sleeves with wide armholes and full skirts. It is also helpful if the dress opens all the way down the front.
8. Coats: one-half or three-quarter-length coats are more practical than full-length coats for patients in the wheel chair or on crutches.

Footwear:

1. Socks and stockings: for methods of putting on see page 72. Stockings for women: service-weight nylon is suggested (see also garter belt

above). Socks for men: no elastic on top will facilitate putting on as well as prevent cutting off the circulation. To prevent pressure sores, patients with sensory disturbances must be careful that their socks or stockings do not wrinkle in their shoes.

2. Shoes: for method of putting on see Fig. **23.** For type of shoes see "Braces" in Chapter VII.

Accessories:

1. Gloves: In the wintertime, woolen gloves with a leather palm are helpful in handling crutches.
2. Pocketbooks: Shoulder bags are easier to carry when using crutches than other kinds of pocketbooks or briefcases (Fig. **43C**).

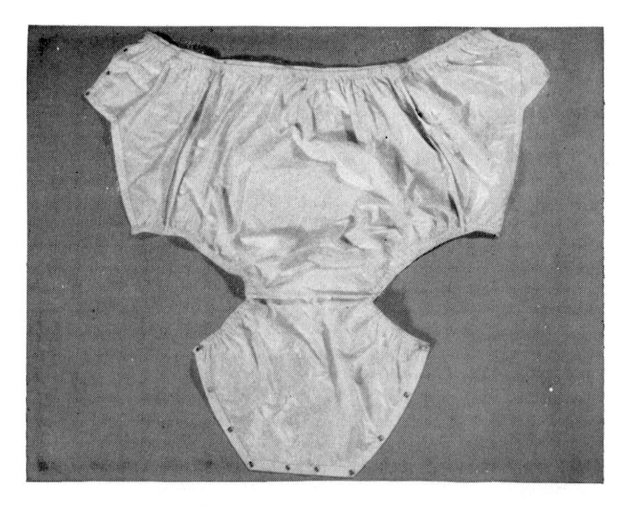

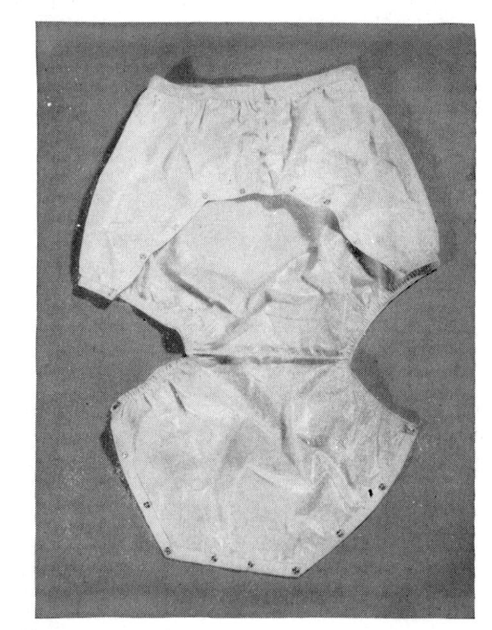

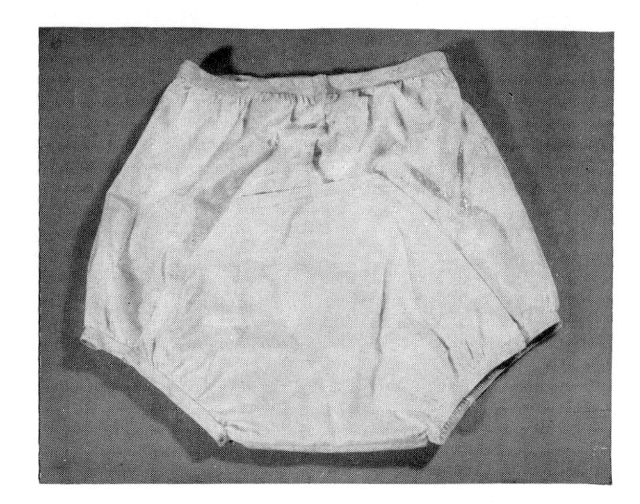

PUTTING ON AND TAKING OFF SLACKS

When choosing specific methods, the same considerations in regard to flaccid or spastic lower extremities apply as in "Putting on Shoes."

Fig. 24A. PUTTING ON AND TAKING OFF SLACKS WITHOUT BRACES

Preliminary exercises: rolling over and moving sideward—supine; sitting up; sitting balance; push-ups in sitting.

Putting on slacks:

Starting Position: Sit in bed and slip pants over legs. For different positions, see Figure **23.**

Instructions:

1. Lie down and roll to left and pull up slacks...

2. ...roll to right and pull up slacks. Repeat as often as necessary until slacks can be fastened around waist.

Taking off slacks: Reverse entire procedure. (Read pictures in reverse sequence.)

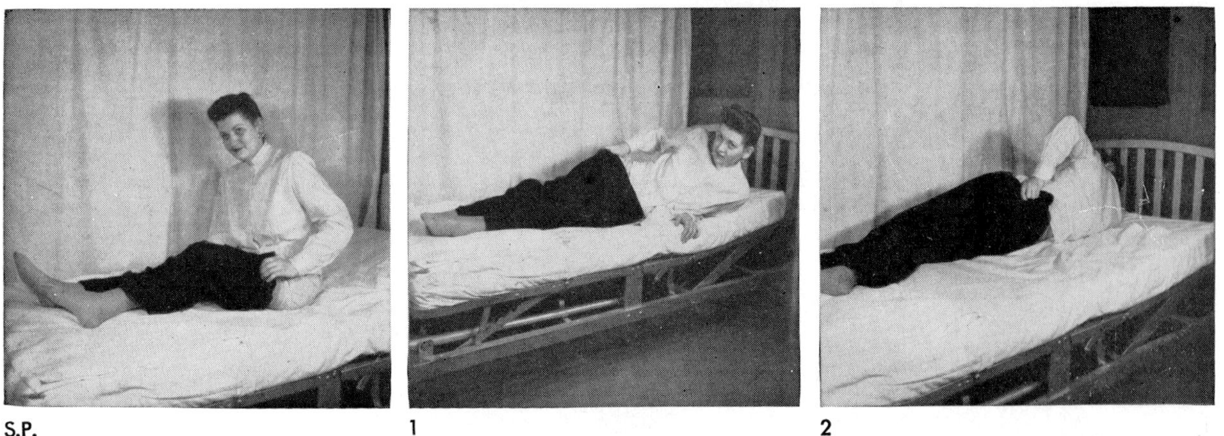

S.P. 1 2

Fig. 24B. PUTTING ON AND TAKING OFF SLACKS OVER BRACES

Preliminary exercises: putting on and taking off slacks; putting on and removing braces (Fig. 25).

Instructions: The same method as in Figure **24A** can be used. If patient is very spastic or needs help for some other reason, the following method is indicated:

1a, 2a. Slip on pant legs while sitting with knee joints of brace locked.

3a. Push up on small sandbags, so that therapist can pull slacks up for you.

4a. If you have difficulty bending forward, use a stick to slip slacks over legs.

Helpful remarks: For some patients it is easier to leave knee joint of brace unlocked as they slip pant leg over front of shoe. Then knee joint of brace is locked and as leg is raised with one hand, pant leg is pulled over heel of shoe with other hand. Now knee joint of brace is unlocked and same procedure is repeated with other leg (no picture shown). Pants are then pulled over bent knees (see **S.P.**) and activity is finished as in instructions 1 and 2 (Figs. **24A**·1 and **24A**·2).

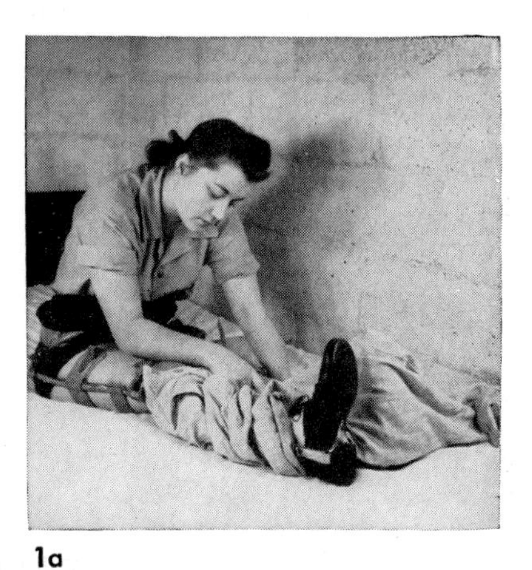

1a

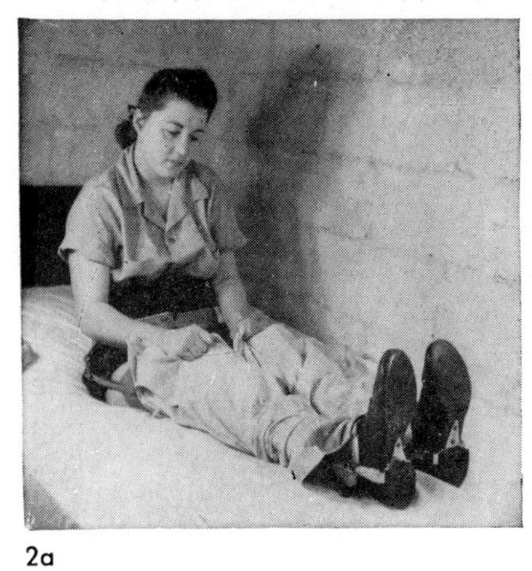

2a

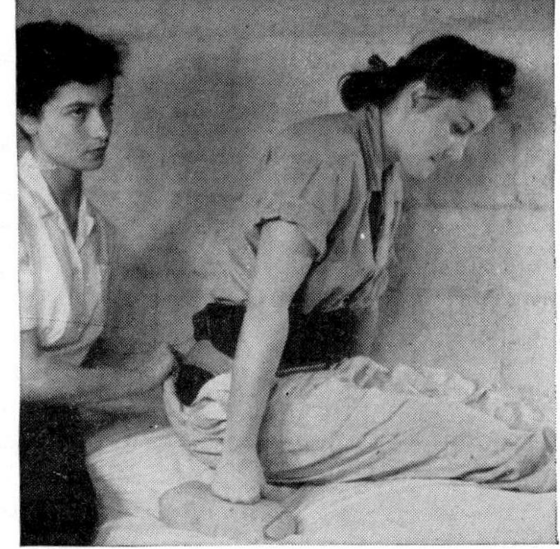

3a

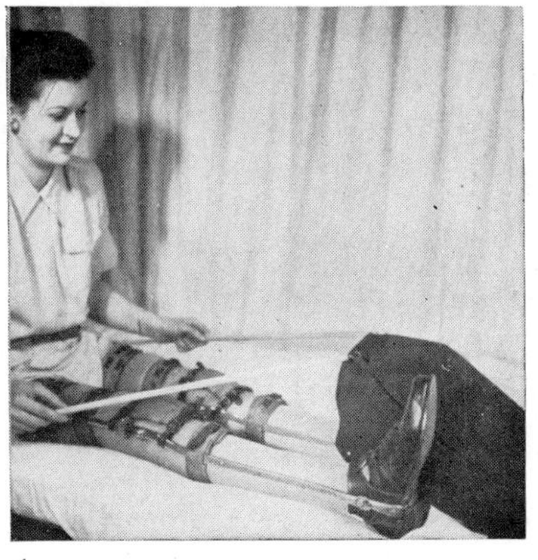

4a

Fig. 25. PUTTING ON AND REMOVING BRACES

The following methods are used for double long leg braces with a pelvic band. This procedure can be easily applied and modified for putting on any other kind of brace.

Preliminary exercises: rolling over; moving sideward —supine; sitting up; sitting balance; push-ups in sitting.

Putting on braces—method 1:

Starting Position: Lie on back with braces on your right. (**S.P.**)

Instructions:

1. Roll to left side, pull brace toward you so that pelvic band is about at height of hips. Roll and...

2. ...wiggle back into brace, so that you lie in it. Grasp pelvic band on each side and pull on it, wiggling hips, until buttocks are in right position, so that hip locks are at side of thighs and pelvic band is around waist. Finish procedure as shown in Figures 25·3a–5a.

Putting on braces—method 2:

Starting Position: Sit in bed with braces on your right. (**S.P.a.**) Arrange so that pelvic band is placed at height of hips.

Instructions:

1a. Place left hand near left hip on bed, right hand outside pelvic band on bed, or for better lifting on small sandbag. Push on both hands and...

2a. ...lift body into braces. Wiggle until you sit well in brace with hip locks at side of hips. Place right leg on top of brace.

3a. Unlock left knee lock and put left foot into shoe. Tie shoelaces while knee is still bent, then push down on knee and lock knee lock; fasten all straps, including kneepad.

4a. Unlock right knee lock, put right foot into shoe. Tie laces while knee is still bent. Tie laces in back. (Shoe has been cut in back to make it easier to put foot into shoe.)

5a. Push down with right hand (or both) on side or above knee, in order to extend it and lock knee lock. Fasten kneepad, all straps, and pelvic band. (You may have to lie down to fasten pelvic band.)

Removing braces: Reverse entire procedure. (Read pictures in reverse sequence.)

Helpful remarks:

4. To prevent heels from slipping out of shoe, it is better to lace shoes while knee is still bent.

Variation: Some patients find it easier to put on and remove braces while sitting in wheel chair.

Fig. 25. PUTTING ON AND REMOVING BRACES

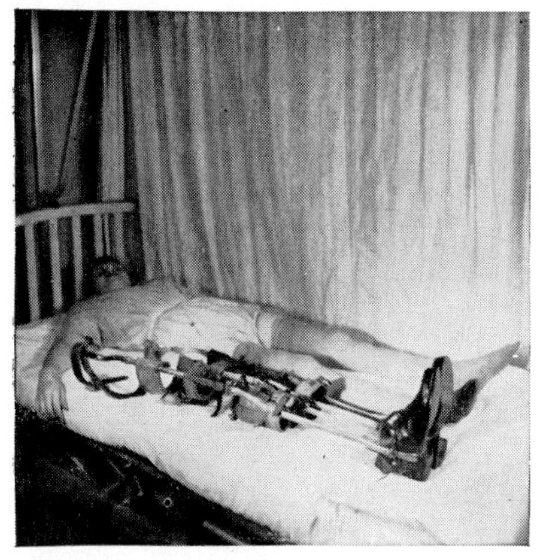
S.P.

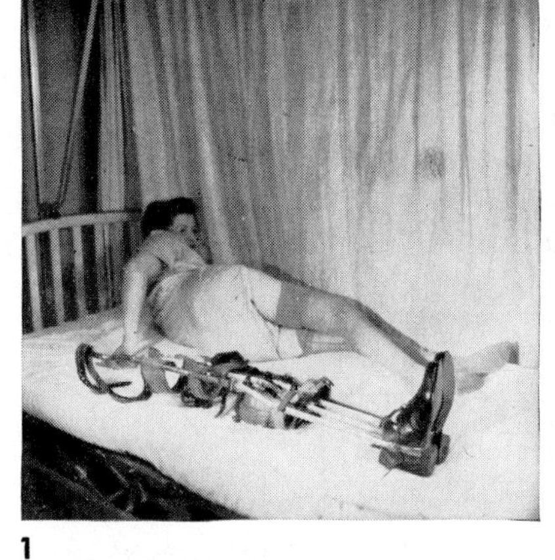
1

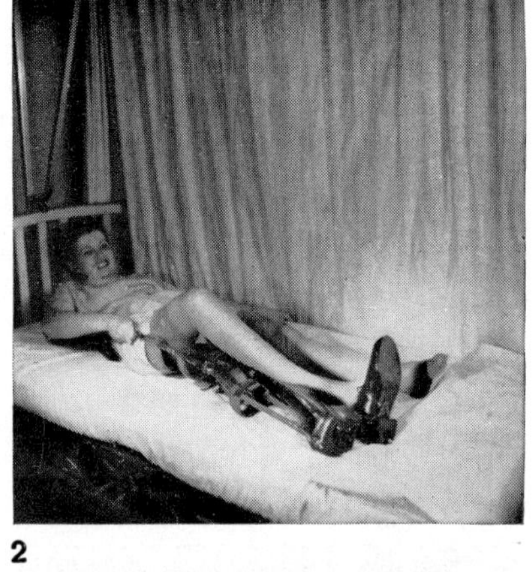
2

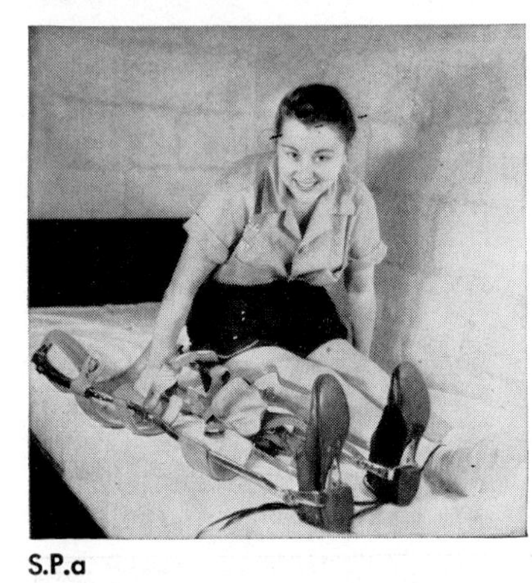
S.P.a

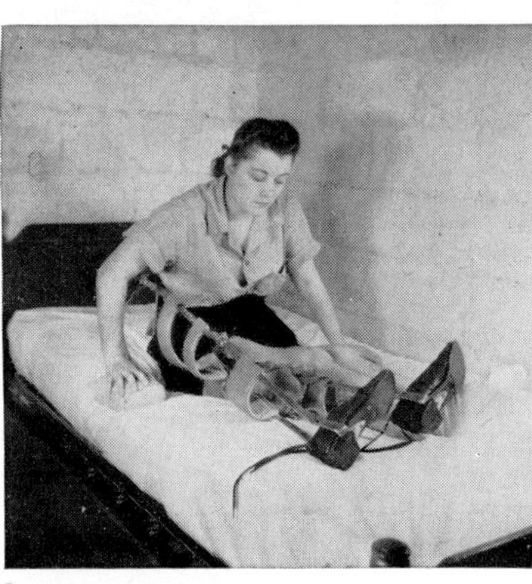
1a

2a

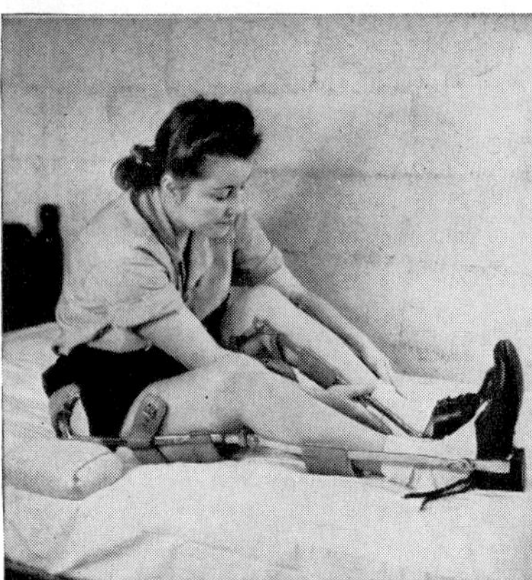
3a

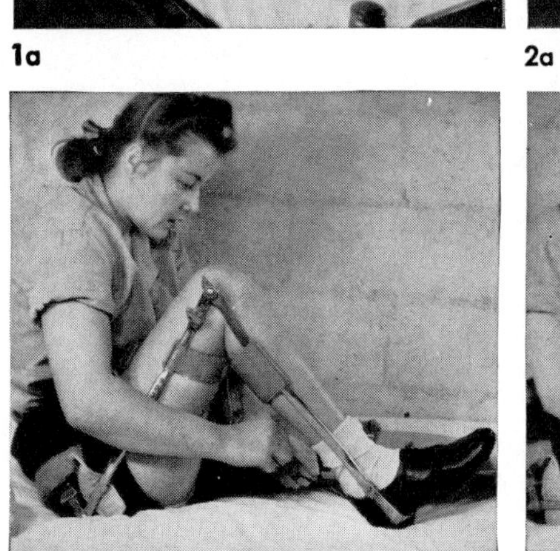
4a

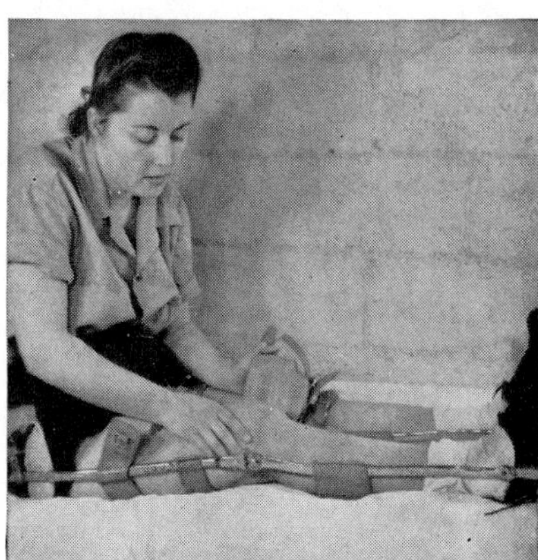
5a

Eating and Hand Activities

When considering eating and hand activities for patients with normal upper extremities, the problems are good posture and proximity of wheel chair to table. The following suggestions for furniture and wheel-chair adjustments may be helpful:

For eating, writing, etc., if the armrests of the wheel chair are not removable, the *table should be high enough* to allow the chair to slide under; otherwise the patient will not be near enough to the table (Fig. 26·1). *Removable armrests* (Fig. 26·2) or *desk arms* (Fig. 26·3) will permit use of most tables and still ensure good posture. In crowded rooms a *lapboard* (Fig. 26·4) will substitute for a table. A good reading lamp properly placed and a tilted board on the table are suggested for reading and writing activities. Telephone, radio, and light switches in the room should all be placed within easy reach.

Fig. 26. EATING AND HAND ACTIVITIES

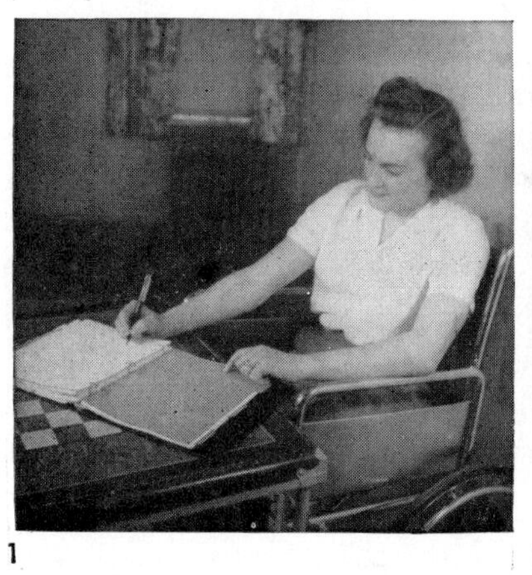

1

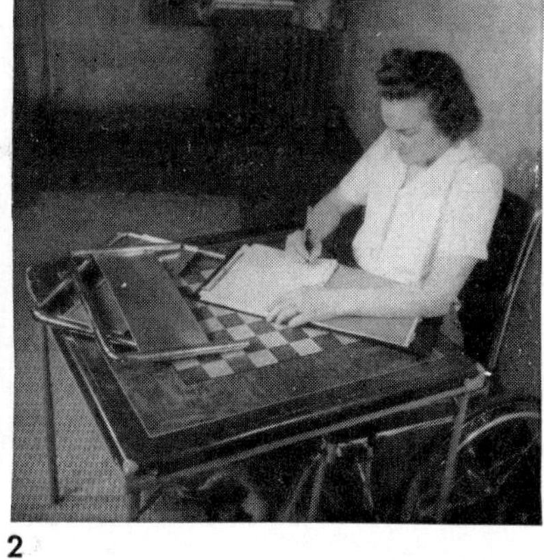

2

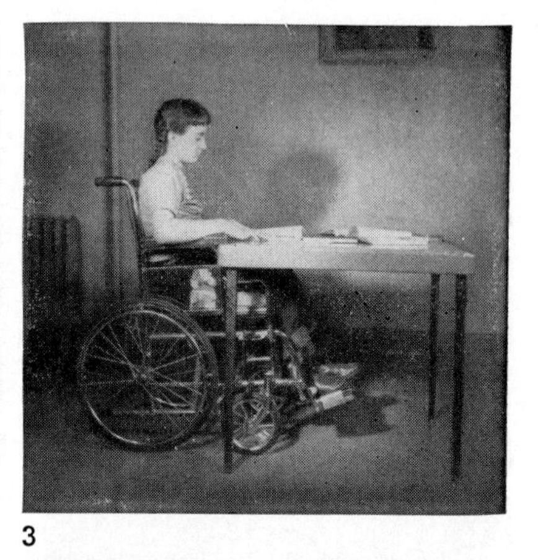

3

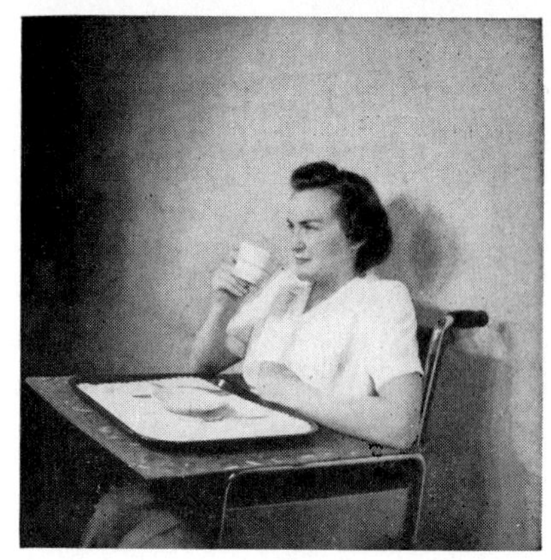

4

Travel in the Wheel Chair

A wheel-chair patient need no longer be confined to his room but can travel in his wheel chair in and out of doors. This involves the problem of stairs, inclines, and curbs as well as using a transportation medium.

1. **From wheel chair to car and back.**
   a. **Wheel chair facing car** (Fig. 27A). If the wheel chair has nonremovable armrests, it is placed facing the car.
   b. **Wheel chair alongside car** (no picture shown). If the armrests are removable, the wheel chair can be placed alongside the car.
   c. **Using board—wheel chair with nonremovable and removable armrests** (Fig. 27B). A board is used to bridge the gap between wheel-chair seat and car seat.

   The patient should learn to get in and out of the car in the gym and practice on as many different models as possible, including taxis outdoors.
2. **Up and down curb in wheel chair** (Fig. 28).
3. **Up and down stairs in wheel chair** (no picture shown).

   Help will always be needed for curbs and stairs.
4. **Up and down incline in wheel chair** (no picture shown).

Fig. 27A. FROM WHEEL CHAIR TO CAR AND BACK—wheel chair facing car

Preliminary exercises: sitting balance; moving forward and back while sitting; push-ups; control of wheel chair, from bed to wheel chair; from wheel chair to chair and back.

Equipment: wheel chair, car model in gym, later car outside.

From wheel chair to car:

Starting Position: Sit in wheel chair facing car. Unlock and open door.

Instructions:

1. Open door wide and move chair as close as possible. If there is a running board, try to slide footrests under it. Lock brakes. Slide to edge of seat. Place right hand on front seat of car and left hand behind you on wheel-chair seat.
2. Turn body facing wheel chair and push on both hands lifting...
3. ...body and shift to front seat of car.
4. Turn body again so that you sit behind steering wheel. Adjust legs.

From car to wheel chair: Reverse entire procedure. (Read pictures in reverse sequence.)

Precautions: To prevent tipping of chair, all four wheels should be well up on curb. If lower extremities are very spastic, therapist should guide them to prevent bruising feet and toes. Until sufficient skill and confidence are gained, therapist is ready to give support.

Helpful remarks:

1. It helps to roll door window down so that patient can hold on to window frame when shifting body on to seat.
4. For some patients it is easier to put legs into car before shifting to car seat and out of car when shifting to wheel-chair seat.

Patient should learn to fold wheel chair and place it in car while sitting on front seat, and also to lift wheel chair out of car and place it in street.

WHEEL CHAIR—alongside car (no picture shown—position as in Fig. **16F**)

If wheel chair has removable armrests, it is placed alongside car and patient slides and lifts himself sideways on to front seat and out. In general it is easier to get on to front seat, but the same procedure holds for back seat. Choice will depend on construction of car doors.

For more variations see next pages.

Fig. 27A. FROM WHEEL CHAIR TO CAR AND BACK—wheel chair facing car

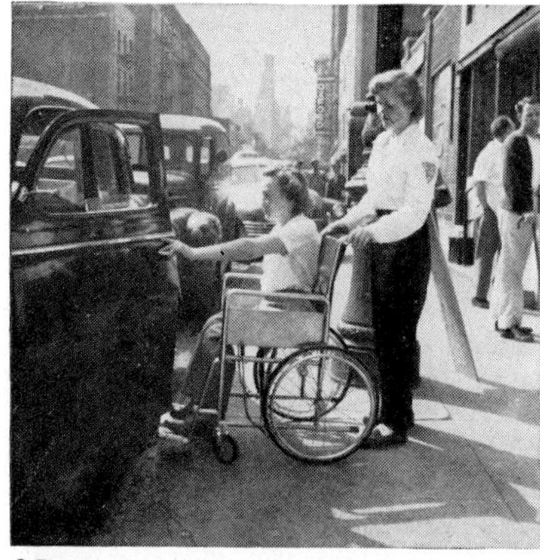
S.P.

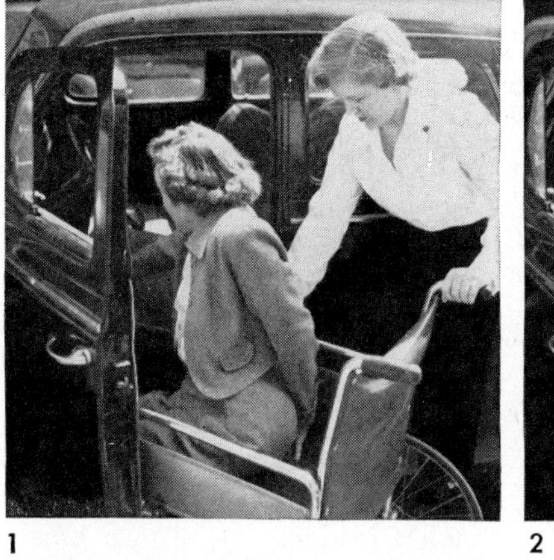
1

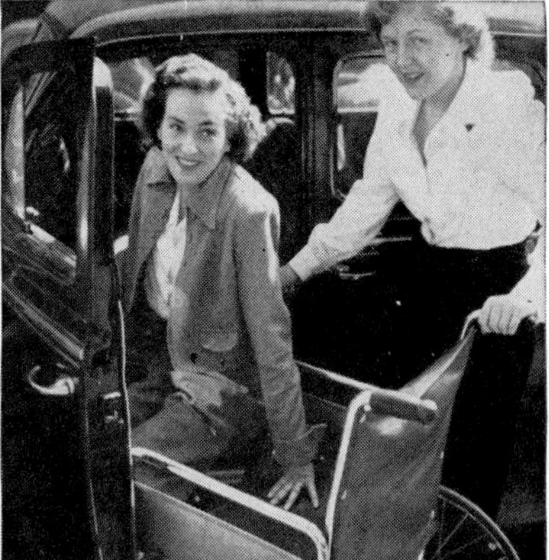
2

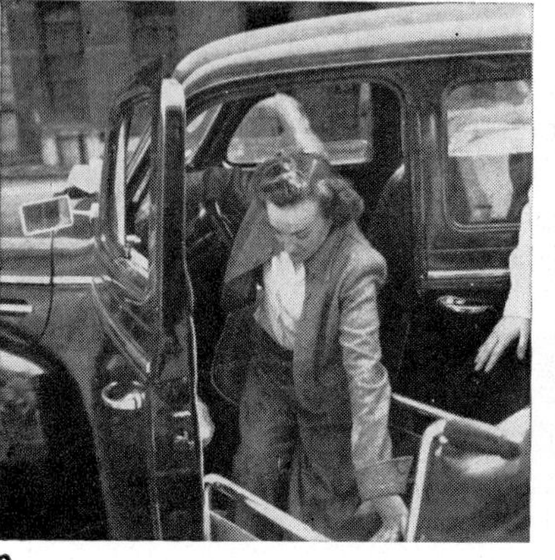
3

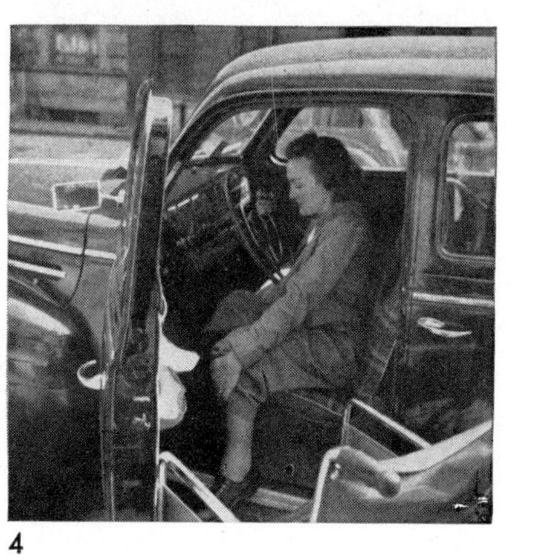
4

Fig. 27B. FROM WHEEL CHAIR TO CAR AND BACK —using board

A board is used to bridge gap between wheel chair and car. This method is helpful for patients with and without braces (*a*) if they do not have sufficient strength and/or balance to push up and lift themselves across from wheel chair to front seat or (*b*) if wheel chair it is impossible to bring near enough to car.
Equipment: wheel chair, car, board.

From wheel chair to car—wheel chair with nonremovable armrests:

Starting Position: Sit in wheel chair with brakes locked. Lean toward left, also have both legs as much to left as possible so that therapist can place board under your...

Instructions:

1. ...buttocks while you push up on hands. If you cannot push, lean as much as you can toward left and let therapist assist you so that you...

2. ...sit down on board. Turn forward so that knees can bend. Unlock brakes. Move wheel chair close enough to car so that other end of board can be placed on front seat. Lock brakes. Place both hands on board and slide sideways on to front seat. Adjust legs as you sit behind wheel.
Board can be easily removed now while you lean toward right.

From car to wheel chair:

Starting Position: Sit behind wheel. (**S.P.a.**) Wheel chair faces car at right angles. Brakes are locked. Board is placed with one end on wheel chair with other on front seat of car.

Instructions:

1a. Place right hand near hip on car seat and left hand on board and lift or slide on to board. Therapist may have to hold other end of board down.

2a. Place both hands on board and slide on to wheel chair. Unlock brakes and move wheel chair away so that board can be removed easily.

Precautions: It is important to place board well under buttocks and also well on seat so that a strong bridge is formed.
Helpful remarks:

2, 2a. It is easier to slide board under patient and have him sit on it before moving the wheel chair into place.

From wheel chair to car—wheel chair with removable armrests:

Starting Position: Sit on front seat. (**S.P.b.**) Therapist removes one armrest and places wheel chair along side of car and then places board with one end on car seat and one end on wheel-chair seat.

Instructions:

1b, 2b. Follow same instructions as above.

Fig. 27B. FROM WHEEL CHAIR TO CAR AND BACK—using board

From wheel chair to car—wheel chair with nonremovable armrests

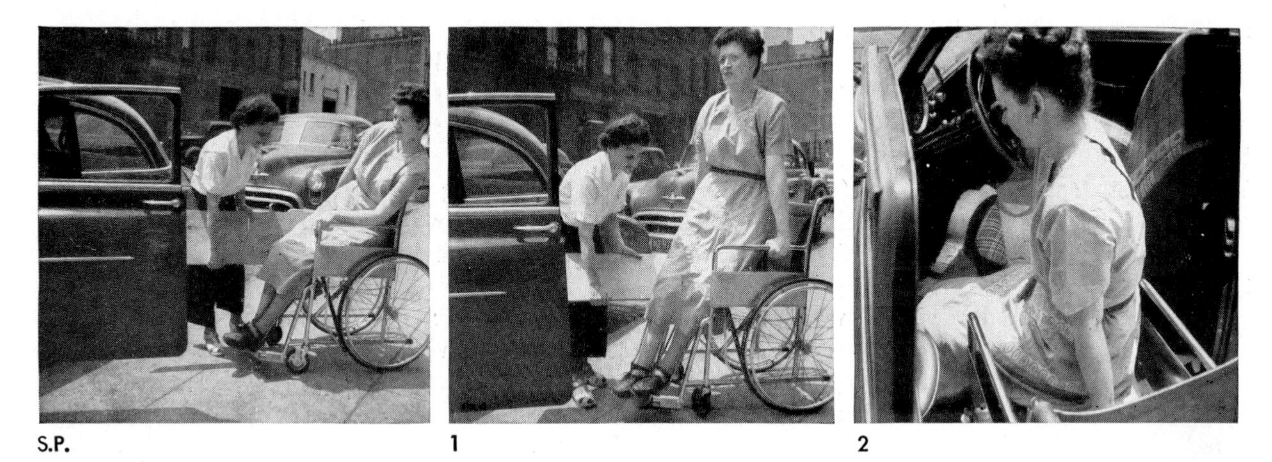

S.P. 1 2

From car to wheel chair

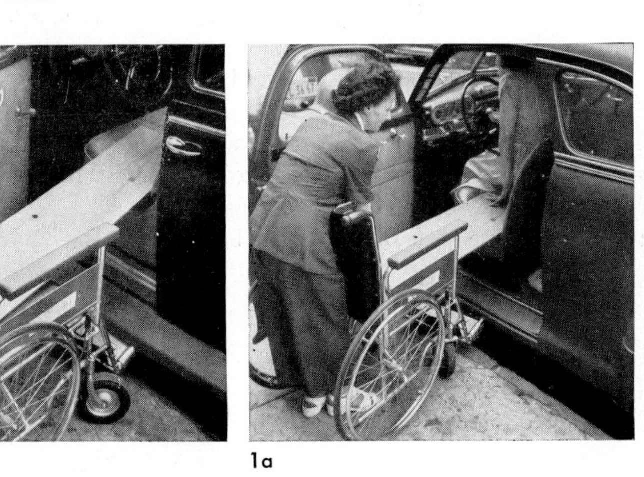

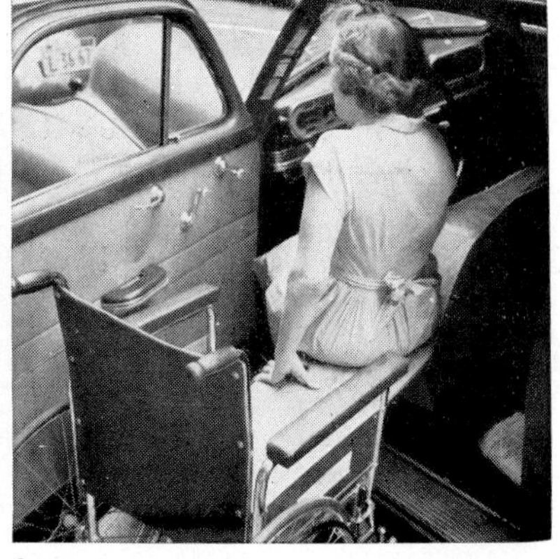

S.P.a 1a 2a

From wheel chair to car—wheel chair with removable armrests

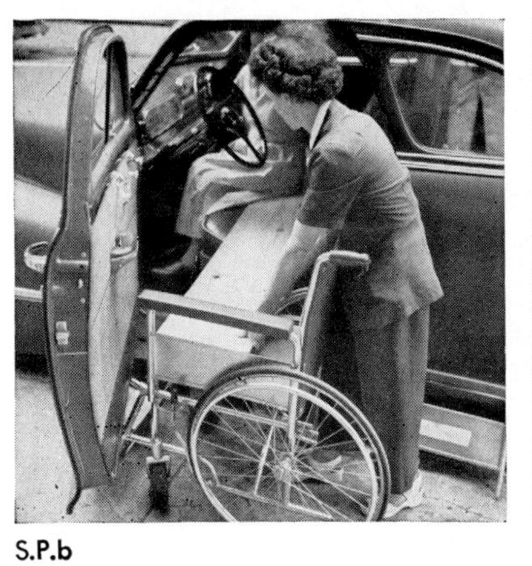

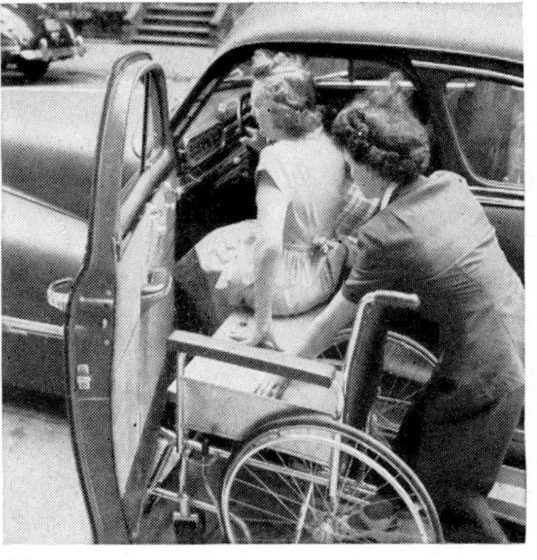

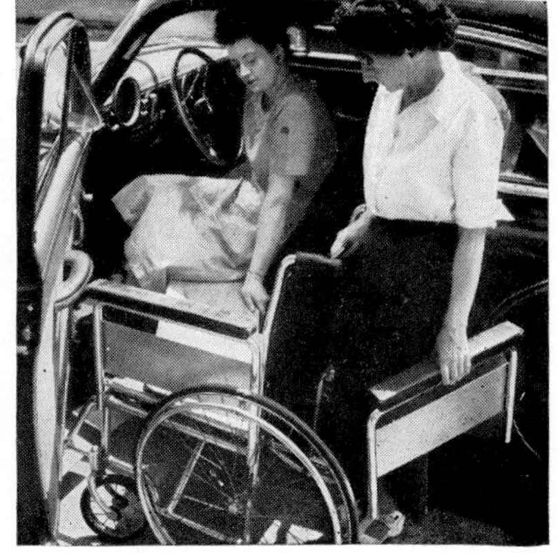

S.P.b 1b 2b

Fig. 28. UP AND DOWN CURB IN WHEEL CHAIR

If big wheels of wheel chair are in back, it is easier for therapist to push wheel chair forward on to curb.

Up curb forward:

Instructions:

1. Therapist steps on tipping lever (Fig. **28**·1a) and exerts downward pressure on chair handles until the chair is tilted back into the big wheels.

2. The chair is rolled forward on big wheels until they touch curb, and now small wheels are lowered on to curb.
By pushing forward and pulling up on chair handles and using knee to exert pressure on back rest of chair, chair is rolled up...

3. ...on curb.

Helpful remarks:

2, 3. Patient can help by grasping hand rims and attempting to roll chair up curb at the same time as therapist exerts pressure with his knee against the back rest.

Down curb backward: Read pictures in reverse sequence.

Down curb forward:

Instructions:

1a. Before chair reaches edge of curb, therapist steps on tipping lever and tilts chair back into big wheels (see instructions above). Then...

2a. ...chair is rolled to edge of curb on big wheels and by...

3a. ...exerting an upward pull on handles, big wheels are slowly lowered on to street and...

4a. ...then small wheels.

Helpful remarks:

3a. Patient can help by using hand rims as a brake while chair is lowered.

Up curb backward: Read pictures in reverse sequence.

Up and down stairs in wheel chair.
A similar procedure as for mounting and descending curbs is followed. Help will always be needed.

Up and down incline in wheel chair.
When ascending incline, you should sit well forward while rolling chair up; when descending incline, you should sit well back, while rolling the chair down.

Fig. 28. UP AND DOWN CURB IN WHEEL CHAIR

Up curb forward. (For down curb backward, read pictures in reverse sequence.)

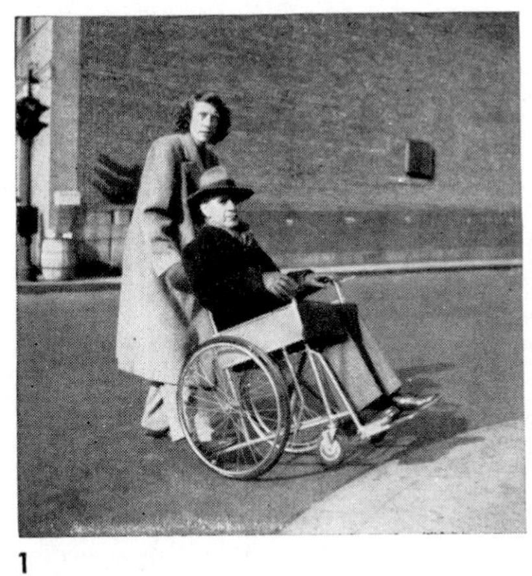

1

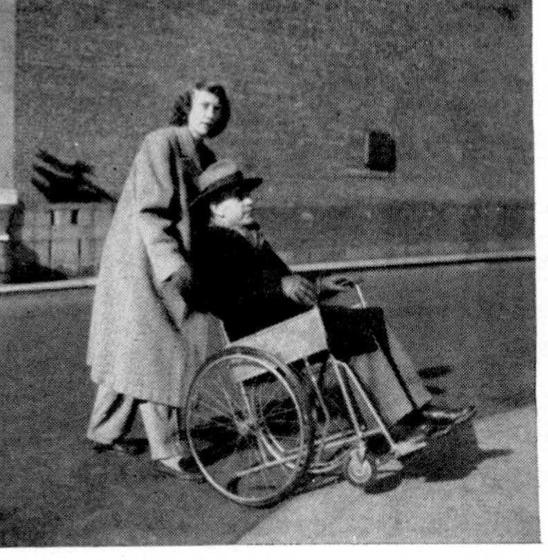

2

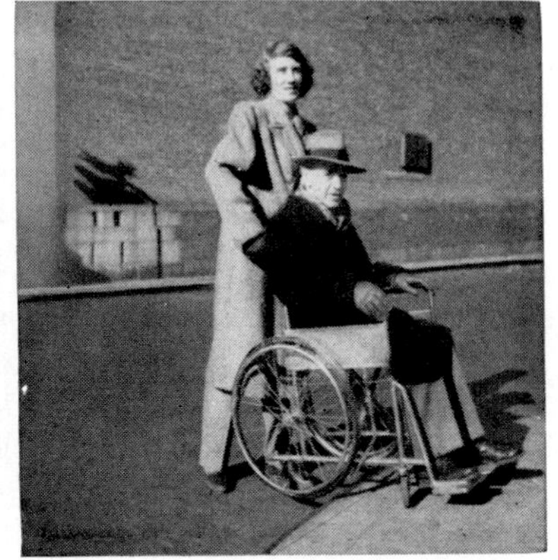

3

Down curb forward

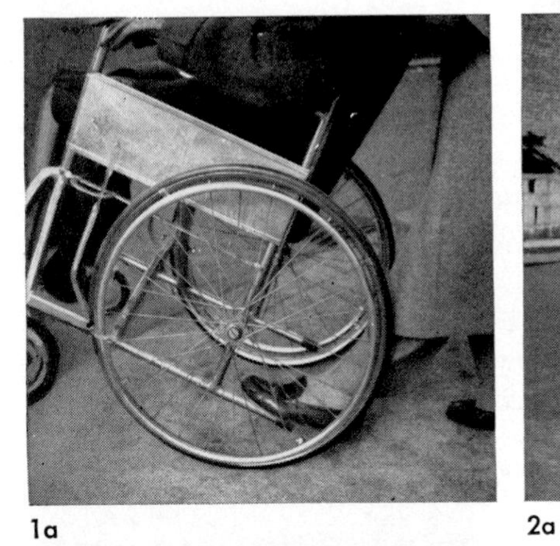

1a

2a

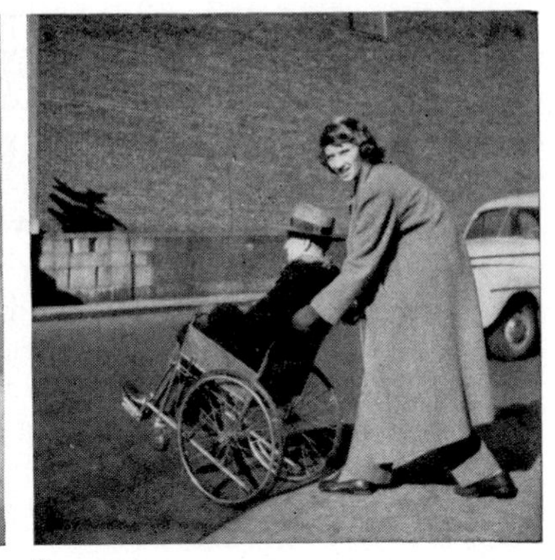

3a

4a

CHAPTER V

Ambulation on Crutches

After the patient has mastered bed, wheel-chair, and mat exercises, he is taught the skills and techniques necessary for crutch walking.

The ultimate goal is to be able to walk not only in the house or the apartment where he lives, on different floor coverings, through doors, in crowded rooms, but also outdoors on different surfaces—gravel, cobblestone, cement, etc.—and in crowds.

In ordinary standing and walking all the weight is on the feet, whereas when standing and walking with braces and crutches, the patient must learn a new way of balancing, since the weight is distributed in the following way: the nearer the crutches (hands) are to the body, the more weight is on the feet (Fig. **39**·1); the farther the crutches (hands) are away from the body, the more weight is on the crutches (hands) as long as the pelvis is tilted forward (Figs. 39·1–3). This applies also to the hands when standing and walking in parallel bars (Figs. **36C**·1 and 3).

The following exercises are planned to train the patient in this method of balancing as well as in the handling of braces and crutches. The exercises proceed from a maximum of support in the parallel bars to a minimum of support on crutches.

The therapist should always be ready to support the patient around the waist when necessary. The patient should be taught to support himself on his crutches (or on his hands in the bars) whenever he loses his balance. Therefore the therapist should avoid grasping his arms or crutches.

In addition to the problem of balance, other factors to be considered in crutch walking are rhythm, endurance, and speed. The patient cannot develop endurance without good rhythm. Smooth rhythmical movements will make for endurance which in turn will bring about speed. Therefore the exercises as well as the gaits should be practiced in units of 2, 4, 6, etc., until 10 units can be done without stopping.

The following exercises should be regarded as the basis for an ambulation training program. Further exercises and variations may be added according to the needs of the patient.

Music and group work will be a great help for all parallel-bar and crutch-balancing exercises, and they should be practiced daily for 20- to 30-minute periods before actual walking on crutches.

Locking and Unlocking Braces (Fig. **29**). It is important that this activity become part of the exercise program. Different methods are shown.

PARALLEL-BAR EXERCISES

To ensure good posture as well as good mechanical advantage for "push-ups," the height of the bars has to be adjusted to the individual patient in the following way: when the patient is standing in the bars the wrists should be dorsiflexed and the elbows bent about twenty-five to thirty degrees (Fig. **36D**·1a).

The patient should learn to *push* rather than *pull* on the bars, since the following parallel bar exercises are a preparation for crutch exercises.

1. **Getting up from and into wheel chair within parallel bars** (Fig. **30**). This is the first step in learning how to handle braces and getting into a standing position.
2. **Standing balance** (Fig. **31**).
3. **Jackknifing** (Fig. **32**).
4. **Push-ups** (Fig. **33**).
5. **Hands forward and back** (Fig. **34**).
6. **Turning around** (Fig. **35**).

These exercises are essential in teaching the patient how to balance in braces and in teaching the motions necessary for walking in braces.

7. **Gaits.**
   a. **Four-point gait** (Fig. **36A**).
   b. **Two-point gait** (Fig. **36B**).
   c. **Shuffle gait** (Fig. **36C**).
   d. **Swing-to gait** (Fig. **36D**).
   e. **Swing-through gait** (Fig. **36E**).

These gaits are first learned in the bars as a preparation for performing them on crutches.

8. **Up and down curb in parallel bars.**
   a. **Hopping up backward, down forward** (Fig. 37A).
   b. **Swinging up forward** (Fig. 37B).

These exercises are more advanced push-ups as well as a preparation for getting up and down curbs on crutches (see Chap. V).

9. **Balancing on crutches in parallel bars.**
   a. **On both crutches** (Fig. 38A).
   b. **On one crutch** (Fig. 38B).

This exercise teaches balancing on crutches within the bars, which provide additional support. Although it is done after the crutches have been measured it is included here for the sake of convenience.

CRUTCHES (p. 106)

The selection and measurement of crutches and crutch stances are described in detail.

CRUTCH BALANCING

The crutch-balancing exercises teach the patient how to balance on braces and crutches. They are practiced against and away from the wall.

1. **Against the wall** (Fig. 40).
   a. **Sideswaying** (Fig. 40·1).
   b. **Lifting one crutch** (Fig. 40·2).
   c. **Lifting both crutches** (Fig. 40·3).
   d. **Pushing up on crutches** (Fig. 40·4).
   e. **Turning crutches out from under arm** (Fig. 40·5).
   f. **Jackknifing** (Figs. 40·6a and b).
2. **Away from the wall** (Fig. 41).
   a to **e**. Same as against the wall.
   f. **Jackknifing** (Fig. 41A).
   g. **Crutches forward and back** (Fig. 41B).

CRUTCH WALKING

Each patient is taught at least two gaits. The selection of the gaits will depend on the patient's condition and his general skill. It is important to practice crutch walking indoors as well as outdoors, over obstacles, for endurance and speed.

1. **Gaits.**
   a. **Four-point gait** (Fig. 42A).
   b. **Two-point gait** (Fig. 42B).
   c. **Shuffle-alternate gait** (Fig. 42C).
   d. **Shuffle-simultaneous gait** (Fig. 42D).
   e. **Swing-to gait** (Fig. 42E).
   f. **Swing-through gait** (Fig. 42F).
2. **Walking in different directions and carrying articles.**
   a. **Sideward** (Fig. 43A).
   b. **Backward** (Fig. 43B).
   c. **Carrying pocketbook, briefcase, etc.** (Fig. 43C).
3. **Walking through door** (Fig. 44).

These activities (2 and 3) are important for indoor as well as outdoor activities and for all elevation and traveling on crutches (see also Chap. V).

Fig. 30. UP FROM AND INTO WHEEL CHAIR*

This exercise is the very first step in learning how to stand on braces.

Purpose: to come to a standing position; to tilt the pelvis forward while standing, in order to lock the hip lock(s).

Preparation for: standing balance in bars and on crutches; getting up and down from chairs on crutches.

Preliminary exercises: sitting balance in wheel chair; push-ups.

Equipment: parallel bars.

Up from wheel chair:

Starting Position: Sit in wheel chair as far to edge of seat as possible; both knees locked. Grasp bars well in front.

Instructions:

1. Pull yourself up...
2. ...keeping trunk forward and throwing weight on feet. Continue...
3. ...pulling until shoulders are in front of hands, then push down on hands and...
4. ...straighten up by throwing shoulders back so that pelvis tilts forward.

Into wheel chair: Reverse entire procedure. (Read pictures in reverse sequence.) Bend elbows slowly as trunk bends forward and pelvis goes back on to seat. Be sure that elbows rest on bars for support (Fig. 30·1).

* Note that Figures 30 through 38 illustrate parallel bar exercises preparatory to crutch balancing.

Precautions: If feet slide forward, all weight has to be shifted to hands so that patient can pull up and over feet nearly simultaneously.

Helpful remarks: Whole exercise should be a continuous motion. When getting up, motion is forward and weight is shifted from hands to feet. When getting into chair, the motion is backward and weight is shifted from feet to hands.

3, 4. *To lock or unlock hip lock,* pelvic tilt forward is essential since brace has to be in perfect alignment so that hip lock can slide up or down side bars. This is brought about in the following way:

4. Patient must stand completely erect with both feet exactly parallel *on one line* and pelvis markedly tilted forward. In this position, lock can be easily put into place with one hand or it may slide into place by itself. If side bars are not in perfect alignment, brace will not lock. Rather than trying to adjust lock by hand, it will be much more helpful to (*a*) check that feet are on one line; (*b*) exaggerate pelvic tilt forward by throwing shoulders back as far as possible. (At first, therapist may have to push patient's pelvis forward to increase pelvic tilt.) For unlocking hip lock, the same position is used. Whenever getting up or down into a chair, locking and unlocking of hip locks must be done in this position.

Fig. 30. UP FROM AND INTO WHEEL CHAIR

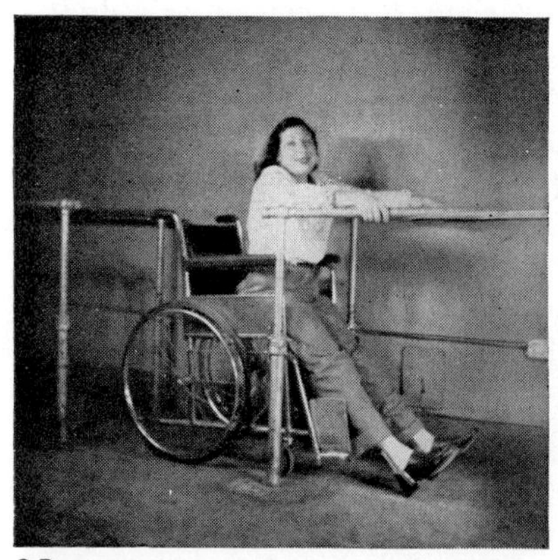

S.P.

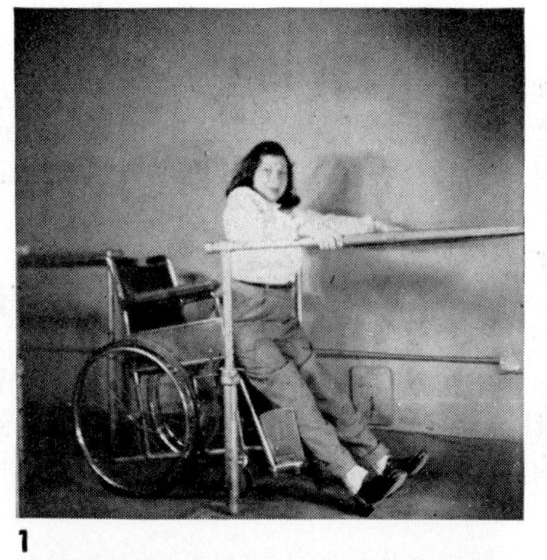

1

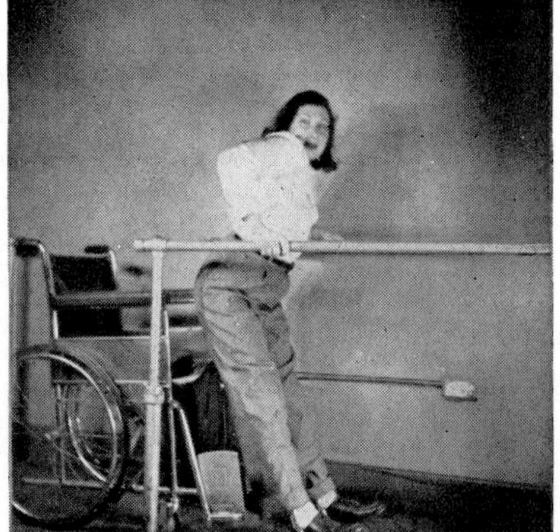

2

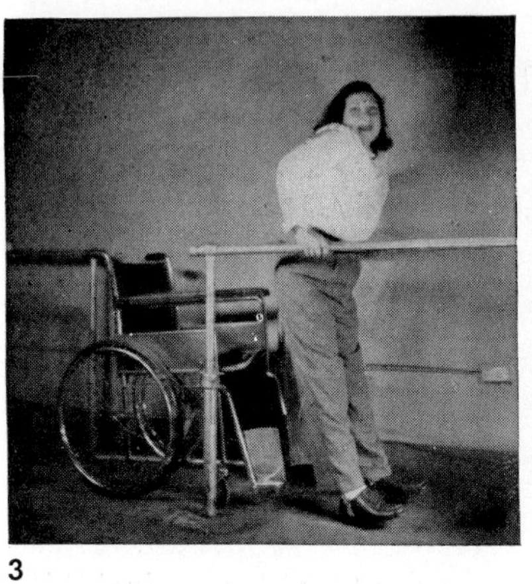

3

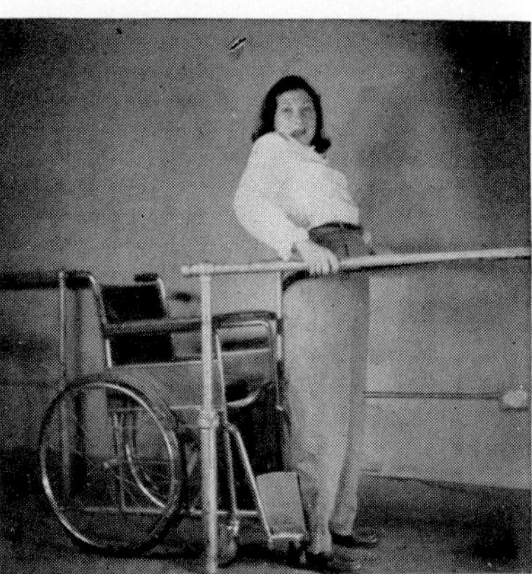

4

Fig. 31. STANDING BALANCE

Purpose: to stand on braces; to shift weight from hands to feet and back.
Preparation for: crutch balancing; crutch walking.
Preliminary exercises: sitting balance; push-ups.
Equipment: parallel bars.

Starting Position: Stand erect in bars holding on to bars.
Instructions:
1. Shift most of weight to feet, grasp bars only for balance. Hold shoulders back, so that pelvis tilts forward. Try to "feel" that weight is on feet. Keep shifting weight from hands to feet and back.
2. Balance and support yourself on both feet and left hand so that right hand can be raised. Replace and repeat with other hand.
3. Shift all weight to feet, exaggerate pelvic tilt forward and raise both hands, hold for a moment, replace and shift weight to hands again.

Precautions:
3. When all weight is on feet and hands are raised, patient must be ready to grasp bars quickly. Therapist stands in front of patient ready to support him around waist.

Fig. 32. JACKKNIFING

Purpose: pelvic control. This term as used here means to control pelvic tilt forward* as well as backward† by pushing on hands and holding shoulders back, in order to maintain standing balance.
Preparation for: all crutch walking and elevation.
Preliminary exercises: standing balance in bars.

Starting Position: Stand erect in bars, holding on to bars, tilting pelvis forward, and placing most of weight on hands.
Instructions:
1a. Lean into hands, bring shoulders forward so that pelvis tilts back slowly (but not beyond control) and feet take more weight.
Straighten up by pushing on hands, bringing shoulders back and arching back so that pelvis can tilt...
S.P. ...forward to starting position.
1a. Repeat Fig. **32**·1a and let trunk bend...
2a. ...forward to horizontal. The pelvis is now markedly buckled, weight is distributed on hands and feet, and you are in a jackknife position. Straighten up...
1a. ...as...
S.P. ...before.

Precautions: Therapist stands in back of patient ready to support him around waist.
Helpful remarks: The exercise is a series of continuous smooth movements, with a gradual shifting of weight in the following way:
S.P. When standing erect, more weight is on hands.
2a. When trunk is bent to horizontal, weight is distributed on hands and feet.
Special Note: Marked imbalance of abdominal muscles in relation to trunk and hip muscles will bring about involuntary "jackknifing" or "buckling" (backward tilt of the pelvis).
In jackknifing as an exercise the patient is made to jackknife deliberately and then taught to straighten up, in order to learn how to overcome and prevent this position.

* Pelvic tilt forward: anterior superior spine of the pelvis moves upward and forward.

† Pelvic tilt backward: anterior superior spine of the pelvis moves downward and backward.

Fig. 31. STANDING BALANCE

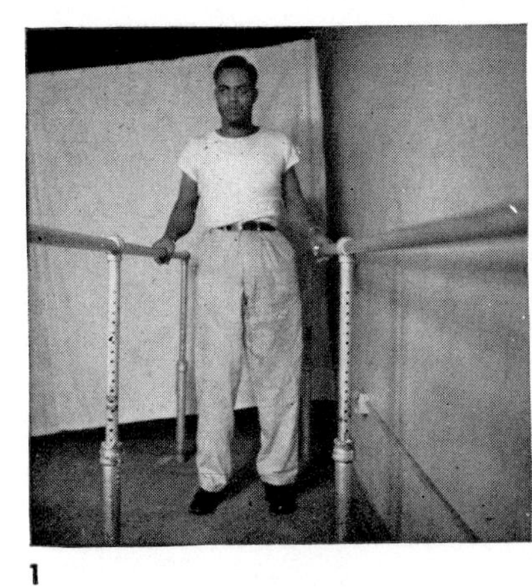

1

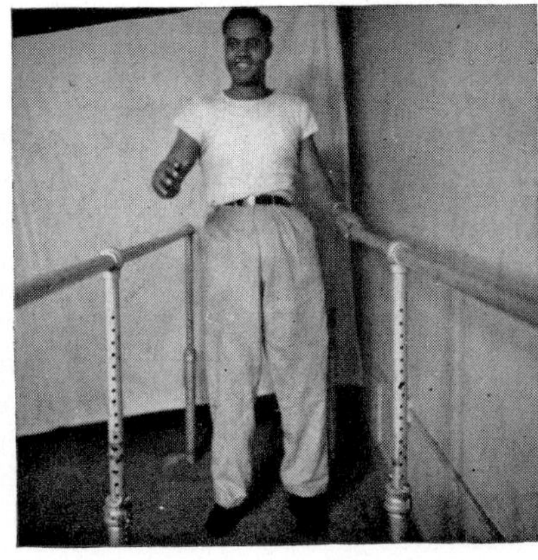

2

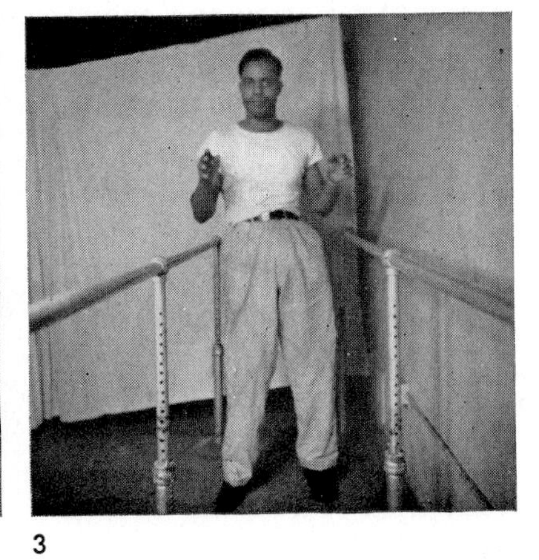

3

Fig. 32. JACKKNIFING

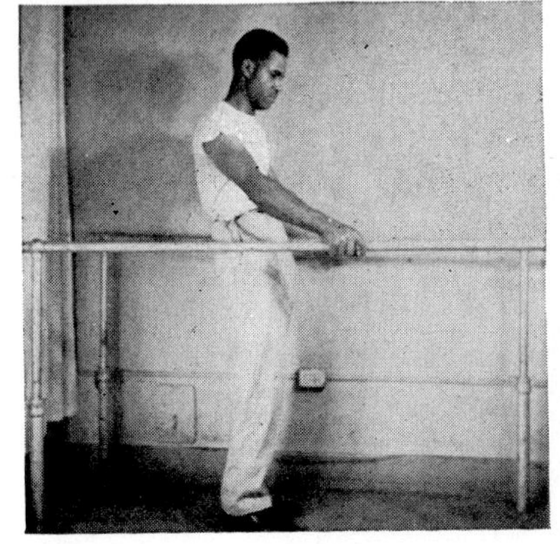

S.P.

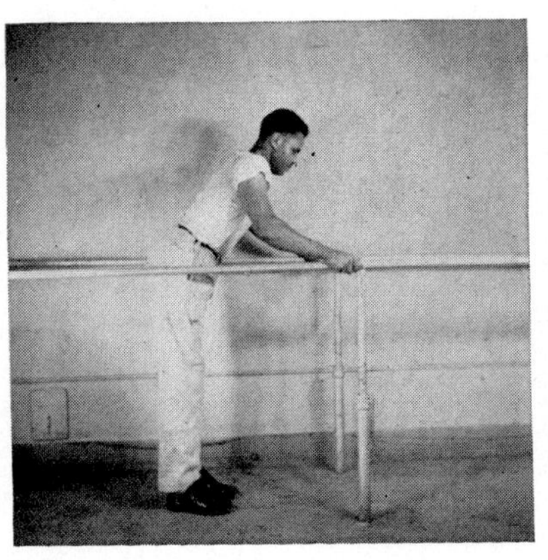

1a

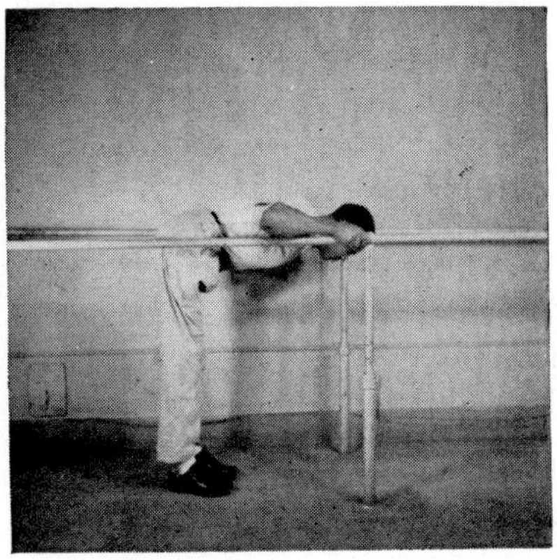

2a

Fig. 33. PUSH-UPS

Purpose: to develop arm and shoulder muscles; to lift body off floor by pushing on hands.
Preparation for: crutch walking; elevation.
Preliminary exercises: sitting balance; push-ups in sitting; standing balance.
Equipment: parallel bars.

Starting Position: Stand erect in bars, hands near hips, slightly in front.
Instructions:
1. Push on hands, straightening elbows and lift body off floor. Depress shoulders throughout exercise. Duck head to gain height.
S.P. Lower body by bending elbows slowly and land on heels first, returning to starting position.

Helpful remarks:
S.P. Slow bending of elbows will aid in smooth landing of heels on floor.
1. To gain more height, push-up can be combined with jackknifing and/or pulling in of abdominal muscles while body is off floor (Fig. **36E**·2b).

Fig. 34. HANDS FORWARD AND BACKWARD

Purpose: to move body and arms forward and back, while pelvis is tilted forward.
Preparation for: swing-through gait.
Preliminary exercises: jackknifing; standing balance in bars.

Starting Position: Stand erect in bars.
Instructions:
1a. Place hands well in front of hips and shift most of weight to hands, keeping pelvis tilted forward. Swing body back on heels and...
2a. ...nearly simultaneously lift hands and grasp bars in back of hips (same distance as they were in front). Shift weight to hands again. Hesitate slightly to ensure good balance and rhythm. Still keeping pelvis tilted forward, swing body forward at ankles and simultaneously bring arms...
1a. ...forward. Grasp bars in front and shift weight to hands again.

Precautions: To prevent buckling, body should at no time be bent forward at waist but only move forward and backward at the ankle joint, while back is arched. Therapist stands in back of patient ready to support him around waist.

Fig. 35. TURNING AROUND

Purpose: to balance on braces.
Preparation for: crutch balancing; crutch walking.
Preliminary exercises: all parallel-bar exercises.

Starting Position: Stand erect in bars.
Instructions:
1b. Push up and, lifting body off floor, turn 90 deg. to your right. Lower body by bending elbows slowly and land on heels first. Bring right hand...
2b. ...forward to grasp bar. Keep pelvis tilted forward and shoulders back so that you are well balanced.
1b. Place right hand behind you on bar, push up lifting body off floor, and turn 90 deg. to your right.
Repeat same exercise to left.

Fig. 33. PUSH-UPS

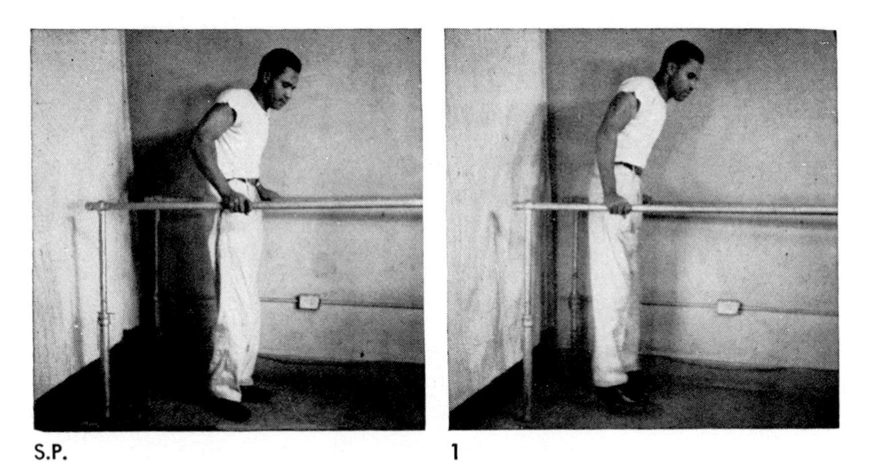

S.P. 1

Fig. 34. HANDS FORWARD AND BACKWARD

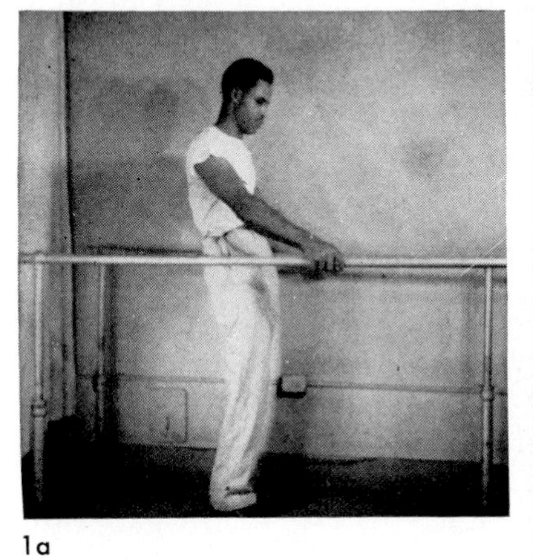

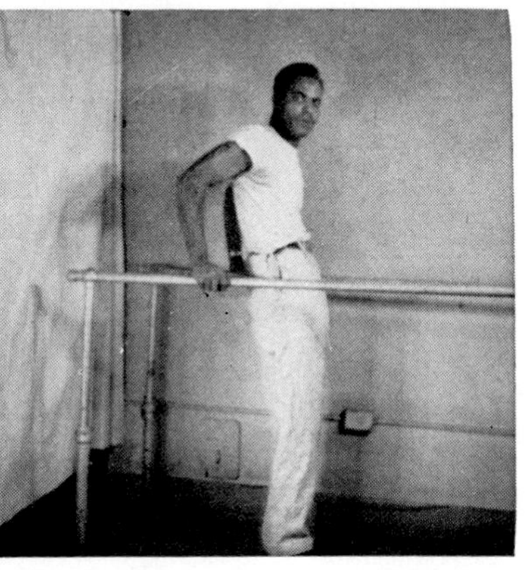

1a 2a

Fig. 35. TURNING AROUND

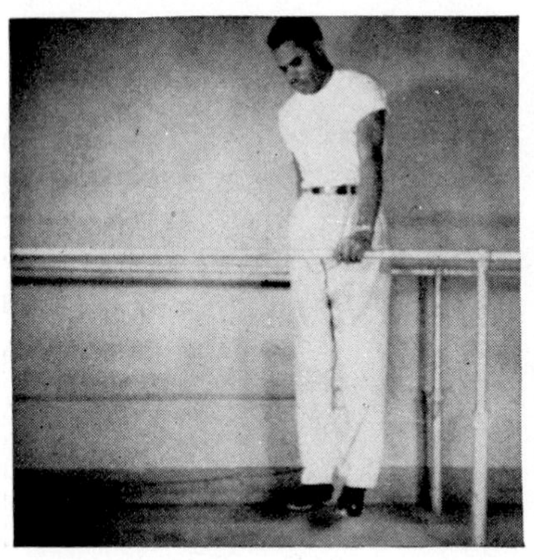

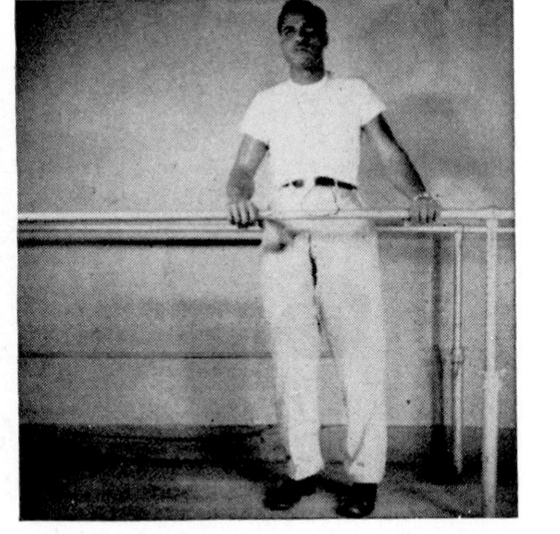

1b 2b

FOUR-POINT AND TWO-POINT GAITS

Both gaits are the preparation for the same gaits on crutches. These gaits can be done only by patients who can bring each leg forward alternately.
1 through **4** represent one unit of the four-point gait.
1a and **2a** represent one unit of the two-point gait.
Each unit is a series of continuous smooth movements, which do not come to a stop unless both feet are on the floor and both hands grasp the bars.

Fig. 36A. FOUR-POINT GAIT

Purpose: to walk by moving one leg forward while standing on other and holding on with both hands to bars.
Preliminary exercises: standing balance in bars.
Equipment: parallel bars.

Starting Position: Stand erect in bars.
Instructions: Count (1) right hand, (2) left leg, (3) left hand, (4) right leg.
1. Place right hand forward and take as much weight as possible on same as well as on right foot, also bend trunk slightly to right.
2. At same time push on left hand in order to lift (or hike) left leg off floor to bring it forward and take a step.
3. Shift weight to left leg. Place left hand in front on bar, shift weight on it, and tilt body to left at the same time pushing on right. . .
4. . . . arm to help lift (or hike) right leg off floor to bring it forward. Take a. . .
1. . . . step and shift weight to right foot. Place right hand forward, etc., and repeat whole sequence for entire length of bars.

Practice gait backward. (Read pictures in reverse sequence.)

Helpful remarks:
4. Pushing on same side as leg is raised and tilting body to opposite side will help bring leg forward.
If patient has no hip flexors, he still can move his legs forward alternately by hiking his legs (using the quadratus lumborum) and also by twisting his trunk.

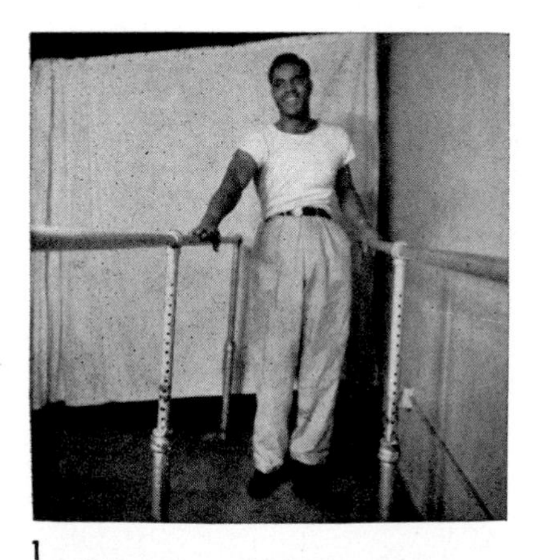

1

2

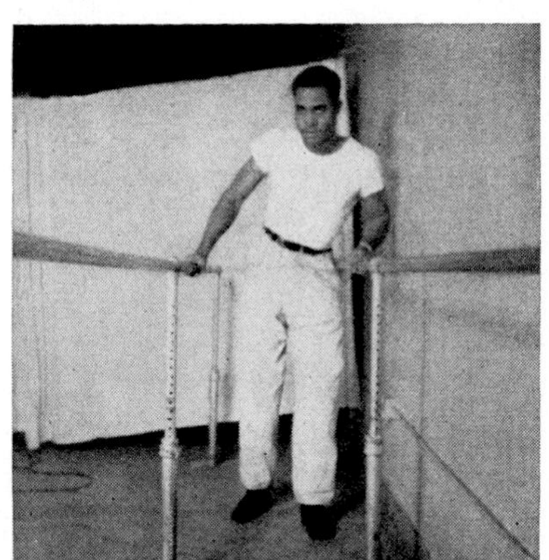

3

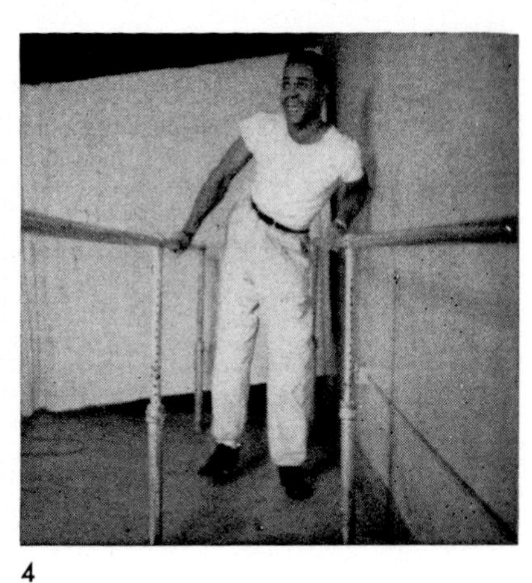

4

Fig. 36B. TWO-POINT GAIT

Purpose: to walk by moving arm and opposite leg forward simultaneously while standing on other leg and holding bar with other hand.
Preliminary exercises: four-point gait in bars.

Starting Position: Stand erect in bars.
Instructions: Count: (1) right hand and left leg, (2) left hand and right leg.
1a. Raise right arm and left leg simultaneously. Weight is evenly distributed between left hand and right foot. Take a step...
2a. ...forward and grasp bar with right hand at the same time. Shift weight to right hand and left foot and repeat with other leg and arm. Walk entire length of bar.

Practice gait backward. (Read pictures in reverse sequence.)

Helpful remarks:

1a. Pushing up on same side as raised leg will help bring leg forward.

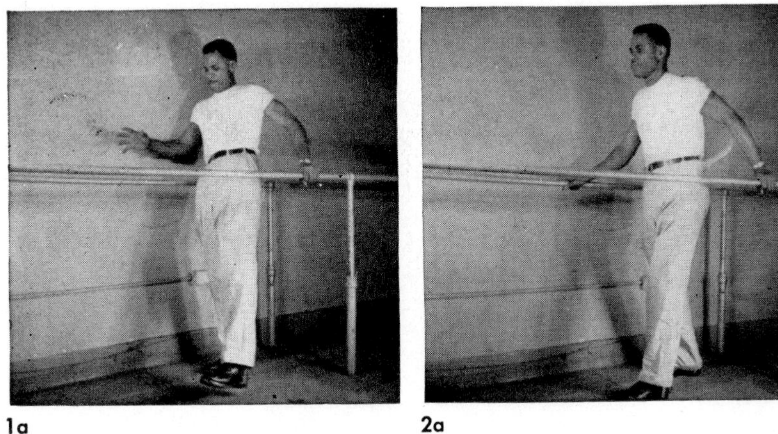

1a **2a**

TRIPOD AND SWINGING GAITS

The shuffle, swing-to, and swing-through gaits within the parallel bars are the preparation for the same gaits on crutches. The three pictures which are shown for each gait represent one unit of a given gait. This unit is a series of continuous smooth movements which should not come to a stop until the hands are well in front and most of the weight is on them. (Figs. **36C**·1, **36D**·1a, **36E**·1b.) These positions again are the end of one sequence as well as the beginning of the next. The gaits should be practiced for the entire length of the bars, forward as well as backward. (For backward gait, read pictures in reverse sequence.) Until sufficient skill and confidence are gained, the therapist should walk back of the patient, ready to give him support around the waist.

Fig. 36C. SHUFFLE GAIT

Purpose: to walk by dragging both legs forward simultaneously.
Preliminary exercises: all preceding parallel-bar exercises.

Starting Position: Stand erect in bars.
Instructions: Count: (1) hands, (2) shuffle.
1. Place hands well in front of hips, lean into...
2. ...hands so that all weight is on same, push on bars and bring body forward by shuffling feet until...
3. ...you stand straight. Keep pelvis tilted forward, shift weight to feet so that you can raise hands forward and place...
1. ...them well in front, shifting weight to hands in order to start new sequence.

Precautions: Pelvis is to be kept tilted forward at all times to prevent buckling.
2. Body should not be brought forward unless shoulders are above or in front of hands, so that there is—not pulling—but pushing on bars while dragging feet forward.

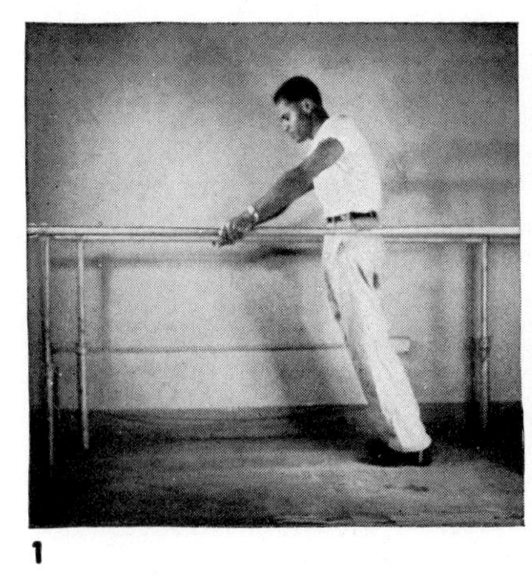

1

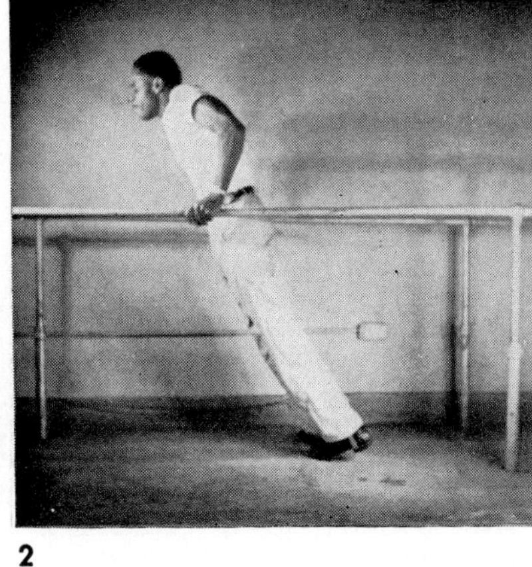

2

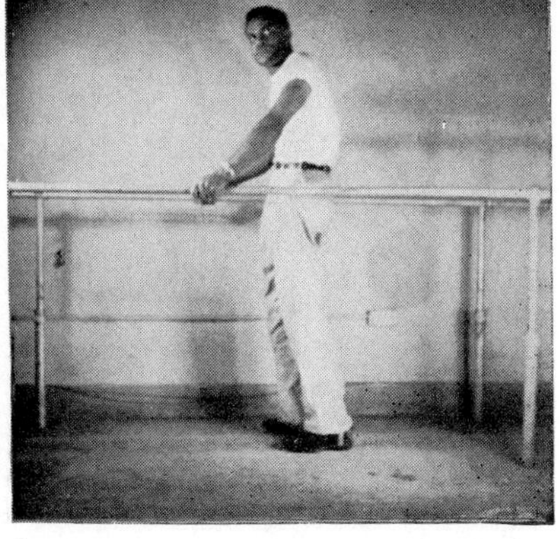

3

Fig. 36D. SWING-TO GAIT

Purpose: to walk by hopping up to hands.
Preliminary exercises: jackknifing; shuffle gait.

Starting Position: Stand erect in bars.
Instructions: Count: (1) hands, (2) hop.
1a. Place hands in front of hips, shift weight to...
2a. ...hands and push up, straightening elbows and ducking head slightly to gain sufficient height, so that feet clear floor.
3a. Lower body by bending elbows and land with heels in between hands. As soon as feet touch floor, bring shoulders back so that pelvis can tilt forward. Shift weight to feet and immediately bring arms...
1a. ...forward, grasp bars and shift weight to hands, in order to start new sequence.

Precautions:
3a. Hands should not be lifted until pelvis is completely tilted forward and weight is on feet.
2a. *Push-up* should not be started until shoulders are above or slightly in front of hands so that there is no pull on bars.

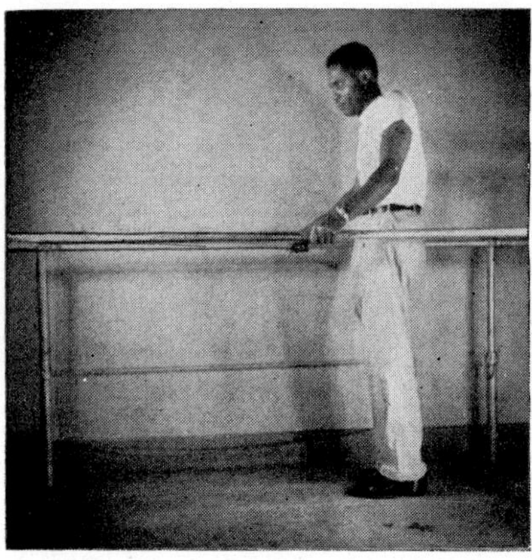

1a

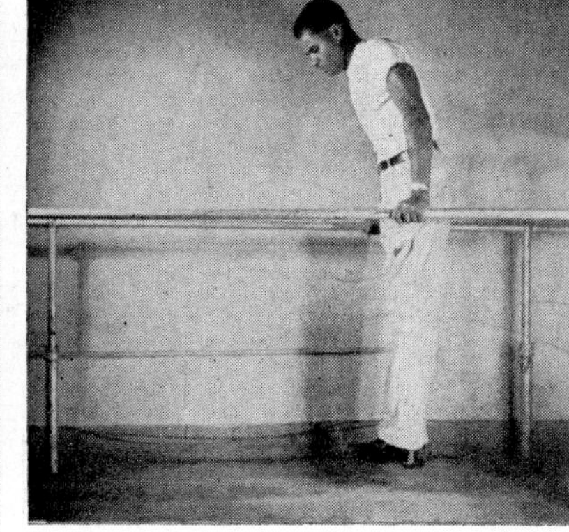

2a

3a

Fig. 36E. SWING-THROUGH GAIT

Purpose: to walk by lifting body off floor and landing in front of hands.

Preliminary exercises: hands forward and back; swing-to gait.

Starting Position: Stand erect in bars.

Instructions:

1b. Place hands in front of hips. Lean into hands and...

2b. ...push body off floor by straightening elbows and ducking head. Pull abdominal muscles in and/or jackknife if possible, to gain more height so that feet clear floor and swing through your hands, heels landing in front...

3b. ...of hands. As soon as feet touch floor, arch back, so that pelvis will tilt forward. Swing body forward at ankles, simultaneously raise hands forward...

1b. ...and grasp bars in front. Shift weight to hands so that you are ready for the next sequence.

Precautions:

2b. Push-up should not be started unless shoulders are above or in front of hands so that there is no pull on bars. Body should not be brought too far forward nor up. Feet land as far in front...

3b. ...as they were in back. To prevent buckling, body should move forward only at the ankle joint and not at waist. This forward movement should not be started until back is arched completely and weight is on feet.

3b. If one foot lands in front of other, this may be a sign that this leg is shorter and a lift has to be put under this shoe. (For more details see "Braces" in Chap. VII.) It may also indicate that patient is pushing harder on one arm than on other.

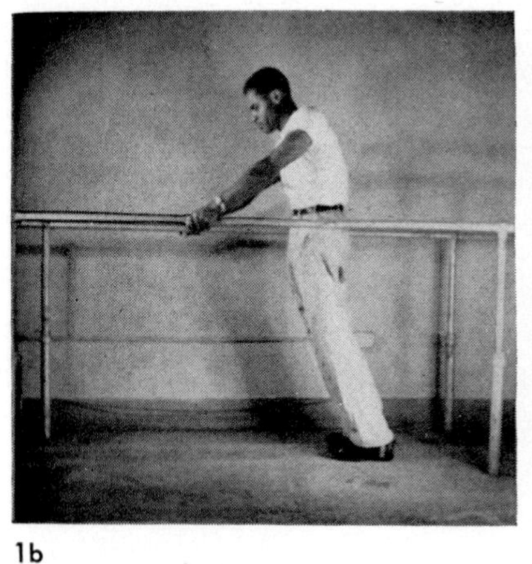

1b

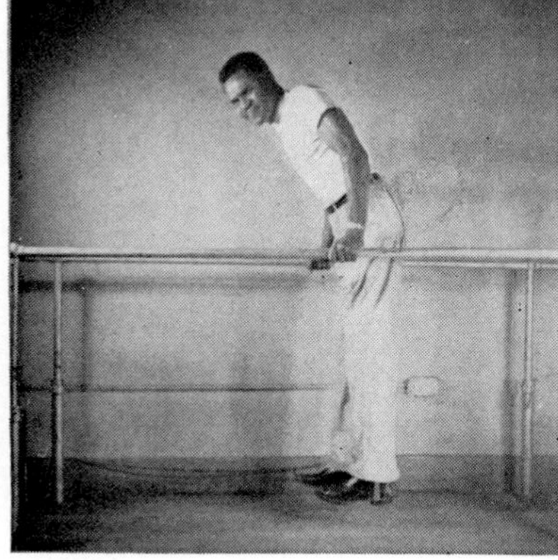

2b

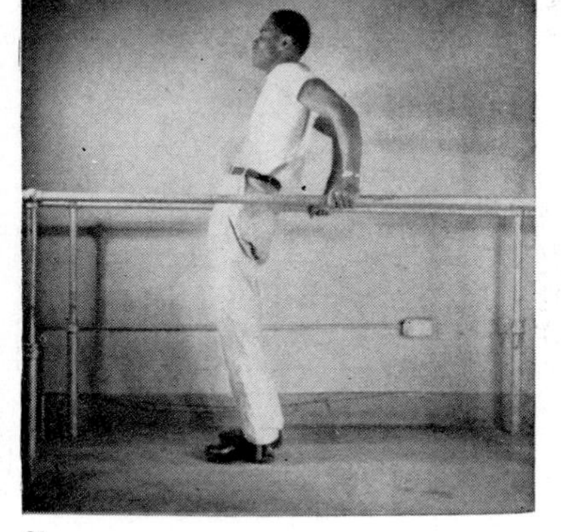

3b

Fig. 37A. UP AND DOWN CURB IN PARALLEL BARS—hopping up backward

Hopping up backward is the easiest method, since it eliminates catching toes on edge of curb.

Purpose: high push-up backward combined with jackknifing; pelvic control.

Preparation for: getting up on curb with crutches.

Preliminary exercises: all parallel-bar exercises.

Equipment: parallel bars, curbs of graduated height.

Starting Position: Back up with heels against curb so that heels actually touch curb. Hands grasp bars in back of hips (or beside hips). Pelvis is markedly tilted forward, and most of weight is on feet.

Instructions:

1. Quickly shift all weight to hands by throwing trunk forward and simultaneously duck head, push-up, and jackknife so that you gain sufficient height to clear curb and hop up and back so that you...
2. ...land with heels first and most of feet on curb. As soon as heels touch curb, tilt pelvis forward. Lean on hands...
3. ...move feet back on curb and straighten up completely.

Hopping down curb: Reverse entire procedure. (Read pictures in reverse sequence.)

Precautions: It is important to push up high enough so that curb is cleared and also to have all weight on hands all the time until heels land on curb. If feet slip, strong pushing on hands must be continued to give support.

Helpful remarks:

S.P. In order to gain sufficient momentum when hopping up curb, back is markedly arched at first and...

1. ...then pelvis quickly buckled during push-up. When hopping down, pelvis is buckled first and then tilted forward.

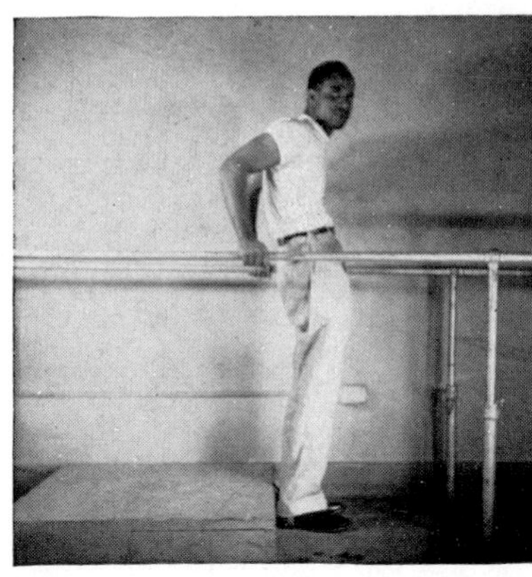

S.P.

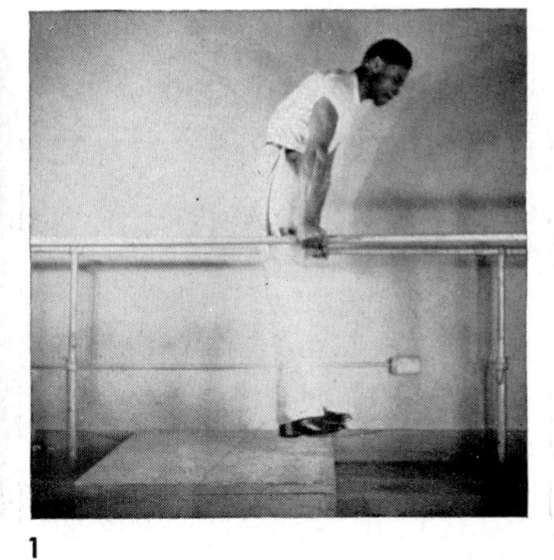

1

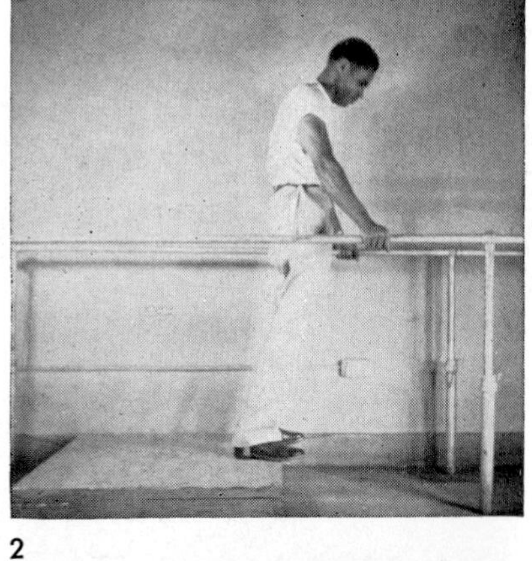

2

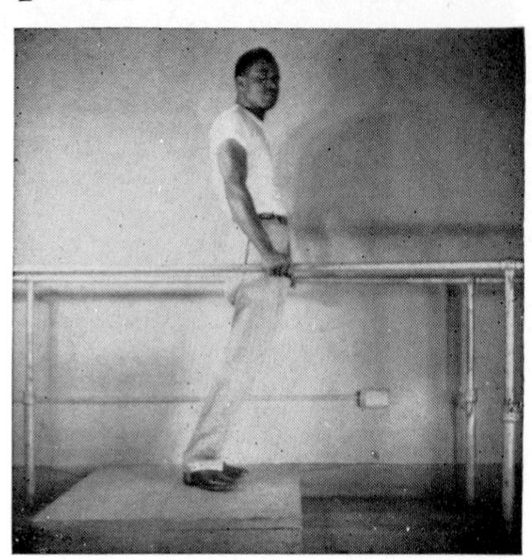

3

Fig. 37B. UP AND DOWN CURB IN PARALLEL BARS —swinging up forward

This method is more difficult than getting up backward, since a higher push-up is needed to prevent catching of toes on edge of curb.

Purpose: high push-up forward combined with jackknife; pelvic control.

Preparation for: swinging up on curb on crutches.

Preliminary exercises: swing-through in bars.

Starting Position: Stand erect in bars with hands well in front. Distance from curb must be well tried out so that when swing-through is completed (Fig. **37B**·2a) feet will be well up on curb. Lean well into hands. . .

1a. . . .push up high, simultaneously duck head and jackknife to gain sufficient height and swing legs through hands so that. . .

2a. . . .heels land on curb. As soon as heels land. . .

3a. . . .quickly tilt pelvis forward. Weight is now evenly distributed on hands and feet. Hesitate slightly in this position to ensure good rhythm and balance. Swing body forward at ankles and simultaneously bring hands forward. Shift weight to hands.

Helpful remarks:

2a, 3a. See Figure **34.**

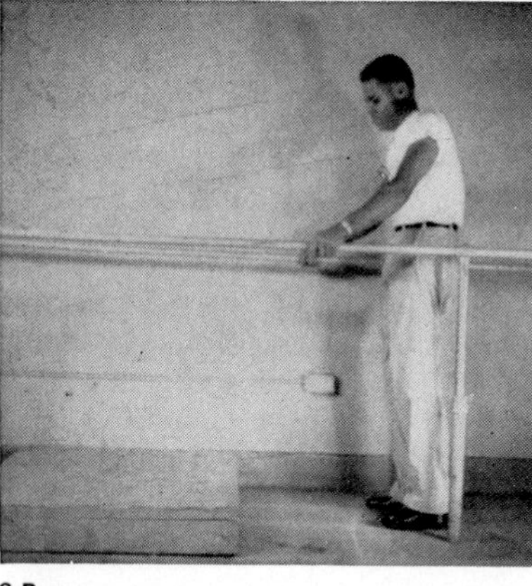

S.P.a

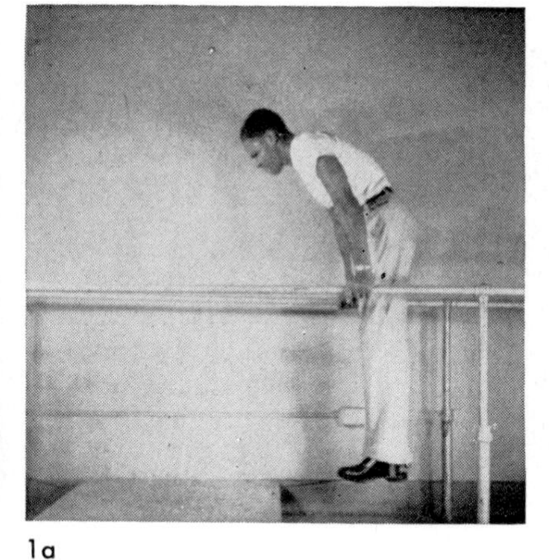

1a

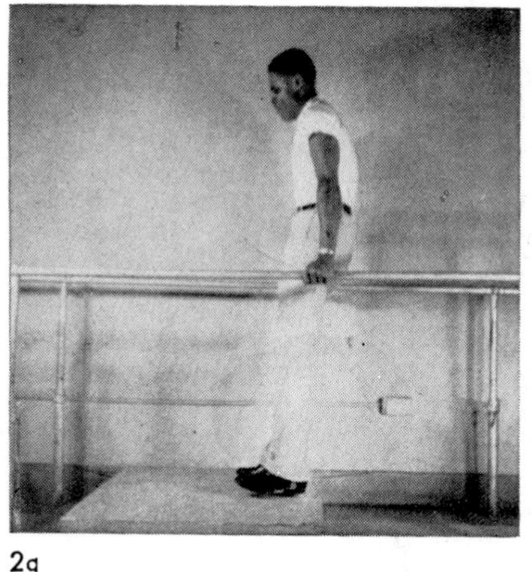

2a

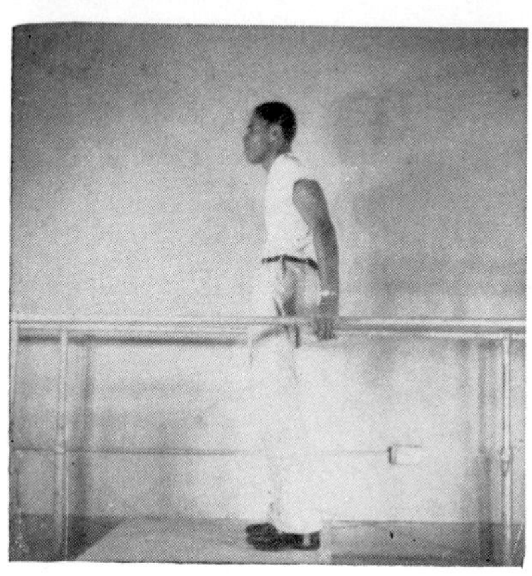

3a

BALANCING ON CRUTCHES IN PARALLEL BARS

After crutch-balancing exercises against the wall and away from the wall have been practiced, the following exercises are done. They are included here with the other parallel-bar exercises only for the sake of convenience.

Fig. 38A. BALANCING ON BOTH CRUTCHES

Purpose: to balance on crutches and braces while shifting weight from crutches to feet and back.
Preparation for: crutch walking.
Preliminary exercises: all parallel-bar exercises, crutch balancing.

Starting Position: Stand in a good tripod position with one crutch under each arm within bars (for details see "Tripod Position," p. 108).
Instructions:
1. Lean into crutches and bring shoulders forward so that pelvis rolls back but not beyond control.
S.P. Straighten up by pushing strongly on both hands, bringing shoulders back so that pelvis tilts forward.

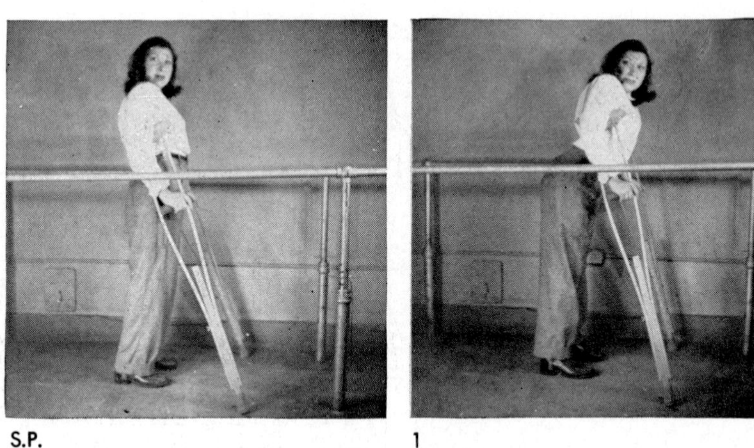

S.P. 1

Fig. 38B. BALANCING ON ONE CRUTCH

Preparation for: getting down on chairs and up.
Equipment: chair with foam-rubber cushion in bars.

Starting Position: Stand in bars facing chair with crutch under right arm. (**S.P.a.**) Grasp bar with left hand for balance (not for support) while weight is on right crutch and both feet.

Instructions:

1a. Slowly shift more weight into crutch, releasing bar and...

2a. ...bend trunk slightly forward trying to touch chair with left hand.

3a. As you touch chair, left hand will take some weight. Leave some weight on heels in order to be able to lift right hand and crutch.

To straighten up: Reverse entire procedure. (Read pictures in reverse sequence.)

3a. Shift weight from left hand into right crutch...

2a. ...release left hand. Push on crutch to straighten up, bringing shoulders back so that...

1a. ...pelvis tilts forward. Shift more weight to heels as you return...

S.P.a. ...to starting position.

Precautions: Therapist should stand behind patient ready to support him around waist.

Variations: In developing skill and balance, all crutch-balancing exercises as done against wall and away from wall can be practiced within parallel bars.

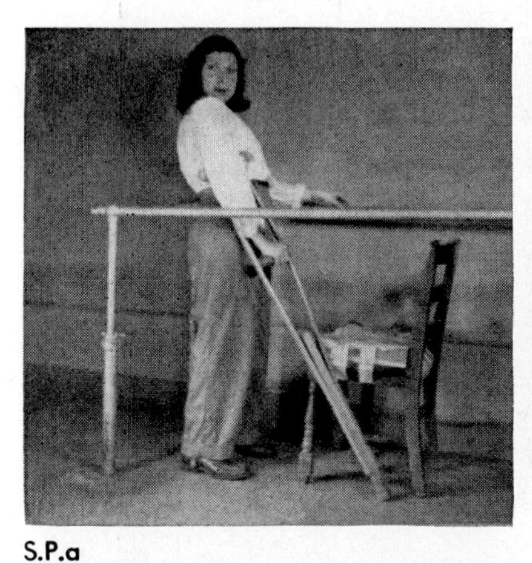

S.P.a

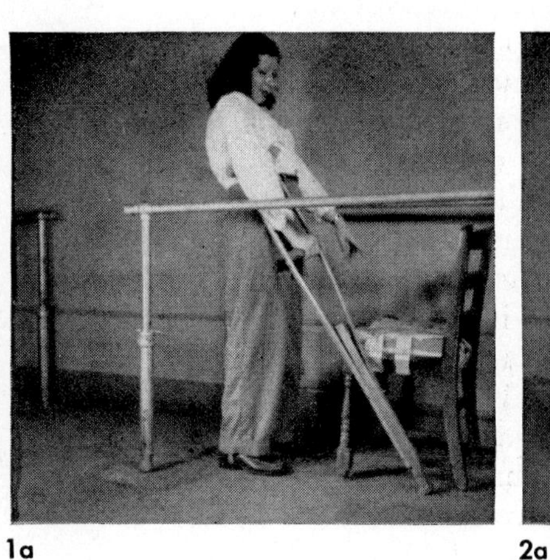

1a

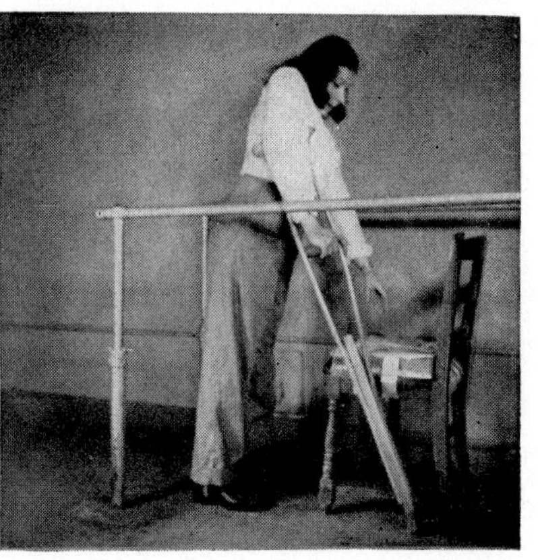

2a

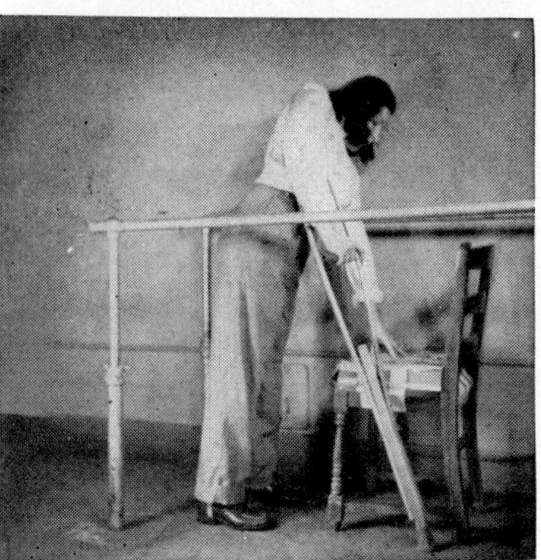

3a

Crutches*

Just as the sportsman must practice to acquire skill in using the tennis racquet, golf club, or skis, so the disabled person must acquire skill in using his wooden or metal crutches. The ability to use crutches efficiently requires a systematic program with competent instruction. This program should include (*a*) the proper selection of the crutches and correct measurement, (*b*) a muscle test to judge the patient's joint movements and strength, (*c*) exercises to develop the muscle groups needed for crutch management, and (*d*) determination of the crutch gaits best suited to meet the patient's needs.

SELECTION OF CRUTCHES AND THEIR ACCESSORIES

Underarm crutches with double uprights and hand bars are the most commonly used crutches today. Since it is not always possible to determine how long a pair of crutches should be and just where the hand bars should be placed, it has proved best to begin with a pair of extension crutches. These crutches can be adjusted to meet the needs of the patient. If the patient is permanently disabled and will need the crutches for many years, or perhaps for life, the extension crutches should be replaced with the standard type of crutches made of oak or hickory. There are new aluminum extension crutches on the market which seem to be so satisfactory that they can be used permanently.

Each shoulder piece should have a rubber cover over it to prevent the pressure of the hard wood in the axillary spaces. A rubber tip always covers the base of each crutch to prevent slipping. The 1½-in. (3.8 cm.) suction tips are the best, as they will remain in contact with the ground at whatever angle the crutch is placed. Small thin crutch tips should never be used as they do not make good contact with the ground.

Canadian crutches are extended canes which give support above the elbows, but do not extend into the axilla. They are useful if the patient has good control of the trunk, pelvis, and upper extremities. If he has trunk weakness and poor triceps, he will not be able to use them in performing many activi-

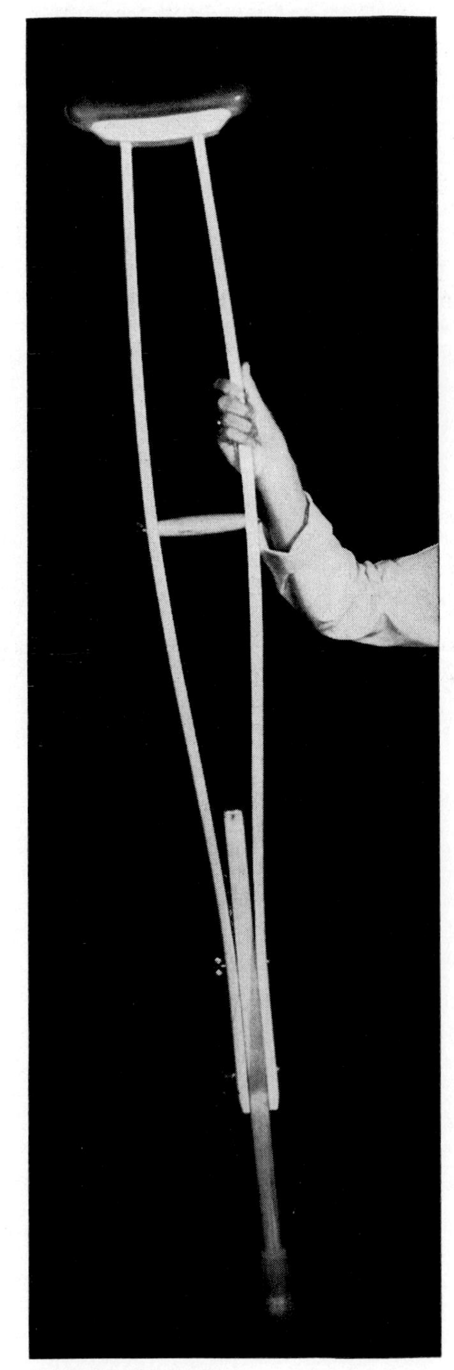

EXTENSION CRUTCH

* Adapted from DEAVER, G. G., What Every Physician Should Know about the Teaching of Crutch Walking, *J.A.M.A.*, Vol. 142, pp. 470–472, Feb. 18, 1950. See also DEAVER, G. G., and MARY ELEANOR BROWN, "The Challenge of Crutches," Institute for the Crippled and Disabled, New York, 1947.

ties essential for daily living, particularly opening and closing doors, going up and down stairs and curbs, and getting up from chairs. When a hand is needed, it must be taken off the crutch. This is hazardous with trunk or triceps weakness, because there is no way of supporting the trunk once the hand is released from the crutch.

It is also difficult for users of Canadian crutches to develop endurance, because they have no opportunity to rest on their armpits and thereby relax the arms and hands, which must be used all the time the crutches are being used. It is only for exceptional patients that the Canadian crutches should be recommended.

MEASURING FOR CRUTCHES

In measuring a patient for crutches, the height of the crutches and the level of the hand piece are primary considerations. If the crutches are too long, they force the shoulders up and the patient has no way of pushing his body off the floor. If the crutches are too short, the patient leans forward too far and stands poorly. There are numerous methods that may be recommended for measuring the patient for crutches.

Three procedures with the patient lying supine in bed are suggested in this chapter:

1. The crutch length is measured from the anterior fold of the axilla to a point 6 in. (15 cm.) out from the lateral side of the heel.
2. The crutch length is measured from the anterior fold of the axilla to the lateral side of the heel, and 2 in. (5 cm.) are added.
3. If the patient wears braces and crutches, the crutch tips and tops are placed on the crutches and the crutch length is then measured from the anterior fold of the axilla and about two to three fingers below the apex of the axilla to the lateral side of the heel of the shoe.

Fitting the crutches in the supine position is only a working basis, to gage the approximate crutch length. In order to make the final adjustments for correct crutch length, the patient must be in the standing position.

For maximum support the patient stands on the crutches either in parallel bars or against the wall with one therapist in front for support. He may also stand away from the wall with one therapist in front and one in back ready for support. The crutches should now be so adjusted that the patient can assume a good crutch stance.

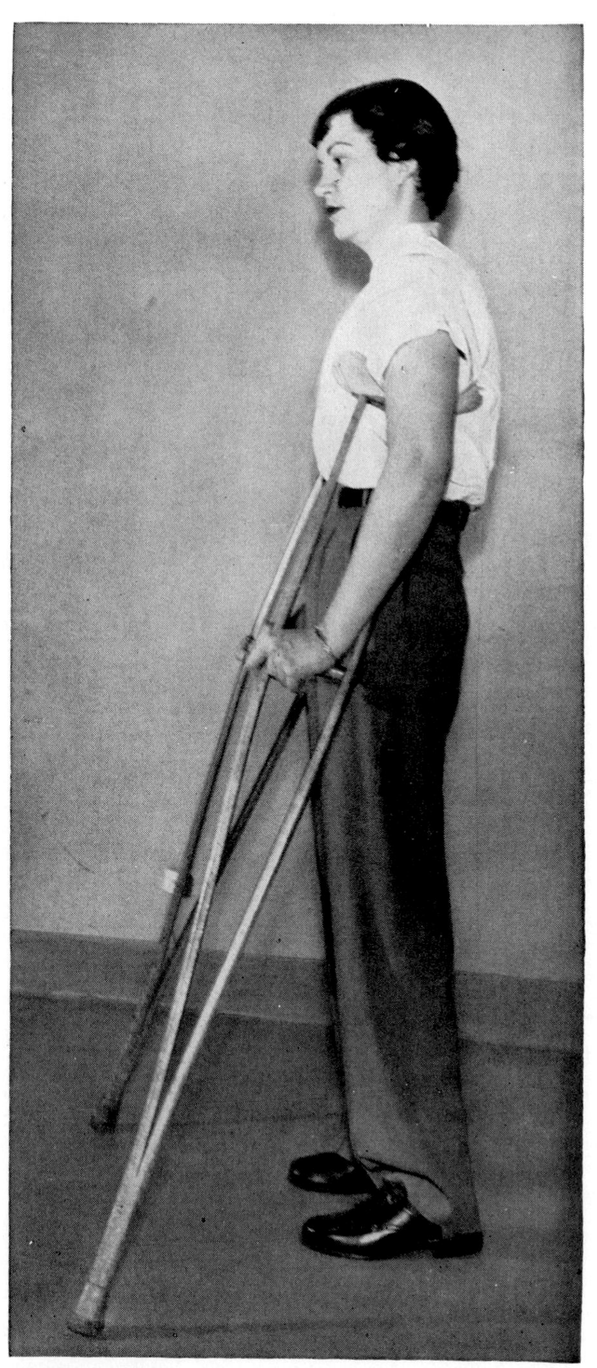

CRUTCH STANCE

CRUTCH STANCES

The ideal crutch stance (Fig. **39**·1) is a position in which the head is up straight and tall and the pelvis is held as much as possible over the feet. The crutches are placed about six to eight inches from the front and from the side of the toes. The elbows are bent 25 to 30 deg., the shoulders are down and not hunched. It should be possible to place about two to three fingers between the crutch tops and the armpit, so that at no time is weight taken by the apex of the axilla. The crutches lean against the ribs and are grasped there by the muscles which form the anterior fold of the axilla and draw the arms toward the body. The disability of the patient may make an ideal position on crutches impossible. If he has no abdominal, back, or hip-joint muscles, the tripod position or an exaggerated tripod position should be assumed.

In assuming a *tripod position* (Fig. **39**·2) the crutches are placed about eight to ten inches in front and from the side of the toes, so that the slanted crutches provide the anterior support.

The weight is brought forward at the ankles,the hips are brought forward without bending, the pelvis is tilted forward, and the shoulders are brought back so that the slanted body provides the posterior support and the apex of the tripod is at shoulder level. The hand bars are so adjusted that the elbows are now slightly bent and the crutch tops about two to three fingers below the axilla. More weight is taken on the crutches than on the feet.

In an *exaggerated tripod position* (Fig. **39**·3) the back is arched more, the crutches placed farther forward, and nearly all weight is taken on the crutches.

As coordination, skill, and strength increase, the crutches as well as the body are less slanted and more and more weight is taken on the feet, so that the ideal crutch stance as described above (Fig. **39**·1) is assumed.

When measuring crutches, it must be remembered that there are no rigid rules and that whatever has been said above should be regarded only as a guide.

The degree in which the body or the crutches will be slanted is dependent on the muscle strength, ability to balance, and the general skill and coordination of the patient. But in addition to this, his general body build must be considered. Patients with wider hips will need a wider base to work from than patients with narrow hips; therefore, the placement of the crutch tips in front and from the side of the toes will vary, which in turn will influence the length of the crutches.

For example: Patients who have hips that are wide in comparison with the rest of the body will place their crutches more to the side; whereas, tall patients with comparatively narrow hips will place their crutches well forward.

In general, shorter crutches, although they seem to be more difficult to handle in the beginning, are much easier to handle when the patient learns to climb stairs and to get up and down curbs, but of course there may be patients who need relatively longer crutches. In no instance should the armpit rest on the crutches.

The permanent crutch length can be determined only by finding a "good crutch stance"—the most efficient crutch stance for a given patient—and then adjusting the crutches accordingly. In other words, it is important to remember that, as the patient becomes more used to his crutches and learns to handle them more skillfully and as he progresses with his walking and climbing activities, the crutch length and the height of the hand bars may have to be readjusted to his particular needs. Therefore, it cannot be emphasized too strongly that the patient's posture should be observed continuously in standing as well as when walking and climbing so that necessary crutch adjustments can be made.

Fig. 39. CRUTCH STANCES

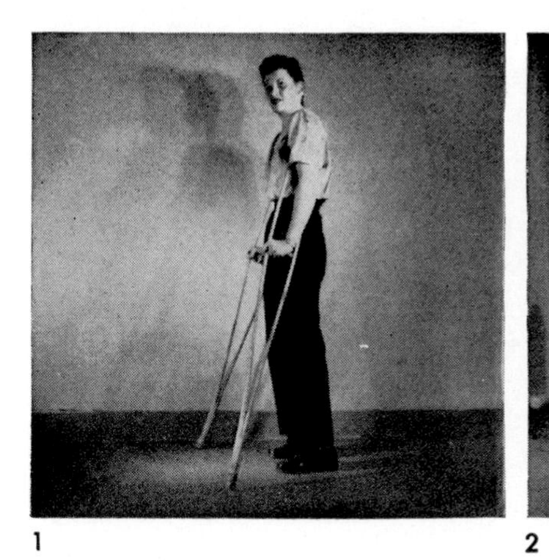

1

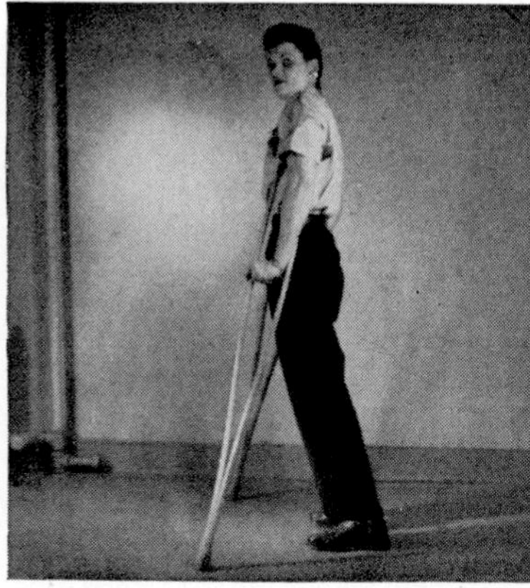

2

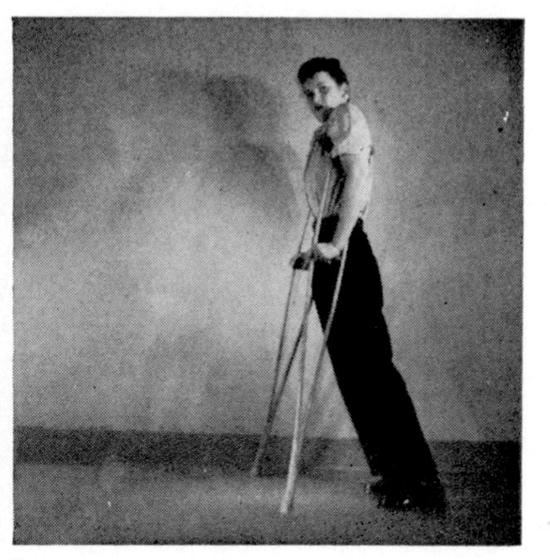

3

CRUTCH BALANCING

The patient has to learn an entirely new system of balancing and of shifting his weight from hands to feet and feet to hands in order to move the crutches or the body.

In order to move one crutch the patient must move all the weight from that crutch to the other crutch and to both feet. If both crutches are moved, the feet must take all the weight. If the feet are moved, the crutches must take all the weight. Therefore the patient has to learn to shift the weight smoothly and maintain his balance while doing so. This is a matter of strength as well as of coordination and timing.

Although patients with spinal-cord lesions may have no sensation below the lesion, they may develop through continuous practice the ability of "knowing" when the weight is on their feet.

At first, crutch-balancing exercises are practiced *against the wall* for maximum safety, and after sufficient skill and confidence are gained, the exercises shown in Figures **40**·1 to **40**·5 are practiced *away from the wall.*

Fig. 40. CRUTCH BALANCING AGAINST WALL

Purpose: to handle crutches; to balance on crutches and braces, shifting weight from crutches to feet and feet to crutches.

Preparation for: crutch balancing away from wall.

Preliminary exercises: all parallel-bar exercises.

Starting Position: Stand against wall with shoulders and heels touching wall; crutches about six to eight inches in front and from side of toes; pelvis tilted forward; elbows slightly bent; wrists dorsiflexed; tops of crutches two to three fingers below axilla (**S.P.**, front view; **6a**, side view). (See also crutch stances, p. 108.)

Instructions: Perform each of the following movements and return to starting position.

1. *Sideswaying.* Sway to left, shifting weight to left crutch and foot; leave no weight on right crutch. Repeat to right.

2. *Lifting one crutch.* Balance and support yourself on both feet and left crutch so that you can lift right crutch forward and up. Hold, then replace, and repeat with left crutch.

3. *Lifting both crutches.* Shift all weight to feet, exaggerate pelvic tilt foward, raise both crutches forward, and replace. (Be sure shoulders touch wall.)

4. *Pushing up on crutches.* Shift all weight to hands, push on crutches, straightening elbows until body is off floor. Lower body by bending elbows slowly and land with heels first, returning to starting position. (Move crutches forward quickly when heels touch floor, to maintain balance. This is important when standing away from the wall.)

5. *Turning crutch out from under arm.* Balance and support yourself on both feet and one crutch. Release grip of right crutch, turn hand completely around so that back of hand is toward crutch as you grasp hand bar again. Shrug shoulder slightly and turn crutch out and forward from under arm. Shift weight to right crutch, repeat turning out with left crutch.

6a. *Jackknifing.* Lean into crutches, bring shoulders forward and bend forward at waist, so that only buttocks are against wall.

6b. Push with buttocks away from wall, continue pushing on hands, straighten elbows, bring shoulders back, so that pelvis tilts forward and you stand straight (see Fig. **32**).

Precautions: One therapist stands in front or two therapists stand, one on each side of the patient, ready to give support. Support is given around waist and never by holding on to crutches.

Fig. 40. CRUTCH BALANCING AGAINST WALL

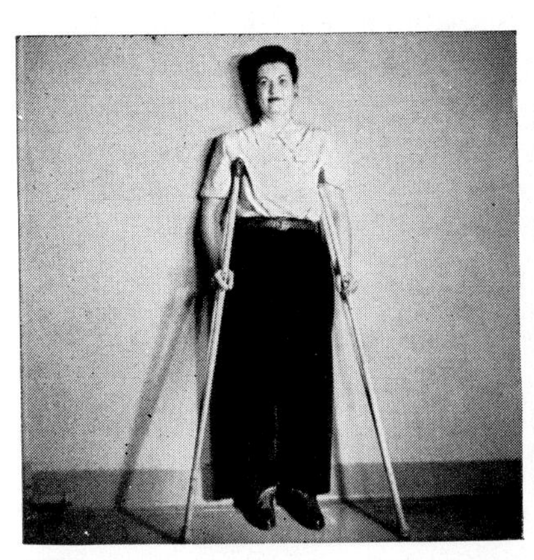

S.P.

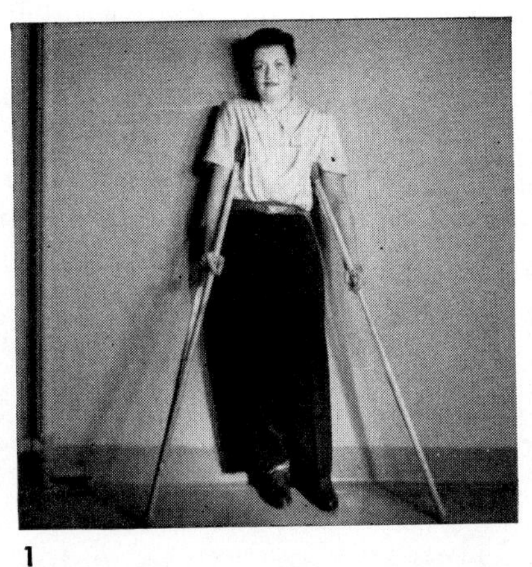

1

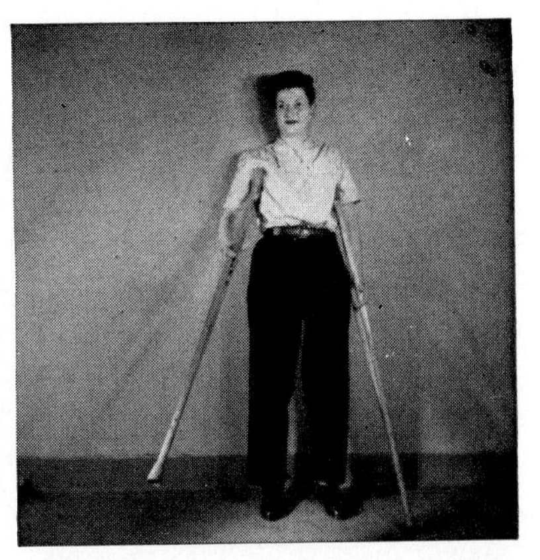

2

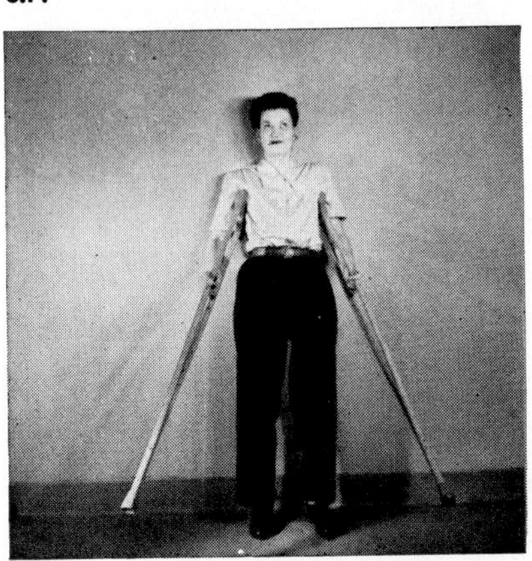

3

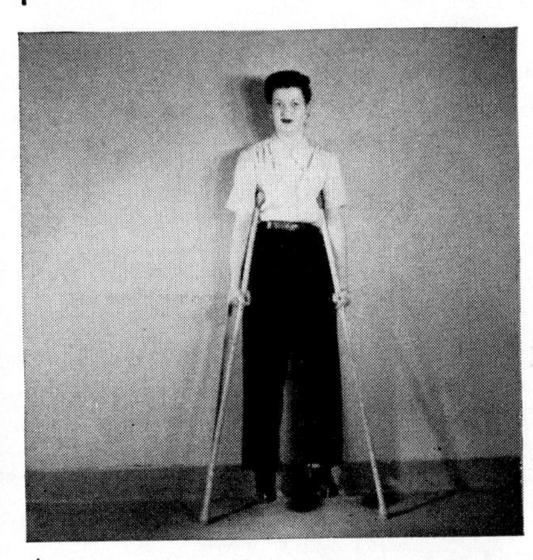

4

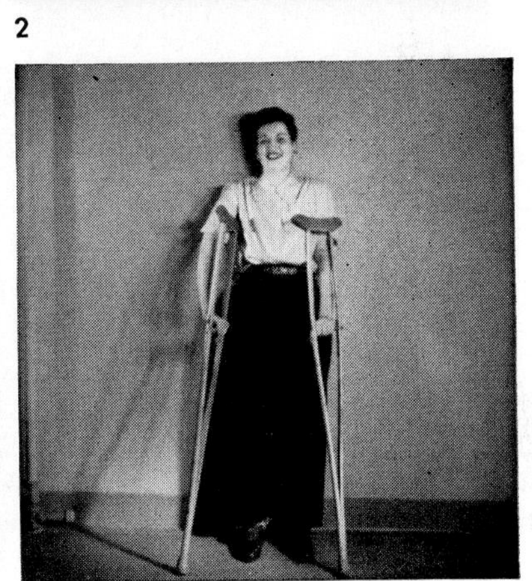

5

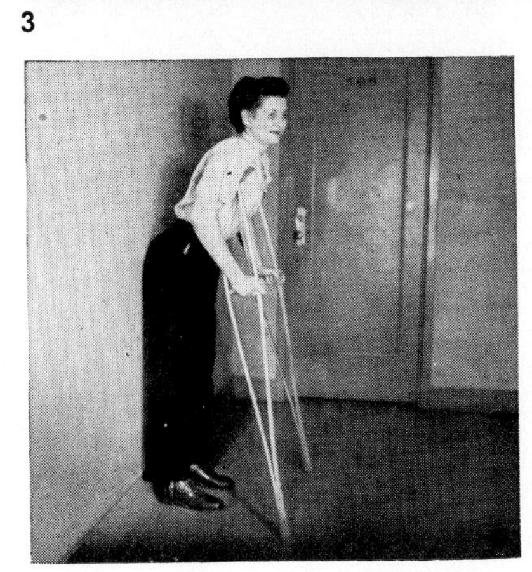

6a

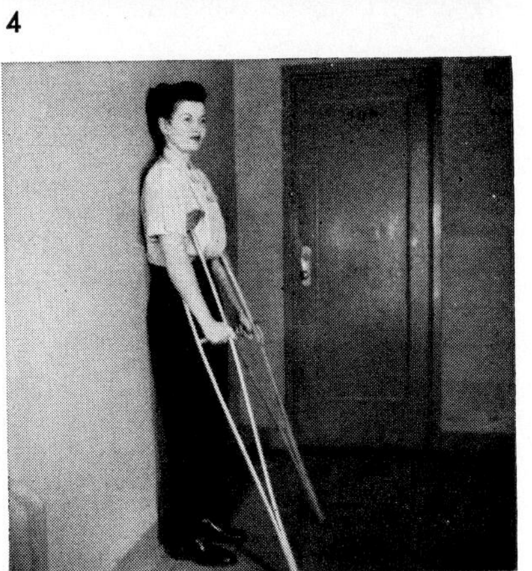

6b

CRUTCH BALANCING AWAY FROM WALL

Once crutch-balancing exercises against wall are mastered, crutch balancing away from wall is practiced. In the beginning, two therapists, one in back and one in front, are ready to give support around waist. Later only one therapist will be needed in back of patient until sufficient skill and confidence are gained, so that patient can practice exercises by himself. Support is always given around waist and never by grasping crutch.

Preparation for: crutch walking; getting in and out of chairs.

Preliminary exercises: crutch balancing against the wall.

Starting Position: tripod position. Stand with crutches about six to eight inches in front of and to side of toes; pelvis is tilted forward; shoulders are back; wrists are dorsiflexed, so that elbows are slightly bent; crutch tops are two to three fingers below axilla.

Instructions: Same as in Figure **40·1** to **40·5**.

In addition to these exercises the ones described below are practiced.

Fig. 41A. JACKKNIFING

Purpose: to control pelvic tilt backward as well as forward by pushing on hands and bringing shoulders back.

Starting Position: tripod position.

Instructions:

1. Lean well into crutches and, keeping elbows straight, bring...

2. ...shoulders forward so that pelvis rolls back and...

3. ...over feet. You are now in a jackknifed position with weight on crutches and feet.

To straighten up: Reverse entire procedure. (Read pictures in reverse sequence.)

2. Push on crutches, keeping elbows straight bring shoulders...

1. ...back so that pelvis can...

S.P. ...tilt forward.

Precautions:

2. If crutches are too near feet, pelvis will roll back beyond control. To prevent falling in this position, back has to be arched quickly, shoulders brought back, crutches moved forward, and weight thrown on them almost simultaneously. Same must be done when buckling occurs involuntarily when standing or walking on crutches and braces.

Helpful remarks: (see Fig. **32**). The only time body is bent voluntarily at waist is when patient has to bend forward in order to grasp armrest when getting in and out of wheel chairs. Crutches then must be well in front so that weight is distributed between crutches and feet (see Fig. **45A**).

Fig. 41B. CRUTCHES FORWARD AND BACKWARD

Purpose: to move crutches forward and back while keeping pelvis tilted forward.

Preparation for: Swing-through gait.

Starting Position: tripod position.

Instructions:

1a. Lean well into crutches and keeping pelvis tilted forward...

2a. ...swing body back on heels. Almost simultaneously swing crutches back...

3a. ...behind feet (same distance as they were in front). As soon as crutches touch floor shift weight on them, bringing shoulders back so that pelvis can be tilted forward. Hesitate slightly in this position to ensure good balance and rhythm.

2a. Swing body forward at ankles and simultaneously bring crutches forward into an...

S.P. ...exaggerated tripod position. Shift weight forward to crutches.

Precautions: Pelvis remains tilted forward all the time. Back is arched to prevent buckling, and whole body moves only at ankle joints. The entire exercise is a continuous smooth movement backward and forward (see Fig. **34**).

Fig. 41A. JACKKNIFING

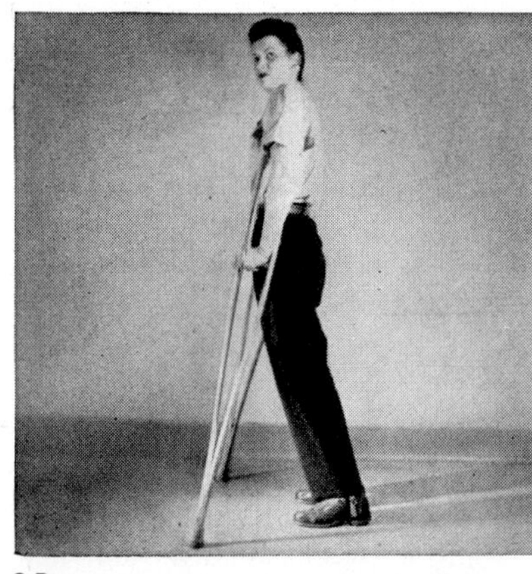
S.P.

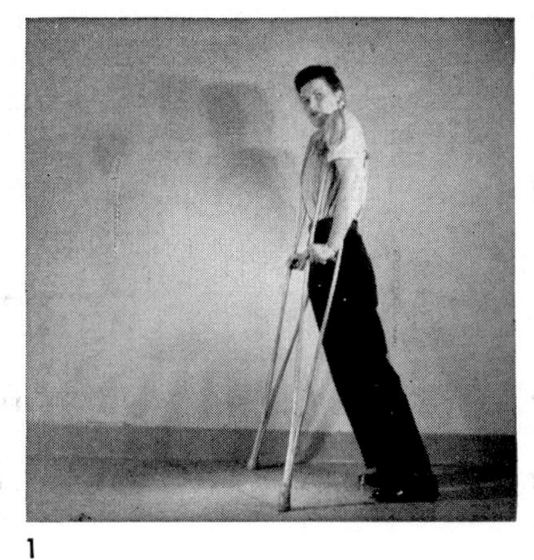
1

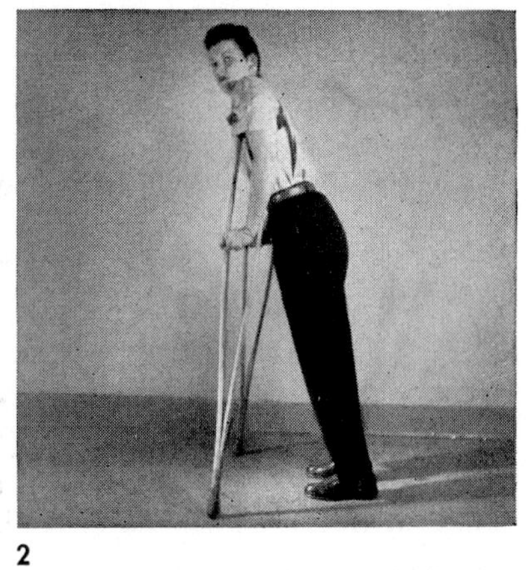
2

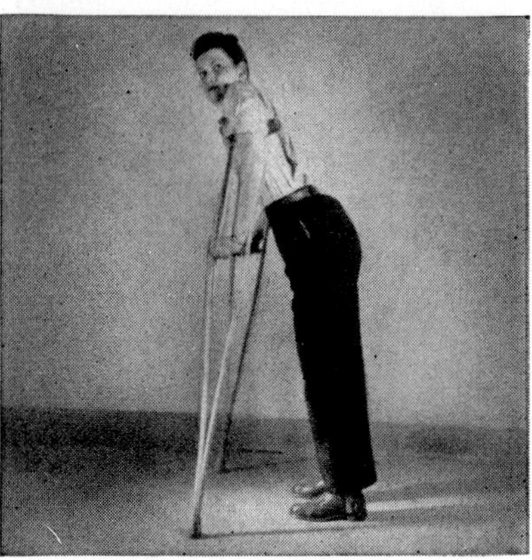
3

Fig. 41B. CRUTCHES FORWARD AND BACKWARD

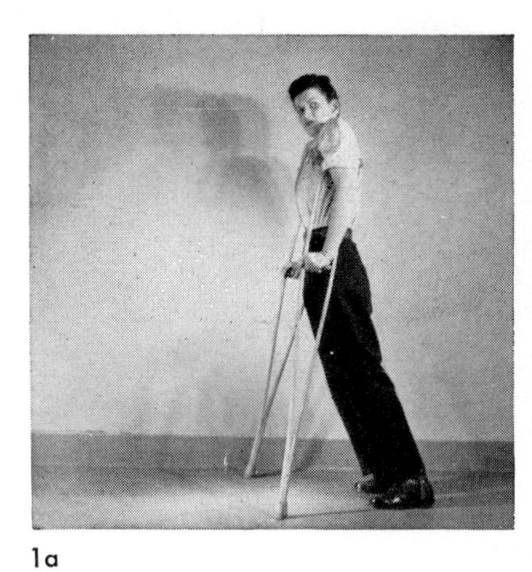
1a

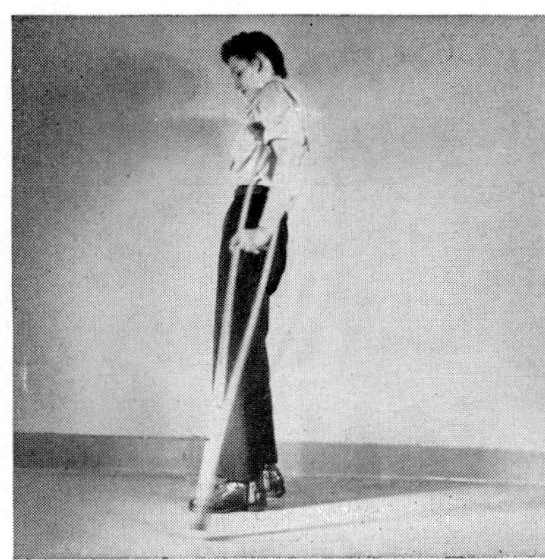
2a

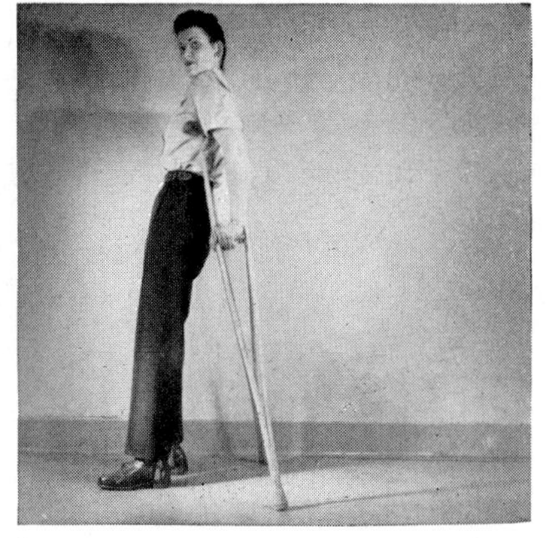
3a

FOUR-POINT AND TWO-POINT GAITS

Figures **42A**·1 to **42A**·4 represent one unit of the four-point gait and Figures **42B**·1a to **42B**·3a one unit of the two-point gait. Each unit is a series of continuous smooth movements, which should not come to a stop unless both crutches and both legs are on the floor.

Special Note: *Endurance and rhythm* must be developed from the start. Therefore all gaits should be practiced in units, starting with two units, then resting, proceeding to four units, then resting, and so on, until 10 units can be done in an even rhythm without rest. Later the patient will traverse the room an ever-increasing number of times. If careful attention is paid from the beginning to good rhythm, speed will develop automatically as endurance increases.

Fig. 42A. FOUR-POINT GAIT

This is a safe slow gait since there are always three points in contact with the ground. Since this gait does not require much space, it can be used in crowds. It can be done only by patients who can bring one leg forward while balancing on the other leg and *both* crutches.

Starting Position: tripod position.
Instructions: Count: (1) right crutch, (2) left leg, (3) left crutch, and (4) right leg.

1. Raise right crutch and...
2. ...place it a few inches in front on floor. Take as much weight as possible on right crutch and right leg, while bending trunk slightly to right. At the same time push on left crutch in order to lift (or hike) left leg off floor and bring it...
3. ...forward to take a step. Shift weight to left leg and...
4. ...bring left crutch forward, put weight on left crutch, tilt body slightly to left, at the same time pushing on right crutch in order to lift (or hike) right leg off floor to bring it forward and take a step. Shift weight to right leg and...
1. ...start new sequence.

Helpful remarks:
2. Pushing on same side as leg is raised and tilting body to opposite side will help in bringing leg forward.

If patient has no hip flexors, he still may be able to move legs forward alternately by hiking them (using the quadratus lumborum) and also twisting trunk.

Fig. 42B. TWO-POINT GAIT

This is a quick gait and should be attempted only after four-point gait has been thoroughly mastered. This gait can be used in crowds since it does not require much space. It can be performed only by patients who can bring one leg forward while balancing on other leg and *one* crutch.

Starting Position: tripod position.
Instructions: Count: (1) right crutch and left leg, (2) left crutch and right leg.

1a. Raise right crutch and left leg simultaneously. Take a step placing crutch on floor at the same time. Shift...
2a. ...weight to right crutch and left leg and repeat with...
3a. ...left crutch and right leg.

Helpful remarks: Pushing on crutch on same side as raised leg will help to bring leg forward.
1a. Weight is on left crutch and right leg when raising right crutch and left leg.

Fig. 42A. FOUR-POINT GAIT

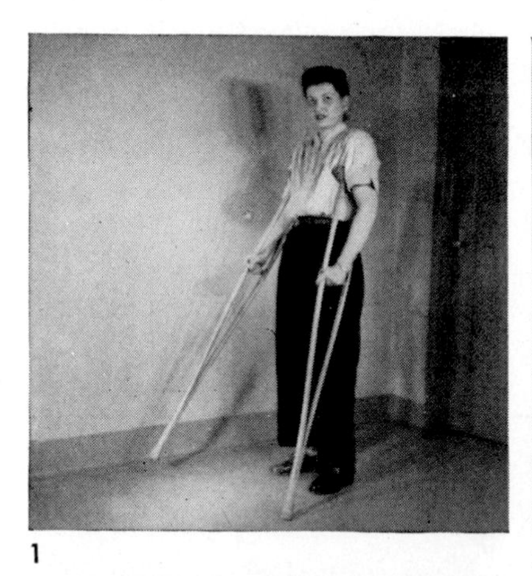
1

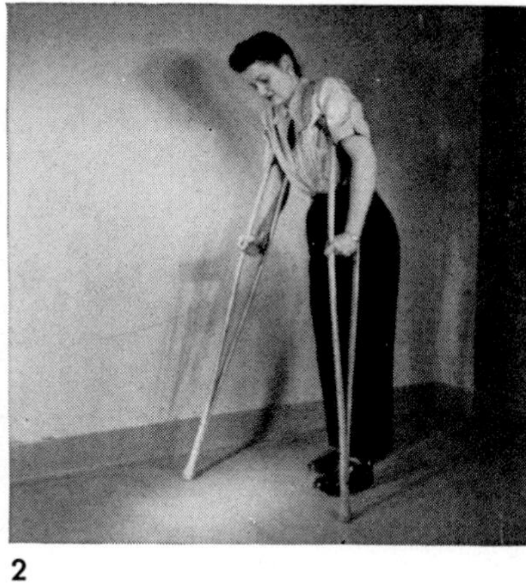
2

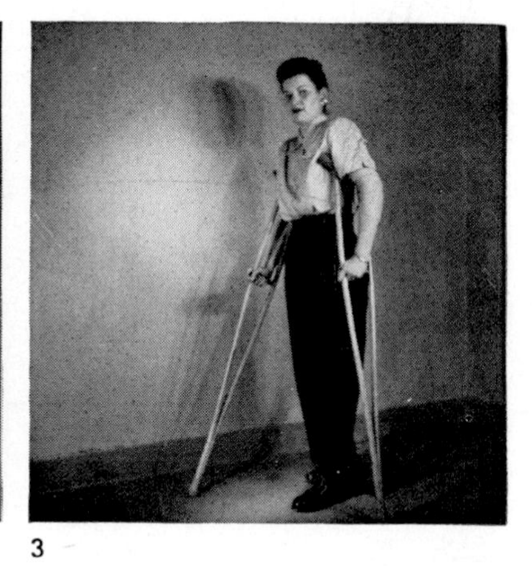
3

4

Fig. 42B. TWO-POINT GAIT

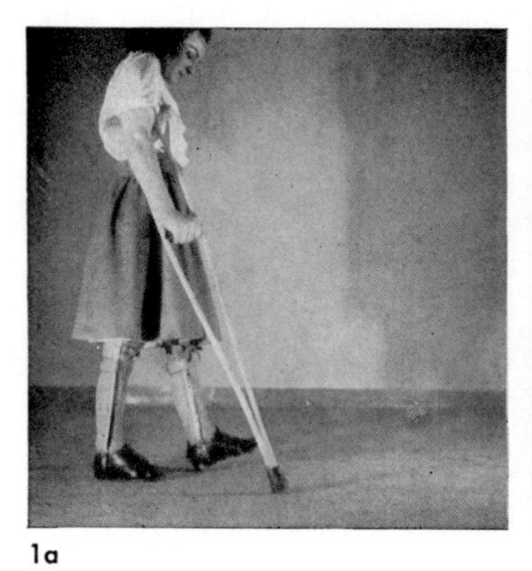
1a

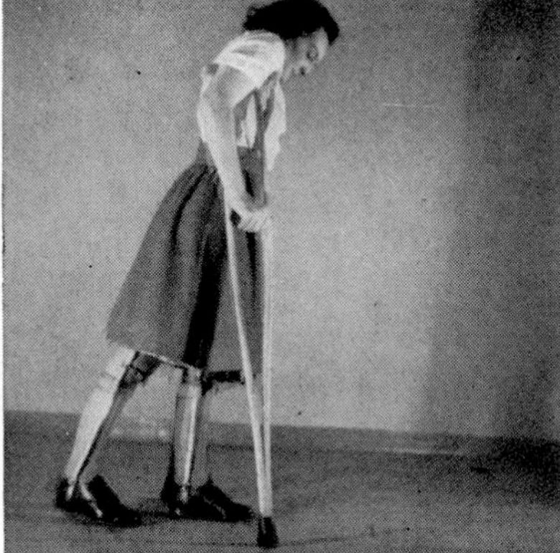
2a

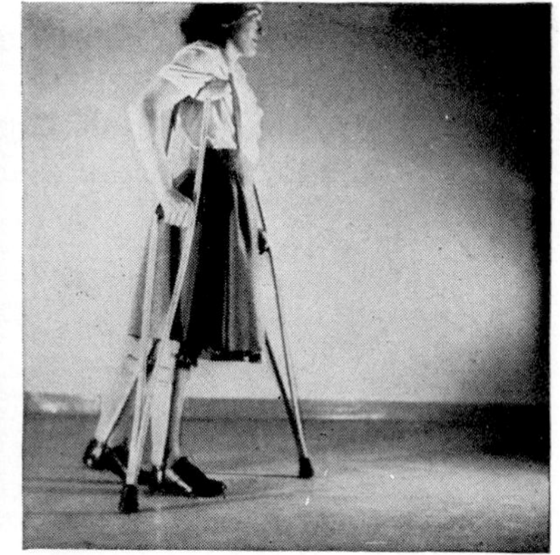
3a

SHUFFLE GAITS

These are slow safe gaits since the feet are always in contact with the ground. They are choice gaits for beginners. Older people may use them exclusively. Since these gaits do not require much space, they can very well be done in crowds. Until sufficient skill and confidence are gained, a therapist walks in back, or if two therapists are necessary, one walks in front and one in back, ready to support the patient around the waist.

S.P. through 4 represent one unit of the shuffle-alternate gait.

S.P.a through 2a represent one unit of the shuffle-simultaneous gait.

Each unit is a series of continuous smooth movements which should not come to a stop unless the weight is in front on both crutches and the patient in a tripod position (**S.P.** and **S.P.a**). This position is the end of one sequence as well as the beginning of the next. To develop endurance as well as speed, gaits should be practiced in sets of two, four, six, etc. (See special note to Four-point and Two-point Gaits, p. 114.)

Fig. 42C. SHUFFLE-ALTERNATE GAIT

Preliminary exercises: crutch balancing.

Starting Position: tripod position. (**S.P.**)

Instructions: Count: (1) right crutch, (2) left crutch, (3) shuffle feet.

1. Raise right crutch and...

2. ...place it a few inches in front. Repeat with left crutch until...

3. ...both crutches are on one line and parallel.

4. Lean into both crutches so that all weight is on crutches and pull body forward, dragging...

S.P. ...both feet to starting position, so that you are ready to start a new sequence.

Fig. 42D. SHUFFLE-SIMULTANEOUS GAIT

Preliminary exercises: shuffle-alternate gait (most patients start immediately with this gait).

Starting Position: tripod position. (**S.P.a.**)

Instructions: Count: (1) crutches, (2) shuffle feet.

1a. Raise both crutches simultaneously and place ...

2a. ...them well forward, shifting all weight to them. Lean into crutches and pull body forward, shuffling...

S.P.a. ...both feet to starting position. You are now ready for a new sequence.

Precautions: To prevent buckling, body is never bent at the waist.

Helpful remarks:

1. While raising one crutch, weight is on other crutch and both feet.

4. All weight must be on crutches so that feet can be dragged forward.

1a. For a moment all weight is on feet while both crutches are raised and *immediately* placed...

2a. ...forward again.

Fig. 42C. SHUFFLE-ALTERNATE GAIT

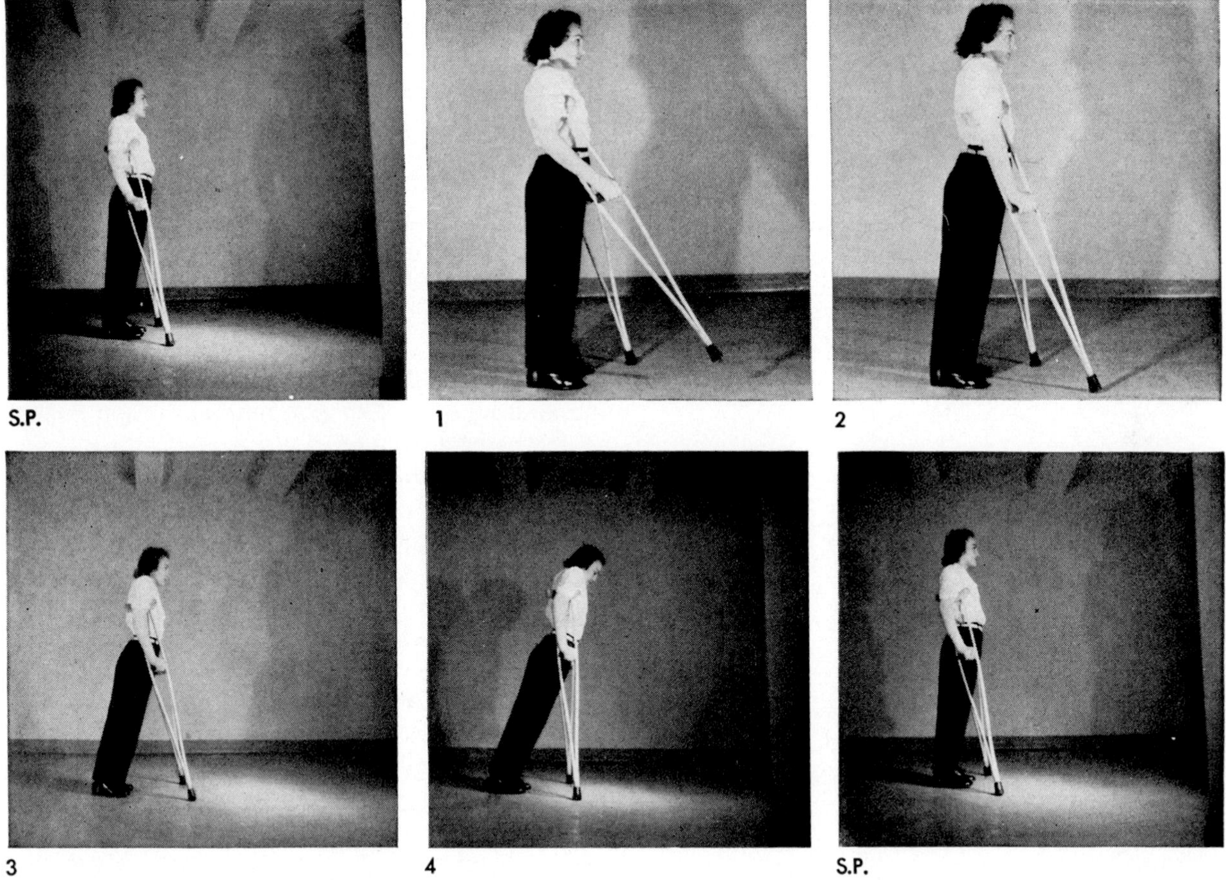

S.P. 1 2

3 4 S.P.

Fig. 42D. SHUFFLE-SIMULTANEOUS GAIT

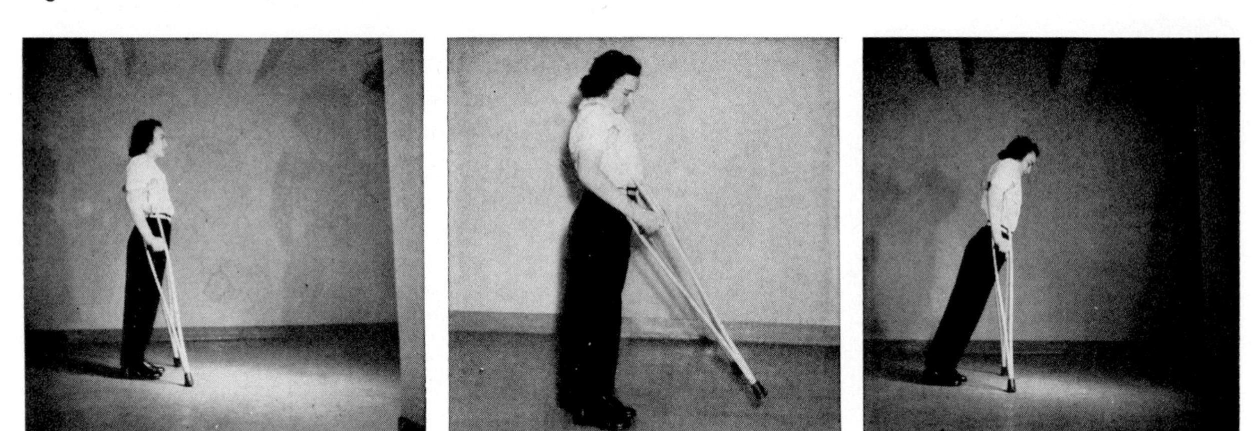

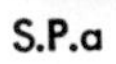

S.P.a 1a 2a

Fig. 42E. SWING-TO GAIT

This is a fairly quick gait since feet clear floor and small obstacles can be hopped over. This gait needs a fair amount of space. Many patients will use this gait exclusively.

Preliminary exercises: jackknifing; push-ups; shuffle-simultaneous gait.

Starting Position: tripod position.

Instructions: Count: (1) crutches, (2) hop.

1. Raise both crutches and place them well in front. Lean into crutches, putting all your weight on them. Push...

2. ...body off floor, straightening elbows and ducking head slightly to gain sufficient height so that feet clear floor.

3. Land heels first in between crutches. As soon as feet touch floor bring...

4. ...shoulders back so that pelvis can tilt forward, shift weight to feet and nearly simultaneously bring crutches...

5. ...forward and...

1. ...place them well in front in an exaggerated tripod position. Shift weight to hands to start new sequence.

2. Push body off floor, etc.

Precautions:

5. Crutches should not be raised until pelvis is completely tilted and weight is on feet.

3, 4, 5, 1. These movements are all performed nearly simultaneously.

Until sufficient skill and confidence are gained, one therapist walks in back of patient or two therapists walk, one in front and one in back of patient, ready to give support around waist.

Helpful remarks:

1–5. Represent one unit of swing-to gait. This unit consists of a series of rhythmical continuous movements which do not come to a stop until weight is shifted forward on both crutches and patient is in an...

1. ...exaggerated tripod position. This position is the end of one as well as the beginning of the next sequence.

To develop endurance, rhythm, and speed, gait should be practiced in units of two, four, six, etc. (See special note to Four-point and Two-point Gaits, p. 114.)

Fig. 42E. SWING-TO GAIT

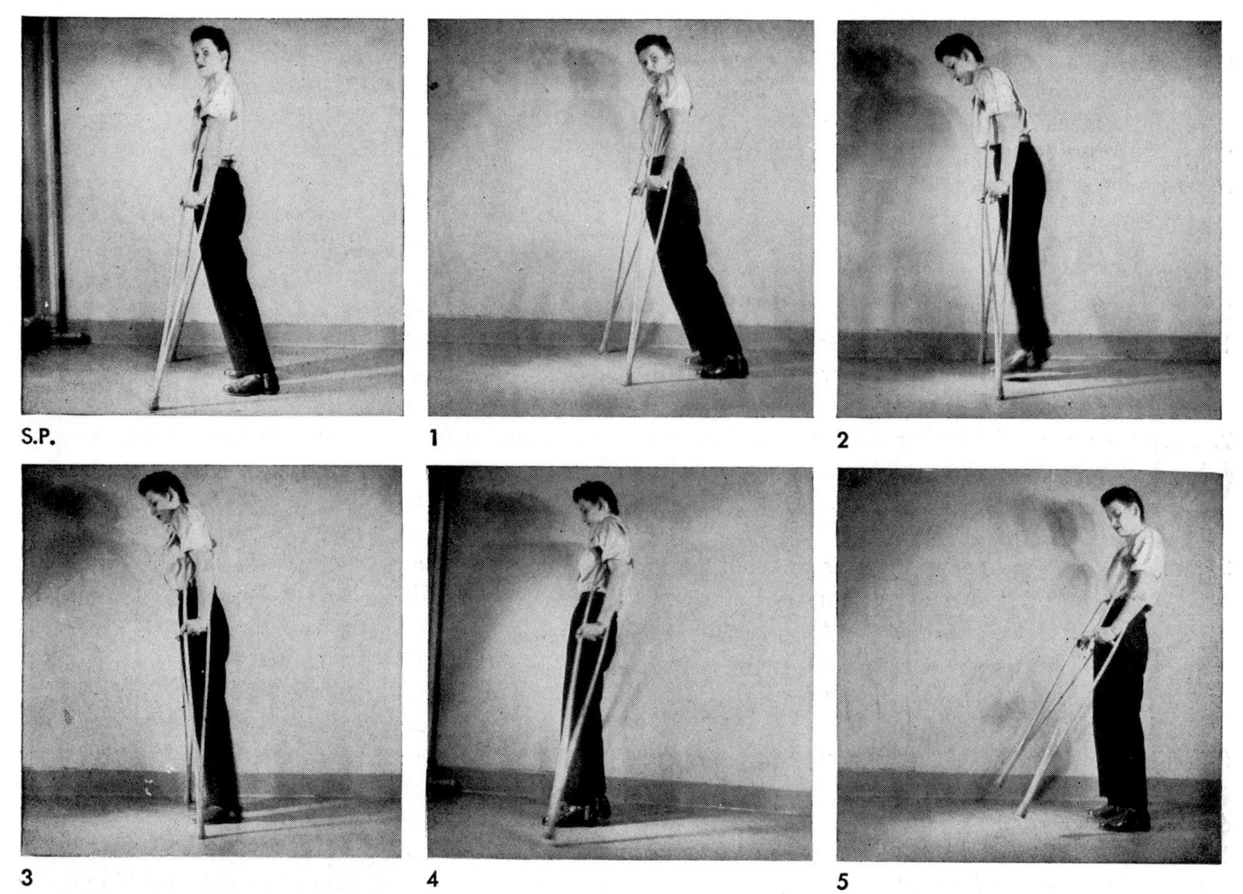

S.P. 1 2

3 4 5

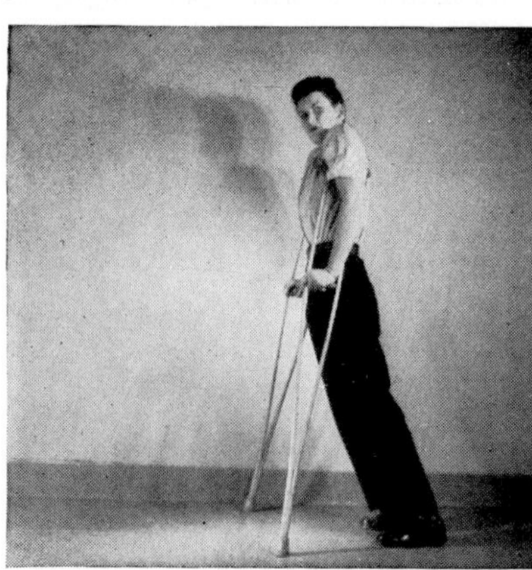

1

WALKING IN DIFFERENT DIRECTIONS AND CARRYING ARTICLES

When walking through narrow doors or getting up from (or down into) a chair, sofa, etc., or car, it is important that the patient be able to walk sideward, and backward as well as forward.

Fig. 43A. WALKING SIDEWARD

Preliminary exercises: crutch balancing; crutch walking.

Starting Position: tripod position. (S.P.)
Instructions:

1. Move right crutch, then left crutch, to right.
2. Lean into crutches and move feet either alternately or simultaneously the same distance to right.

Repeat to left.

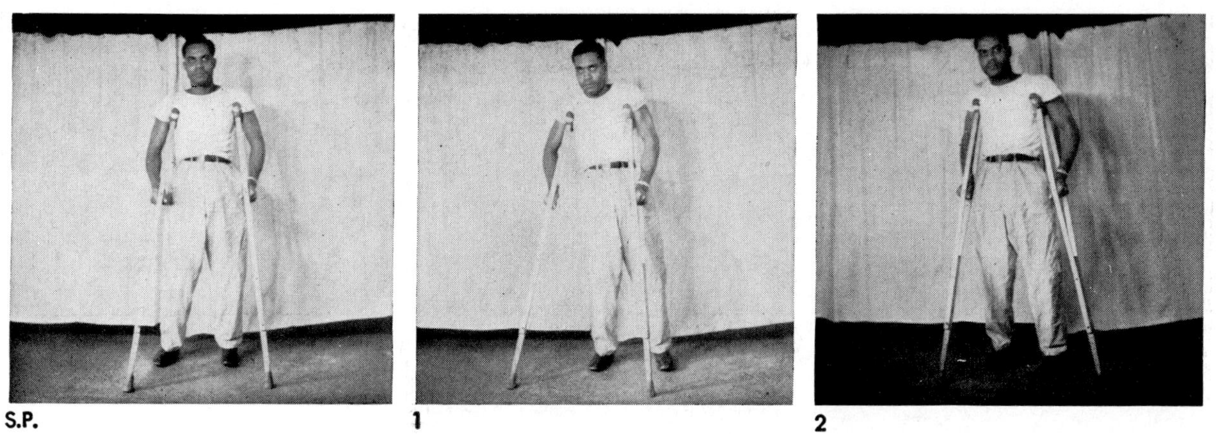

S.P. 1 2

Fig. 43B. WALKING BACKWARD

Starting Position: tripod position. (**S.P.a.**) Arch back and...

Instructions:

1a. ...quickly buckle, shifting all weight on to crutches. Push up and hop...

2a. ...backward. As heels touch floor, tilt pelvis...

S.P.a. ...forward. Move crutches back the same distance and straighten up, returning to tripod position.

Precautions: One therapist walks in back or two therapists walk, one in front and one in back, ready to give support around waist.

Helpful remarks: If patient can move legs alternately, he can take steps backward instead of hopping (see Fig. **42A,** and read pictures in reverse sequence).

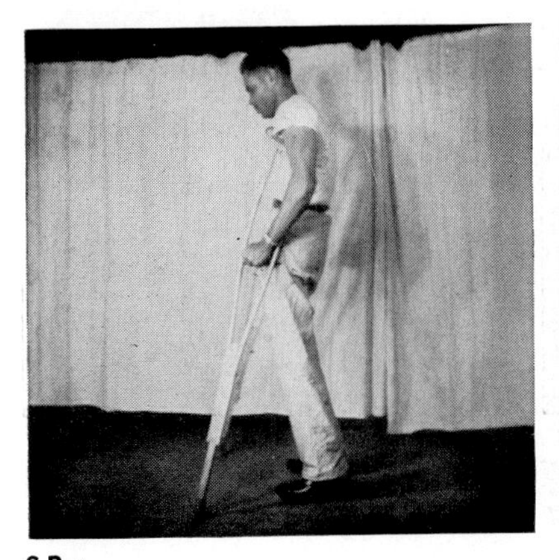

S.P.a

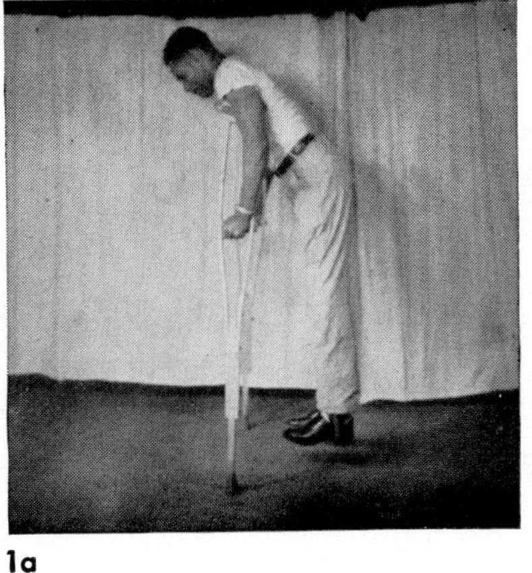

1a

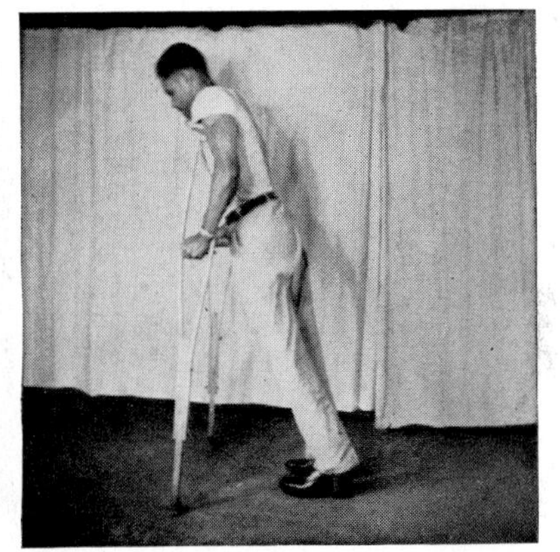

2a

Fig. 43C. CARRYING POCKETBOOK, BRIEFCASE, ETC., WHILE WALKING ON CRUTCHES

It is important that patients practice walking while carrying a pocketbook, briefcase, package, etc. The shoulder-strap type of bag (Fig. **43C**·1) is the most practical, since it leaves the hands free for handling the crutches.

To prevent pressure sores, it is important that patients with sensory disturbances always carry a small sponge-rubber pillow to sit on. This pillow has a cover, large enough to accommodate small articles such as a purse, cigarettes, etc. (Fig. **43C**·2). The cover has a handle for easy carrying.

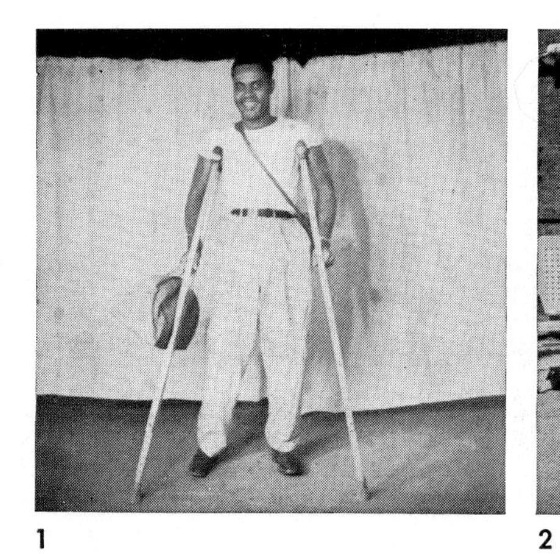

1

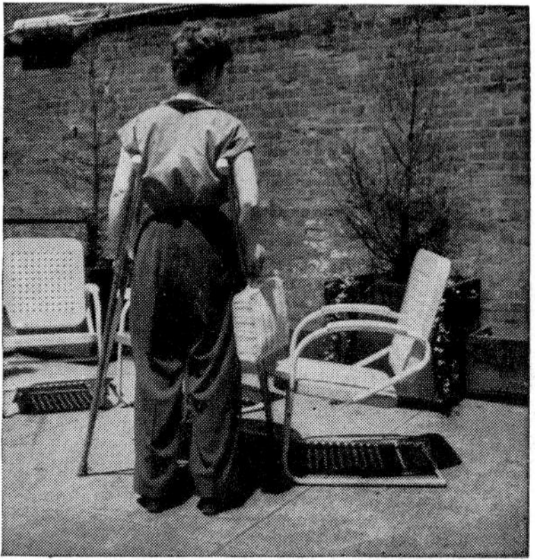

2

Fig. 44. WALKING THROUGH DOOR

Preliminary exercises: crutch walking in all directions.

Starting Position: If door opens toward you and doorknob is on the right, stand, facing door, slightly at an angle, so that you can turn doorknob with one hand while supporting yourself on crutch with other hand and on both feet. Be sure that you are far enough away from door so that when you open it it will not strike your feet.

Instructions:

1. Balance and support yourself on both feet and right crutch while you open door with left hand and...
2. ...immediately grasp left crutch again and place crutch tip against door to keep it open.
3. Take a few steps forward, then turn, so that you can walk through door, trying to keep it just sufficiently open with left crutch. Do not walk too far through, so...
4. ...that you can grasp doorknob and close door with left hand, balancing and supporting yourself on right crutch and both feet.

Precautions: No weight should be placed at any time on doorknob, but patient must balance and support himself on one crutch and both feet.
It is also wise to make sure that nobody is going to open door from opposite side and throw patient off balance.

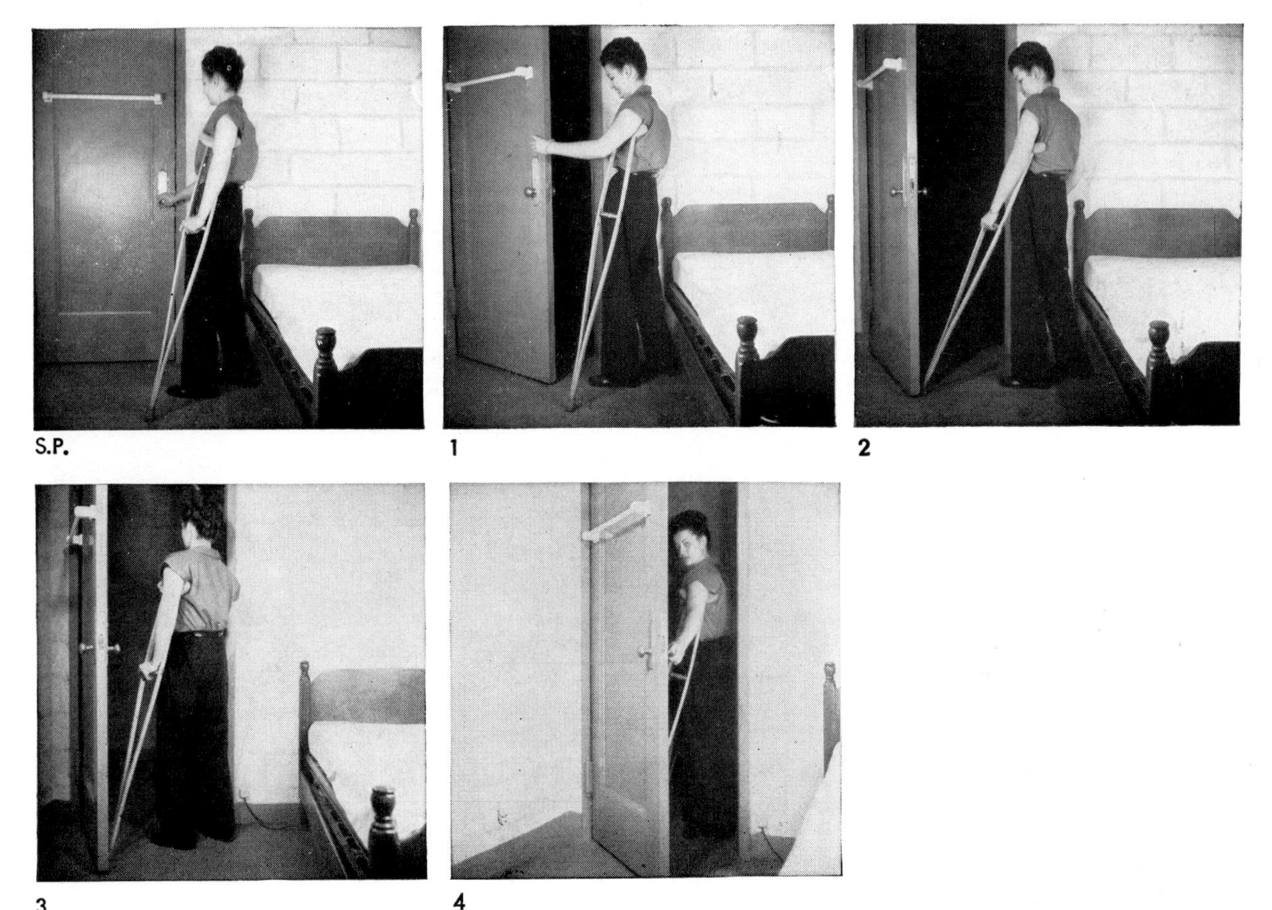

S.P. 1 2

3 4

CHAPTER VI

Elevation and Travel on Crutches

After the patient has learned crutch walking on level ground, he is taught elevation on crutches. The term "elevation" as used in this book pertains to *standing up and sitting down* as well as to *climbing* stairs, ramps, curbs, etc.

STANDING UP AND SITTING DOWN

The following methods are all interchangeable and each can be used for the wheel chair, the chair, the toilet seat, the bed, etc.

1. **Into and out of wheel chair.**
   a. **Both knees locked—facing chair** (Fig. **45A**). The patient locks both knee locks and faces the chair, while sitting down and standing up.
   b. **Both knees locked—profile to chair** (Fig. **45B**). For small patients it is easier to remain in profile to the chair while sitting down.
   c. **Up—legs crossed** (Fig. **45C**). For some patients it is easier to cross their legs before standing up.
2. **Down on and up from straight chair** (Fig. **46**). The same method is used as in getting into and out of wheel chair.
3. **Down on and up from toilet seat.**
   a. **One knee locked** (Fig. **47A**). Patients with long legs may find it easier to lock only one knee.
   b. **Both knees locked** (Fig. **47B**). This is the same procedure as **1a**—only more difficult, since the toilet seat is low.
4. **Up from and down on bed—both knees locked** (Fig. **48**). This is also the same procedure as **1a**—only more difficult, since the bed is low and the mattress soft.
5. **Up from and down on floor.** This is the most difficult of all standing-up and sitting-down procedures, and only very advanced crutch walkers should attempt it.
   a. **Up—one crutch under each arm** (Fig. **49A**).
   b. **Up—pushing on both crutches** (Fig. **49B**).
   c. **Falling** (Fig. **49C**).

Special Note: *Locking and unlocking hip locks* is important for all activities that involve standing up and sitting down (for details see Helpful Remarks, Figs. **30**·3 and **30**·4). A patient wearing a double long leg brace with a pelvic band may need hip locks so that he may lock one or both, as necessary, in order to remain upright when standing or walking. (If he wears, in addition, a spinal brace both hip locks have to be locked.) In this case the patient has to learn to *lock* the hip locks whenever getting out of the wheel chair or car or up from a chair, toilet, or bed, and to *unlock* the hip locks when sitting down.

CLIMBING

Tremendous skill, strength, coordination, balance, and endurance are required for performing climbing activities. Although patients should, if they possibly can, learn to climb stairs and curbs, it will depend entirely on the individual patient how many of these activities he will be able to carry out safely and independently in his daily life. If patients wear hip locks they have to unlock them in order to buckle as much as possible, as buckling helps to gain height.

In all climbing activities the patient must be able to "push up" high enough on his crutches so that he gains sufficient height to clear an average step or curb. Because of the railing on staircases, steps are easier to climb than curbs and are therefore taught first. Standard steps and curbs are about eight inches high and bus steps approximately twelve inches. The patient will practice first on steps and curbs of graduated height, preferably starting from a 1-in. height until he gradually learns to clear the standard height. He will start in the gym and progress to real-life situations, indoors as well as outdoors.

1. **Up and down stairs.**
   a. **Up backward, down forward** (Fig. **50A**).
   b. **Up forward, down backward** (Fig. **50B**).

2. **Curbs and crossing street.**
   a. **Up and down curb—one leg at a time** (Fig. **51A**).
   b. **Hopping up backward** (Fig. **51B**).
   c. **Swinging up forward** (Fig. **51C**).
   d. **Hopping down** (Fig. **51D**).
   e. **Swinging down** (Fig. **51E**).

The time factor has to be considered in curb climbing and crossing the street. In New York City, for example, the green light changes in 22 seconds on an avenue about sixty feet wide. This means that 3 ft. have to be covered in 1 second. On this basis the patient must be trained to go up and down curbs as well as to cover 60 ft. in 22 seconds. He should be able to accomplish this in less than the allotted time in the gym before he tries to cross the street outdoors, since pedestrians and traffic in the ordinary street make it much more difficult. Only advanced crutch walkers should try to cross a street.

TRAVEL ON CRUTCHES

The ideal medium of transportation for a patient with lower extremity involvement is an automobile with hand controls. He should also be taught to use some form of public transportation. For many patients this may not be practical as their usual means of travel, but it may be necessary in case of an emergency.

1. **In and out of car on crutches** (Fig. **52**). The patient should learn to get in and out of an automobile in the gymnasium and should practice on as many different models as possible, including taxis, out of doors.
2. **In and out of bus.**
   a. **In and out of bus forward—one leg at a time** (Fig. **53A**).
   b. **In and out of bus—both legs simultaneously** (Fig. **53B**).

At first the patient should learn in the gym to get in and out of a model bus, or, if this is not available, to ascend and descend 12-in. steps (standard height for bus steps). He should not attempt to board a public bus until he has thoroughly mastered this activity in the gym.

Fig. 45A. INTO AND OUT OF WHEEL CHAIR—both knees locked, facing chair

Preliminary exercises: crutch balancing; crutch walking in all directions.

Into wheel chair:

Starting Position: Wheel chair is placed against wall. Brakes are locked. Stand in front of wheel chair facing same. Feet are in center between footrests.

Instructions:

1. Support yourself and balance on both feet and one crutch while raising footrest with other crutch.
2. Support yourself on both crutches while moving closer to chair (so that you can place crutch against chair [see Fig. **45A**·3]).
3. With most weight on your feet, take weight from right hand into left hand and remove right crutch from under your arm and...
4. ...place it toward right side of wheel chair against wall. Try to keep most weight on your feet as you immediately grasp right armrest for balance and...
5. ...place left crutch against left side of wheel chair. Immediately...
6. ...grasp left armrest with left hand. Support yourself on both hands, bend forward at the waist and buckle so that you are in a jackknife

position and your weight is distributed on your hands and feet. Hesitate in this position for good balance. Move feet forward or backward as necessary. Lean...

7. ...on both hands, transferring *all* weight from feet to hands. Twist and turn body and feet to right, lower body on to seat by bending elbows slowly. There is more weight on left arm, right arm controls speed of movement as you continue turning...

8. ...until you sit...

9. ...straight. Unlock braces, adjust legs and footrests.

Precautions:

3, 4, 5. If too much weight is on one hand while placing crutches, wheel chair will slide sideward. There must be more weight on feet.

6. Buckling will bring more weight over feet and thereby prevent sliding. The taller the patient, the more he will have to buckle.

Tipping of chair will be avoided by pushing *down* on armrests and at the same time pushing chair against wall. At no time should chair be pulled away from wall.

Helpful remarks:

2. This is the position in which patient usually unlocks his hip lock (for details see p. 90).

6. To lower body onto seat, it may be necessary to move feet forward or backward. This can be done in the following ways: (*a*) if legs are moved alternately, weight is on both hands and one foot, so that other foot can be moved; (*b*) if patient cannot move feet alternately, he has to twist body and shuffle both feet simultaneously with all weight on hands. At end of each procedure, weight is again on hands and feet.

7. There is a definite transfer of weight from feet to hands while turning body.

Out of wheel chair: Reverse entire procedure. (Read pictures in reverse sequence.)

Starting Position:

9. Wheel chair is placed against wall. Brakes are locked. Crutches are on each side of wheel chair. Lock braces.

Instructions:

8. Raise footrests. Sit as near to right side of seat as possible. Place right foot slightly forward and outward of left foot and try to maintain this position of feet until you stand and turn (Fig. **45A**·6).

7. Place left hand behind you on right armrest and grasp left armrest with right hand. Shift *all* weight on hands, lifting body off seat. Start transferring weight to feet as you twist and turn body and feet to left until...

6. ...you face the wall. Distribute weight between hands and feet by buckling so that you are in a jackknife position. Move feet toward chair if necessary. Most weight remains on feet as you straighten up and...

5. ...tilt pelvis forward. Use right hand for balance, pick up left crutch...

4. ...and place it under left arm. Straighten up more, tilting pelvis more forward and put some weight on left crutch until you are well balanced.

3. Pick up right crutch and place...

2. ...under right arm.

Take a few steps sideward or backward so that you can walk away from wheel chair.

Precautions: As to sliding feet and tipping of chair, same as above.

Helpful remarks:

8. To avoid catching feet in footrests, it is important to place them in such a way that they can easily turn (Fig. **45A**·7) with rest of body, right foot describing a circle around left. If feet should be caught, all weight must be shifted to hands so that feet can be brought into right position (Fig. **45A**·6).

7, 6. Feet turn either simultaneously or alternately until toes point into same direction as rest of body.

6. In order to reach crutches, patient may have to walk or shuffle closer to chair.

2. Position for locking hip locks (for details see p. 90).

Special Note: In the following methods for standing up and sitting down, if patients wear hip locks they will lock and unlock them using a position similar to that in Fig. **45A**·2.

Fig. 45A. INTO AND OUT OF WHEEL CHAIR—both knees locked, facing chair

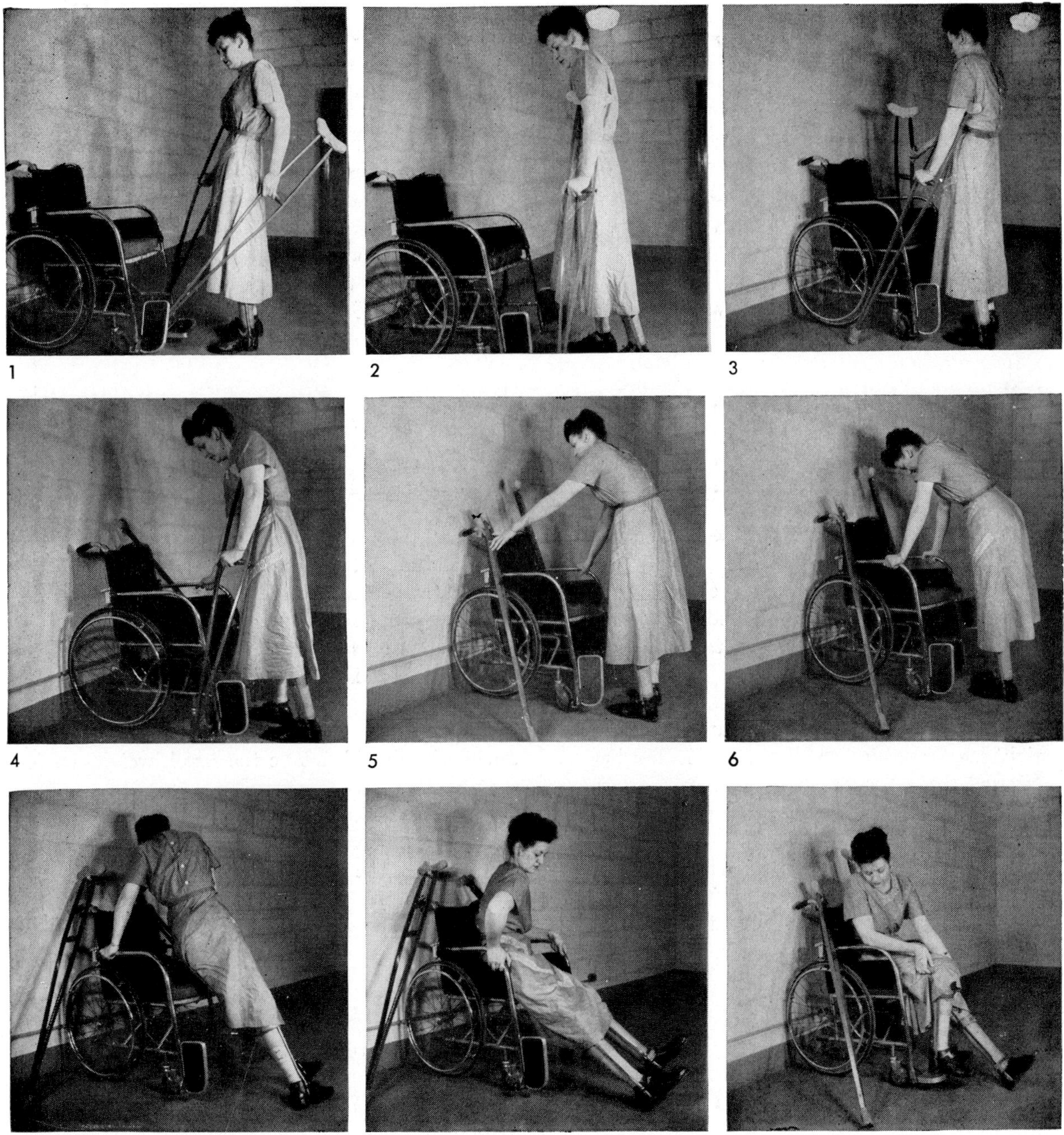

Fig. 45B. INTO AND OUT OF WHEEL CHAIR—both knees locked, profile to chair

This method is easier for small patients since they can grasp wheel-chair arms without bending forward.

Into wheel chair:

Starting Position: Wheel chair is placed against wall. Brakes are locked. Stand in front of wheel chair, facing same.

Instructions:

1. Raise footrest with one crutch while supporting yourself on other crutch.

2. Move closer to wheel chair. Grasp left armrest with left hand and move sideways so that you are off center right and at...

3. ...a slight angle as you turn slightly away from wall. Place right crutch against wall to side of wheel chair, while holding on to left armrest. Repeat with other crutch.

4. Grasp both armrests pivot on your heels so that you stand in profile, with your left side to chair.

5. Slide left hand way back on armrest. Lean on both hands, transferring all weight from feet to hands and twist body to right. Lower body by bending elbows slowly. Weight is mostly on left arm, right elbow controls speed of movement, as you continue turning until...

6. ...you sit. Unlock braces, adjust footrests and legs.

Out of wheel chair: Reverse entire procedure. (Read pictures in reverse sequence.)

Fig. 45C. OUT OF WHEEL CHAIR—legs crossed

Starting Position: Sit in wheel chair (which is against wall). Brakes are locked, footrests up. Slide as near to edge of seat as possible. Lock both knees.

Instructions:

1a. Lift left leg with both hands and cross it over right leg (if turning to right), so that left heel is secured against right ankle. Both legs are as far left as possible, so that they do not become entangled in footrests.

2a. Place right hand behind you on left armrest and left hand on right armrest. Shift all weight to both hands as you lift yourself off the seat turning toward right. Continue...

3a. ...turning until body and toes face wall and weight is distributed between hands and feet. Now transfer most of weight to feet as you place crutches under arms.

Take a few steps sideward or backward so that you can walk away from chair.

Precautions:

3a. There should not be too much weight on feet until they have uncrossed.

For detailed description as to placing of crutches, moving feet, precautions, and helpful remarks, study method in Figure **45A**.

Fig. 45B. INTO AND OUT OF WHEEL CHAIR—both knees locked, profile to chair

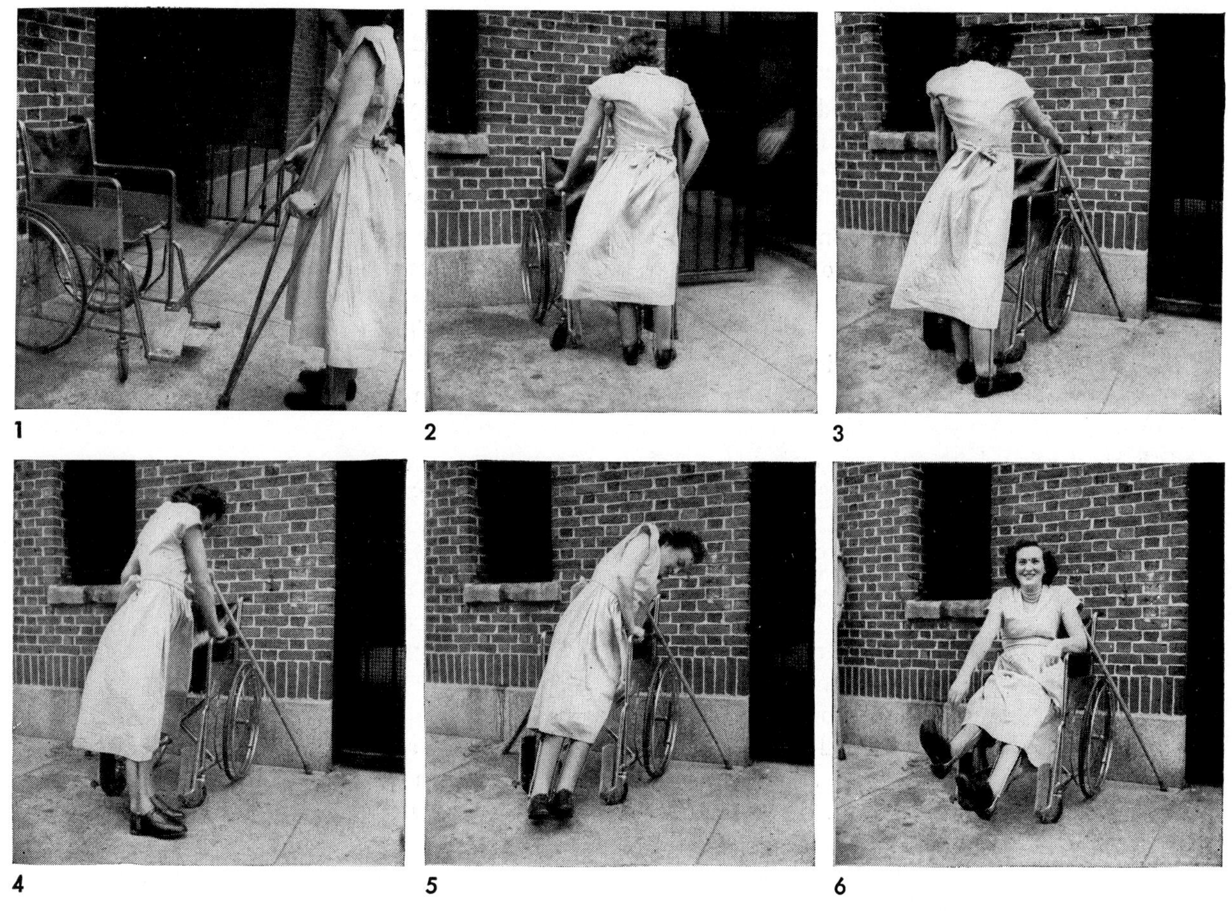

1 2 3

4 5 6

Fig. 45C. OUT OF WHEEL CHAIR—legs crossed

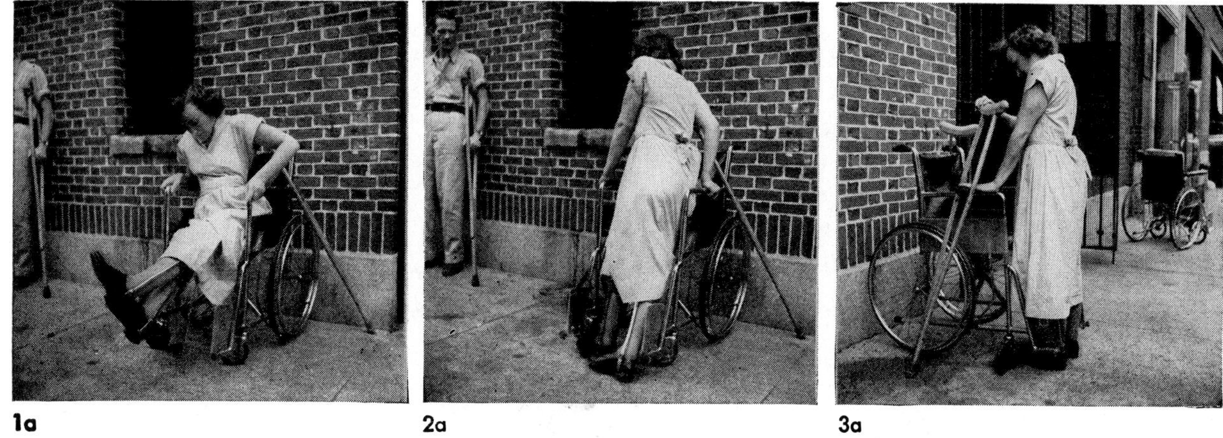

1a 2a 3a

Fig. 46. DOWN ON AND UP FROM STRAIGHT CHAIR—both knees locked

Down on straight chair:

Starting Position: Chair is placed against wall. Stand in profile so that your right side is against wall.

Instructions:

1. Support yourself and balance on both feet and left crutch, so that you can remove right crutch from under your arm and...

2. ...place it...

3. ...against wall toward right side of back rest of chair. Grasp back rest with right hand for balance.

4. With most of weight on your feet, place left crutch on...

5. ...top of other crutch.

6. Bend forward and place left hand on chair seat so that some weight is on hand, but most of weight is on feet.

7. Move left hand forward to edge of seat. Push down on both hands, bend forward at waist and buckle so that you are in a jackknife position (to prevent sliding) and weight is well distributed between hands and feet. Hesitate slightly in this position to ensure good balance. Move feet forward or backward as necessary. Transfer *all* weight from feet to hands and...

8. ...twist and turn body and feet to right. Lower body by bending elbows slowly. There is more weight on left arm, right arm controls speed of movement as you continue turning until...

9. ...you sit.

Unlock braces. Adjust legs, shift position so that you sit with back against back rest of chair.

Precautions: Beginners should always have chair standing against wall.
If chair stands in middle of room (for advanced patients) right hand should be placed on lower rung of back rest or on seat (not on back rest as in Fig. **46**·5) and pressure has to be exerted downward.

Helpful remarks:

3, 4, 5. Back rest should be grasped for balance rather than support while placing crutches.

6. When one hand is on chair seat and one hand on back rest, pressure should be exerted downward to prevent tipping of chair. At no time should chair be pulled away from wall.

Up from straight chair: Reverse entire procedure. (Read pictures in reverse sequence.) For detailed description, see Figure **45A.**

Fig. 46. DOWN ON AND UP FROM STRAIGHT CHAIR—both knees locked

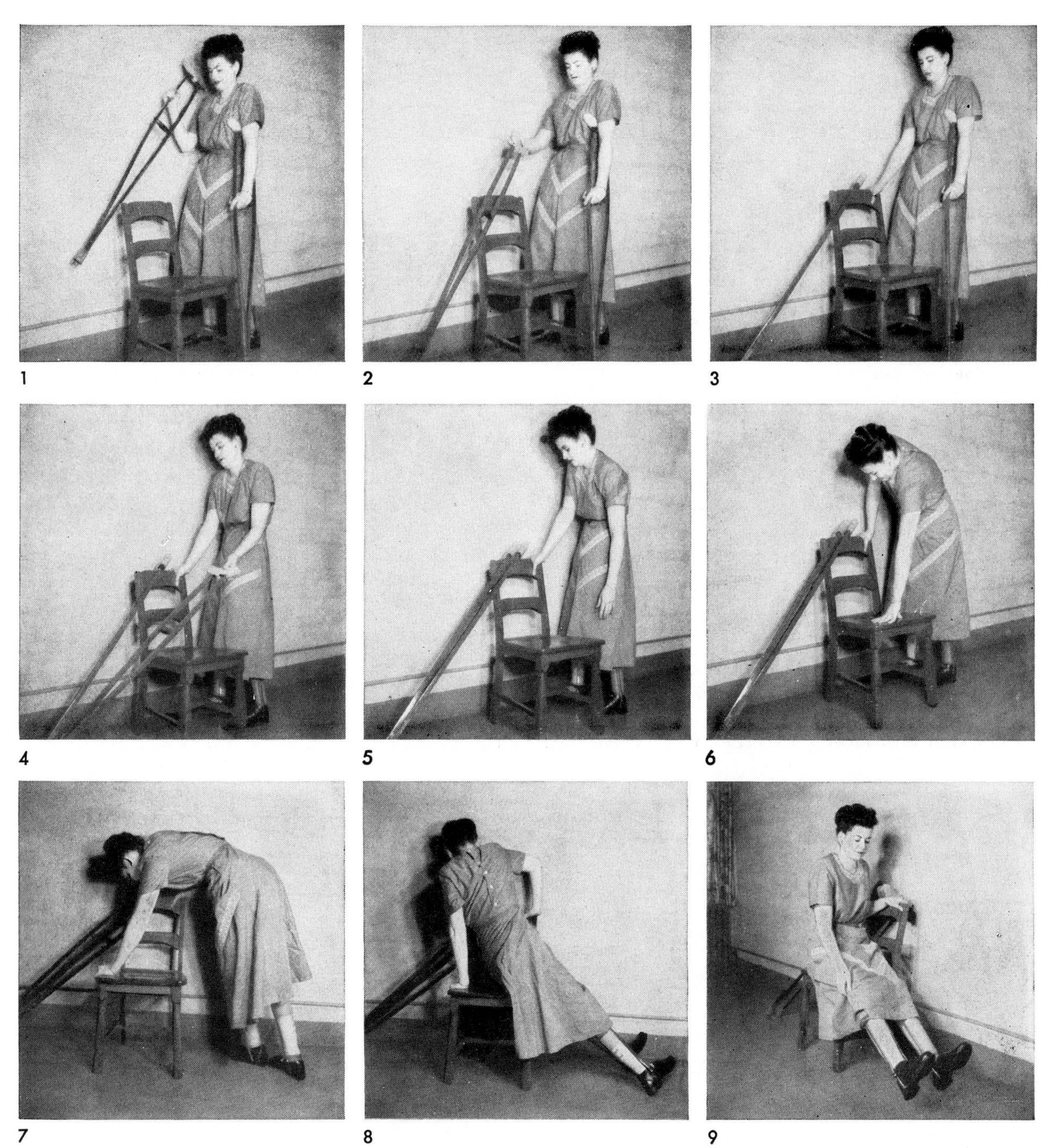

Fig. 47A. DOWN ON AND UP FROM TOILET SEAT —one knee locked

Down on toilet seat:

Starting Position: stand to left of toilet seat facing same.

Instructions:

1. Place left crutch against wall. Balance and support yourself on both feet and right crutch and place left hand on pipe (or toilet tank). Weight is now on both feet and left hand while you place right crutch against...
2. ...wall. Place right hand on far side of toilet seat, lean on both hands, bend sharply forward at waist and move feet backward. Buckle so that weight is distributed between hands and feet and you are in a jackknife position. Hesitate slightly to ensure good balance, then...
3. ...with weight on left hand and left foot, unlock right knee lock with right hand and immediately ...
4. ...replace right hand on toilet seat, still bending forward at waist. Bent right knee rests against toilet seat, and there is no weight on right foot. Transfer...
5. ...all weight to hands and twist body to left. Lower body to seat by bending elbows slowly. Most of weight is on right arm, left arm controls speed of movement. Continue turning until...
6. ...you sit straight. Unlock left knee.

Up from toilet seat: Reverse entire procedure. (Read pictures in reverse sequence.)

Starting Position: Sit in profile with right shoulder to wall. Lock left knee. Right knee remains bent.

Instructions:

5. Place right hand behind you on toilet seat and left hand on pipe or tank. Push up with both hands, transferring some weight from hands to left leg, as you lift body off seat. Right leg (without taking any weight) is resting with bent knee against toilet seat. Continue pushing on arms as you...
4. ...twist and turn body and feet until left shoulder is alongside wall. Bend forward at waist, buckle, so that your weight is distributed between both hands and left foot and you are in a jackknife position. There is no weight on right foot, bent right knee still rests against toilet seat.
3. Hesitate in this position to ensure good balance. Straighten up slightly with weight on left foot and left arm and lock right knee lock with right hand.
2. Replace right hand on toilet seat. Push up on both hands, straightening up and transferring weight into both feet so that pelvis tilts forward and you...
1. ...can replace crutches under arms.

Take a few steps sideward or backward so that you can walk away from toilet seat.

Fig. 47A. DOWN ON AND UP FROM TOILET SEAT—one knee locked

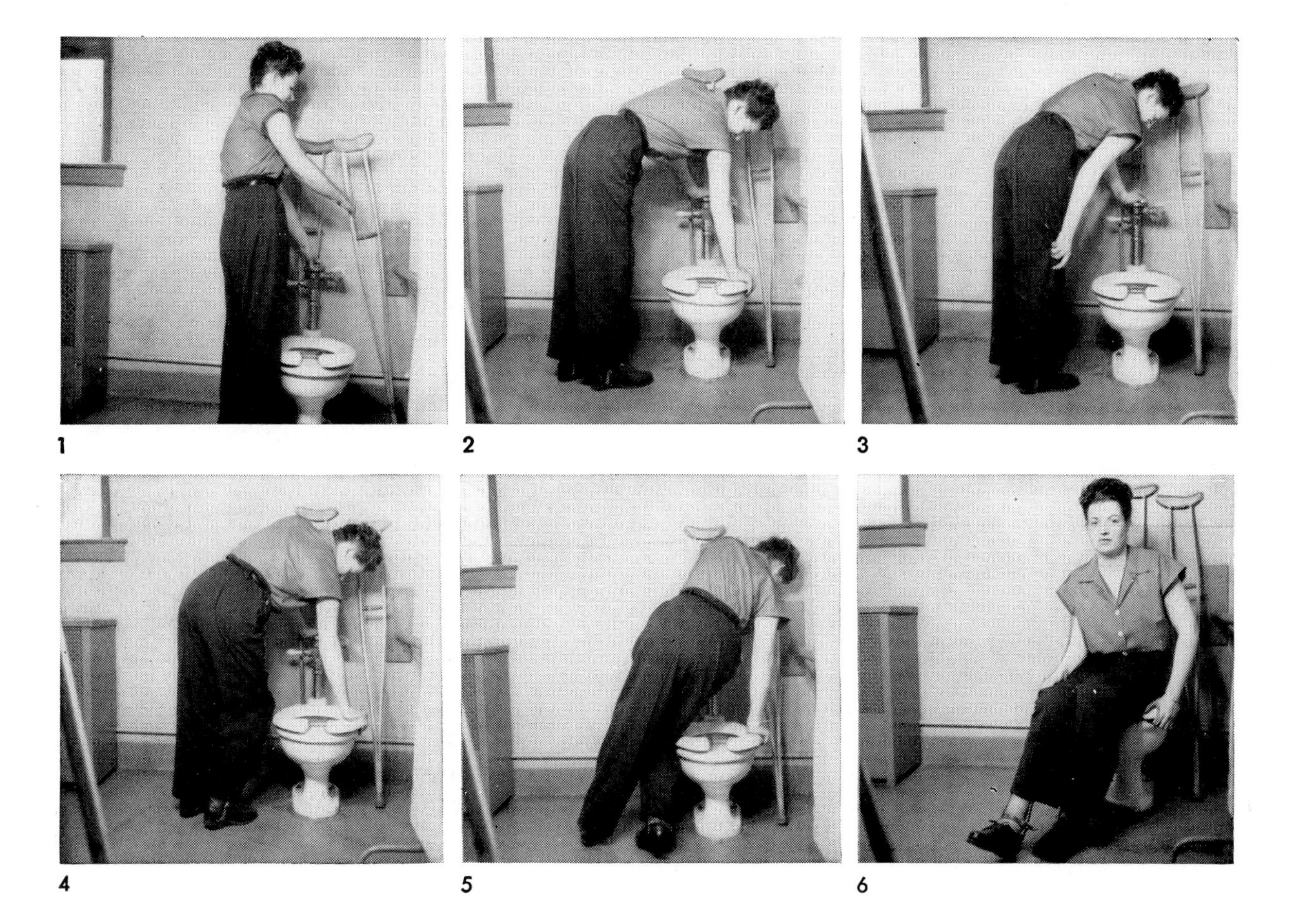

1 2 3

4 5 6

Fig. 47B. UP FROM AND DOWN ON TOILET SEAT —both knees locked

Up from toilet seat:

Starting Position: Sit on toilet seat, facing forward. Lock braces.

Instructions:

1. Place left hand behind you on pipe (or tank) and right hand next to left knee on toilet seat.
2. Put all weight on hands, push up, and lift body off seat. Start transferring weight to feet as you twist and turn body to left until you face wall. Feet turn with body. Distribute weight between hands and feet, by buckling, so that you are well balanced in a jackknife position. Move feet alternately or simultaneously...
3. ...toward toilet, so that you can reach crutches. Transfer more weight to feet as you straighten up and tilt pelvis forward. Place crutches under...
4. ...arms.
5. Turn (or back up or walk sideways), so that you can walk to...
6. ...sink and wash hands.

Down on toilet seat: Reverse entire procedure. (Read pictures in reverse sequence.)

For more detailed description as to instructions, helpful remarks, and precautions, see Figure **45A.**

Special remarks: In regard to adjusting clothes. Some patients adjust their clothes while sitting on toilet. Some find it easier to adjust their clothes standing up. They balance and support themselves leaning against wall or sink, thereby being able to release their crutches in order to have both hands free to handle their clothes.

Fig. 47B. UP FROM AND DOWN ON TOILET SEAT—both knees locked

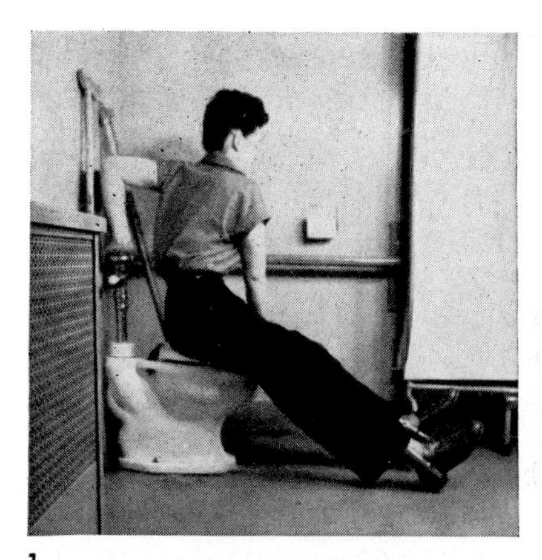
1

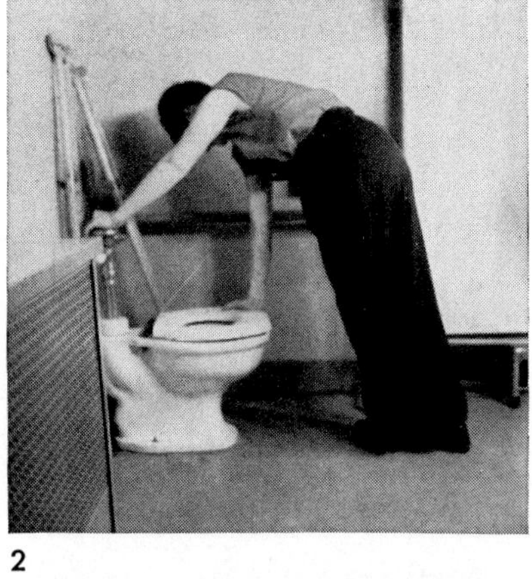
2

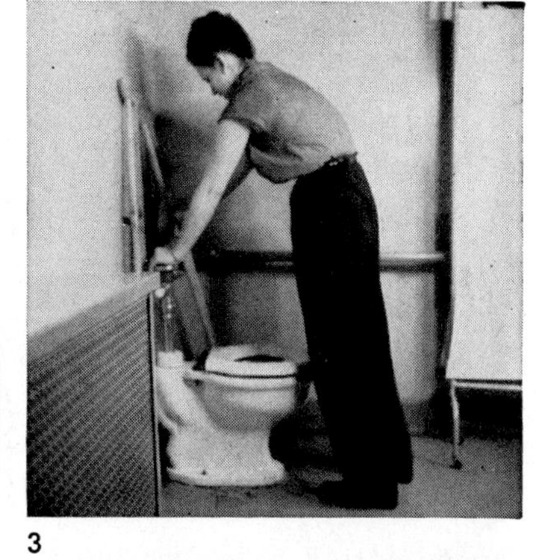
3

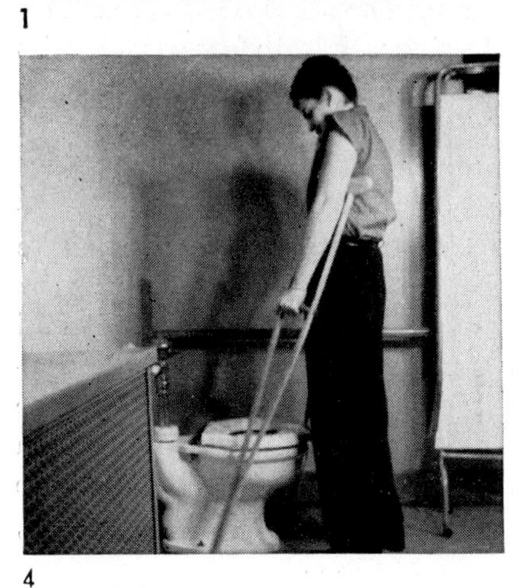
4

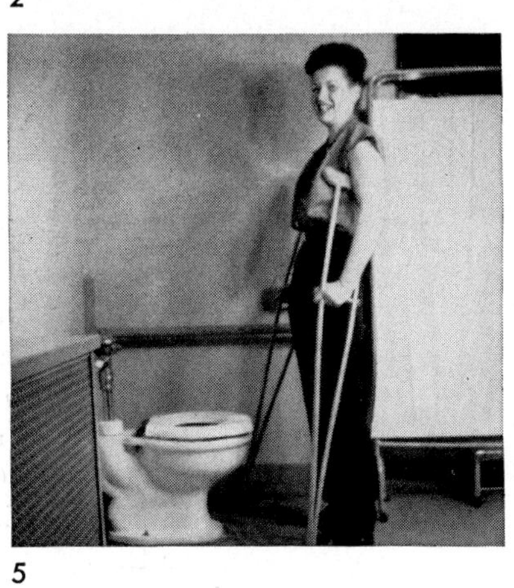
5

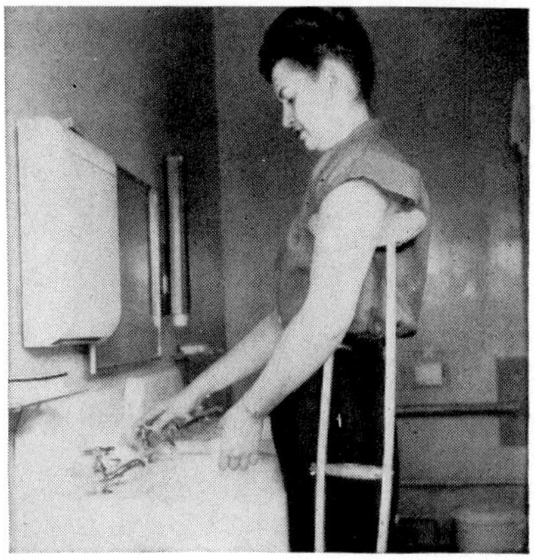

6

Fig. 48. UP FROM AND DOWN ON BED—both knees locked

Up from bed:

Starting Position: Sit near head of bed with both crutches placed on bed to your left (within easy reach). Lock both knees.

Instructions:

1. Sit on bed, as near to edge as possible. Both heels are on floor slightly left off center. Place right foot slightly forward and outward of left foot. Turn body to face foot of bed, place left hand behind you on bed and right hand in front of left knee on bed.
2. Put all weight on both hands and lift yourself off bed. Start transferring weight to feet as you twist and turn body and feet toward left. Move right hand forward on bed, continue pushing on both hands, and turn until you...
3. ...face wall. Buckle so that weight is distributed between hands and feet, and hesitate to ensure good balance.
4. Balance and support yourself on both feet and left hand and straighten up, tilting pelvis forward. Grasp one crutch with right hand, brace top of crutch against right shoulder. Push up on both hands (more so with right hand, since the bed is low) in order to tilt pelvis forward more, so that you straighten up...
5. ...completely and place crutch under right arm. supporting yourself on both feet and right crutch, pick up other crutch and...
6. ...place it under...
7. ...left arm. Turn body toward right so that you face forward. Place crutch tips in front of you, so that you can walk away.

Helpful remarks: If bed is very low, sit as near to head (or foot) of bed as possible so that left hand (or both hands) can be placed on headboard (or footboard) of bed to aid in straightening up and placing crutches under arms.

Down on bed: Reverse entire procedure. (Read pictures in reverse sequence.)

For detailed description as to instructions, precautions, helpful remarks, see Figure **45A.**

Fig. 48. UP FROM AND DOWN ON BED—both knees locked

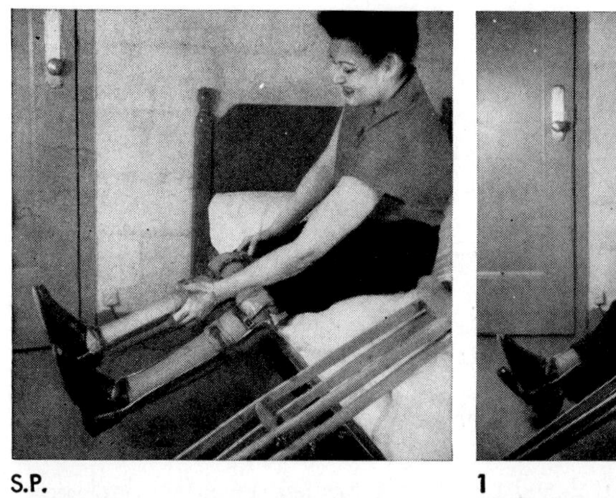

S.P.

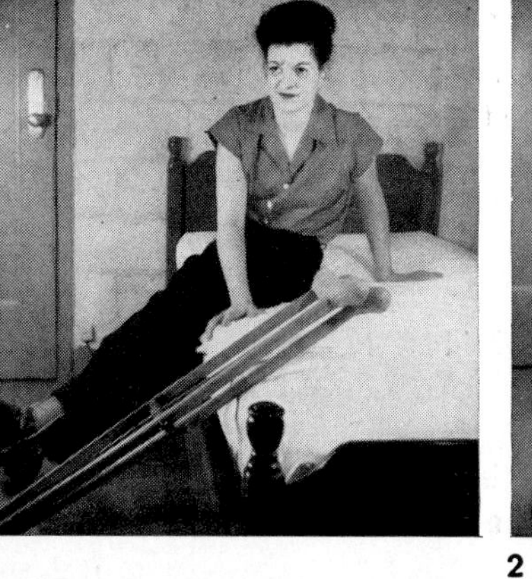

1

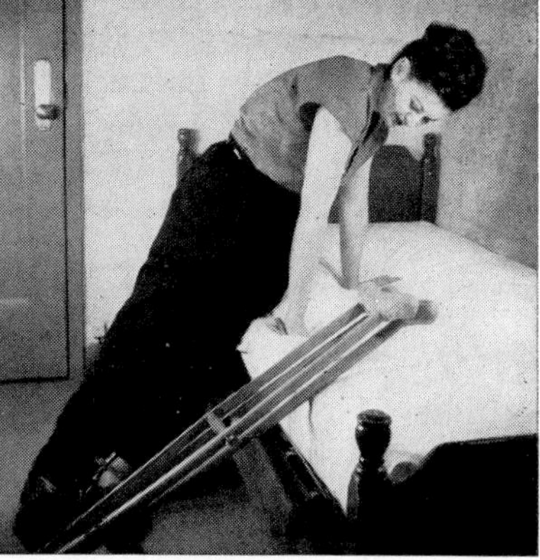

2

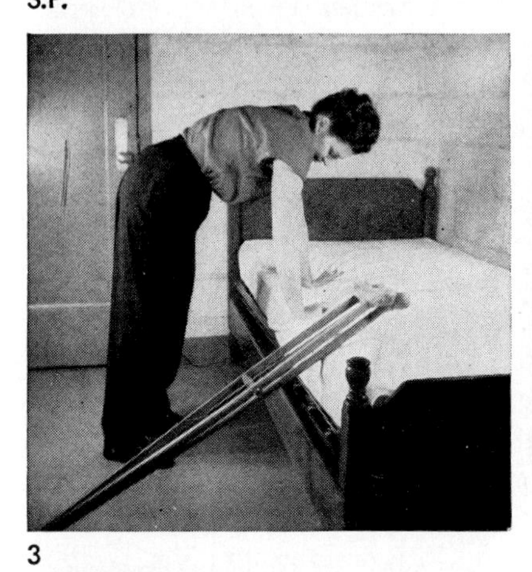

3

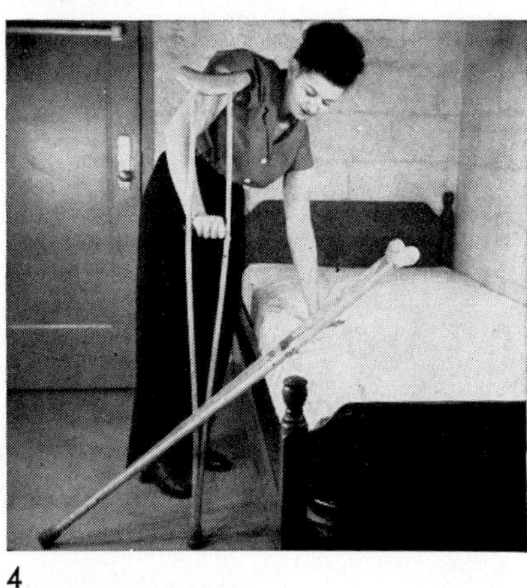

4

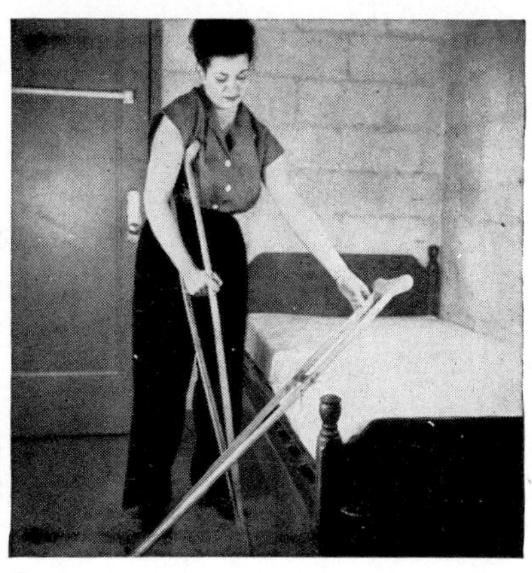

5

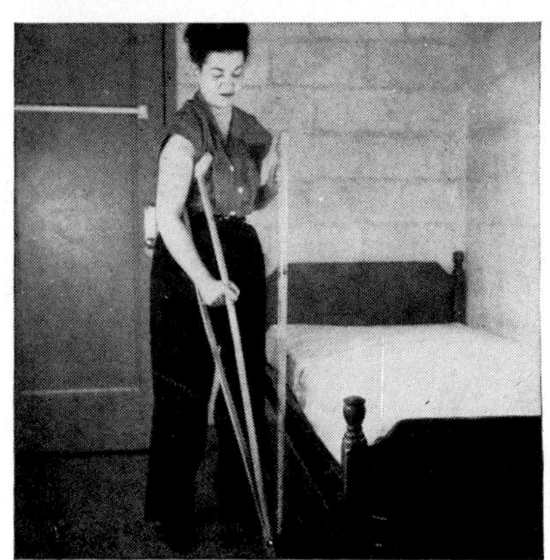

6

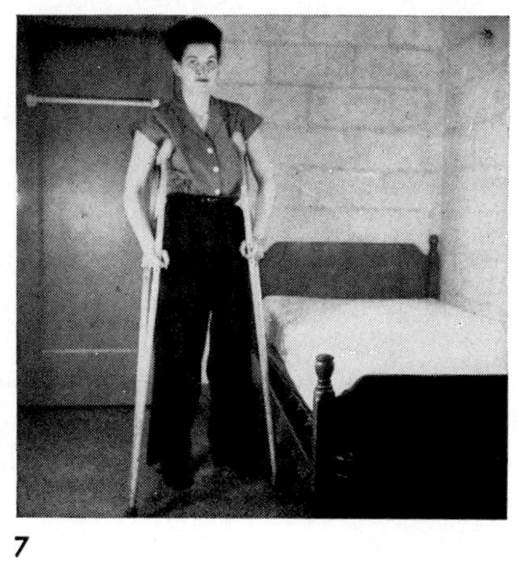

7

UP FROM AND DOWN ON FLOOR

If at all possible, patients should be taught how to get up from floor *using their crutches*. This can be done only by those who can bend forward at the waist and touch the floor with both hands while standing with both knees locked. If patients wear hip locks they must unlock them, so that they will be able to buckle sufficiently while they are getting up or down.

The entire activity requires extraordinary strength of arm, shoulder, and back muscles, as well as a good sense of balance and timing. Patients should be told that if they fall, the safest procedure is to crawl to the nearest post or similar object when in the street, or to the nearest piece of furniture when at home, so that they can pull themselves up. They should also know how to direct others who may try to help them (Fig. **49B**).

Fig. 49A. UP FROM AND DOWN ON FLOOR—one crutch under each arm

Preliminary exercises: crutch walking in all directions; *push-ups;* jackknifing in bars and on crutches.
Equipment: mat.

Up from floor:

Starting Position: Lie flat on stomach. Put crutches in position so that tips point toward head and hand bars are between hips and heels in easy reach when you get up (Fig. **49A**·3).
Instructions:
1. Put all weight on hands, push up and quickly raise pelvis (over heels) walking toward...
2. ...your feet with your hands as close as you can go until pelvis is over and slightly behind feet and most of weight is on hands and feet.
3. Balance well on left hand, grasp right crutch with right hand and...
4. ...brace crutch against right shoulder.
5. Balance on right crutch, grasping left crutch with left hand, and brace left crutch against left arm.
6. Slowly walk crutches toward your feet, with each step transferring more weight into crutches, straightening body up simultaneously until...
7. ...pelvis is tilted forward and weight mostly on crutches.
8. Transferring weight from crutches to feet, walk crutches toward body and straighten up completely. Adjust crutches so that you are in a good tripod position.

Helpful remarks: Some patients find it easier to hold both crutches together in one hand and climb up on them (Fig. **49B**).

Down on floor: Reverse entire procedure. (Read pictures in reverse sequence.)

Starting Position:
8. Stand in an exaggerated tripod position with crutches turned and braced against your arms.
Instructions:
7. Tilt pelvis markedly as you walk crutches...
6. ...forward away from your feet. Start bending at waist...
5. ...until crutches are as far in front as possible, then jackknife sharply in order to bring pelvis over and slightly behind feet, thereby shifting weight to feet.
4. With weight on both feet and right crutch, immediately place left crutch and left hand on floor and shift weight to left hand so...
3. ...that you can release right crutch and place it...
2. ...on floor. Both hands are now on floor. Weight is on hands and feet.
1. Slowly walk forward with hands, transferring weight more and more from feet to hands until...
S.P. ...you lie down by bending elbows slowly.

Precautions: To prevent sliding of feet, pelvis must be brought over and slightly behind feet so that weight is over feet.
Until sufficient skill, strength, and confidence develop, therapist will have to brace his feet against patient's feet to prevent sliding and also give support around waist.
Helpful remarks: Some patients learn to get down on the floor so smoothly and quickly that they may attempt to "fall" (Fig. **49C**).

Fig. 49A. UP FROM AND DOWN ON FLOOR—one crutch under each arm

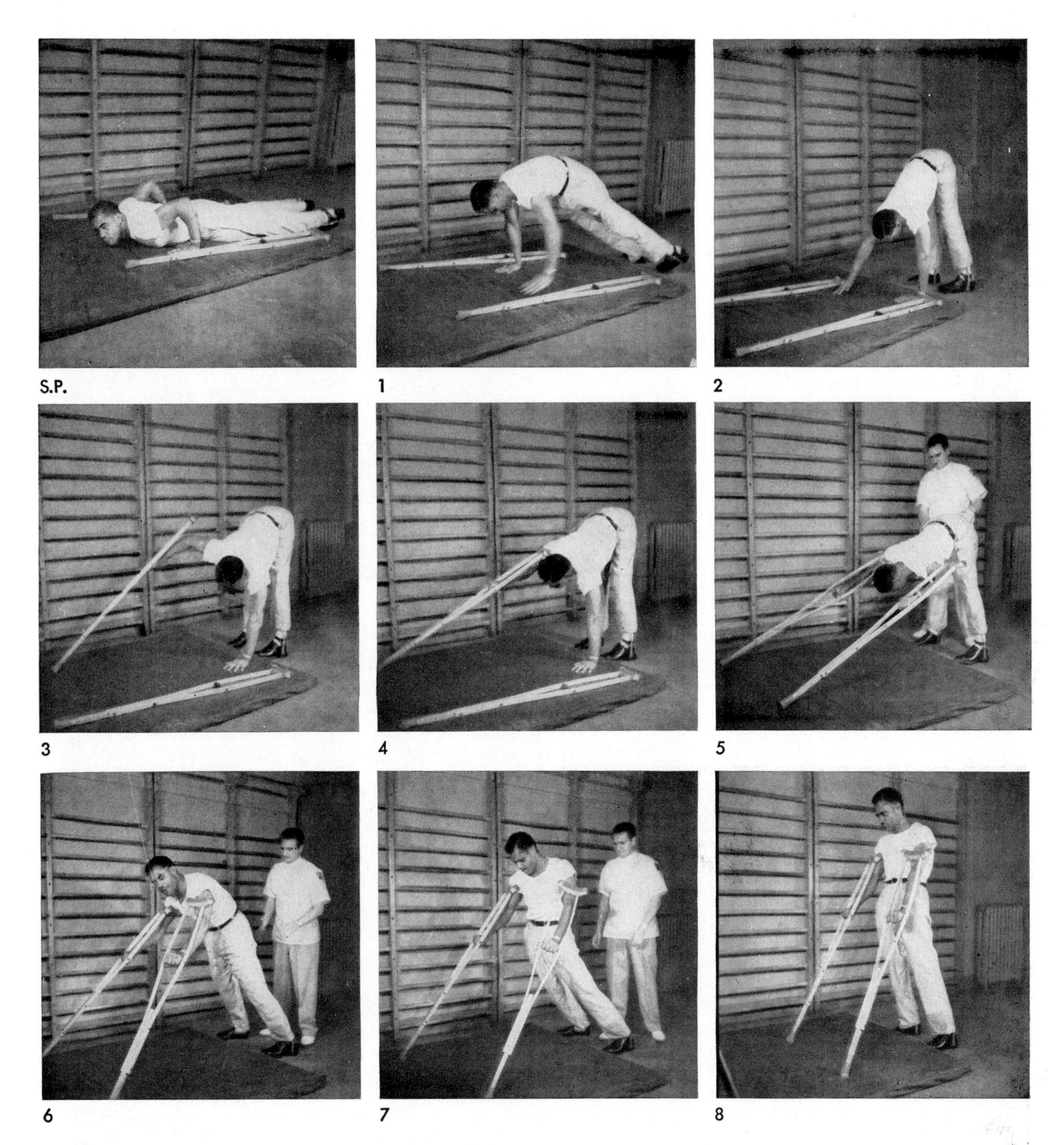

S.P. 1 2 3 4 5 6 7 8

Fig. 49B. UP FROM FLOOR—pushing on both crutches

Getting up from floor (continued)

Precautions: same as for Fig. 49A.

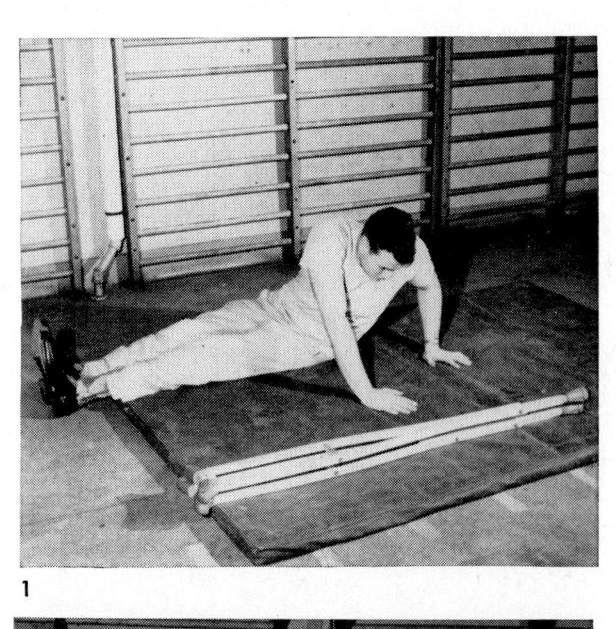

1

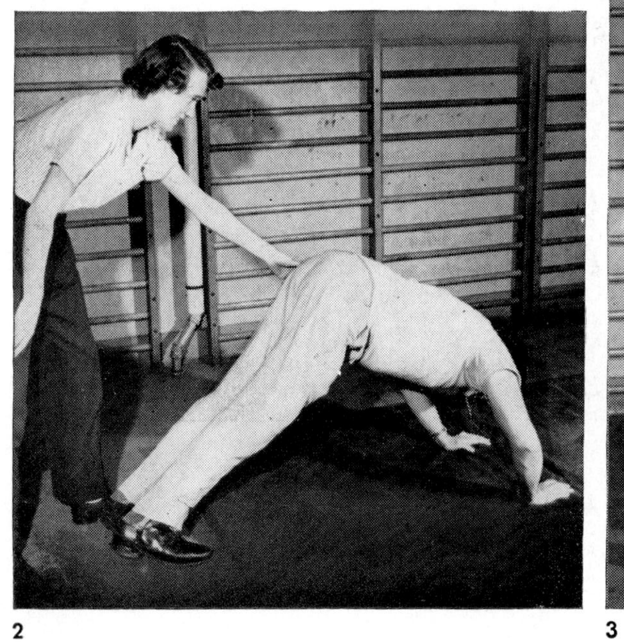

2

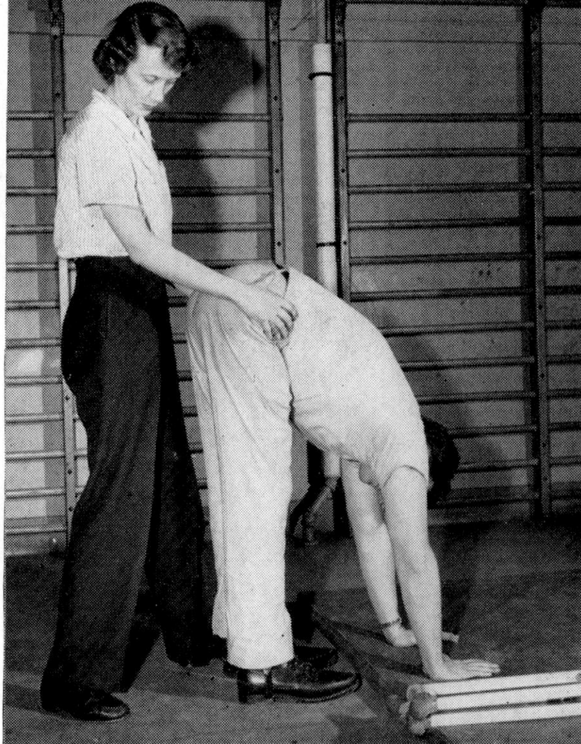

3

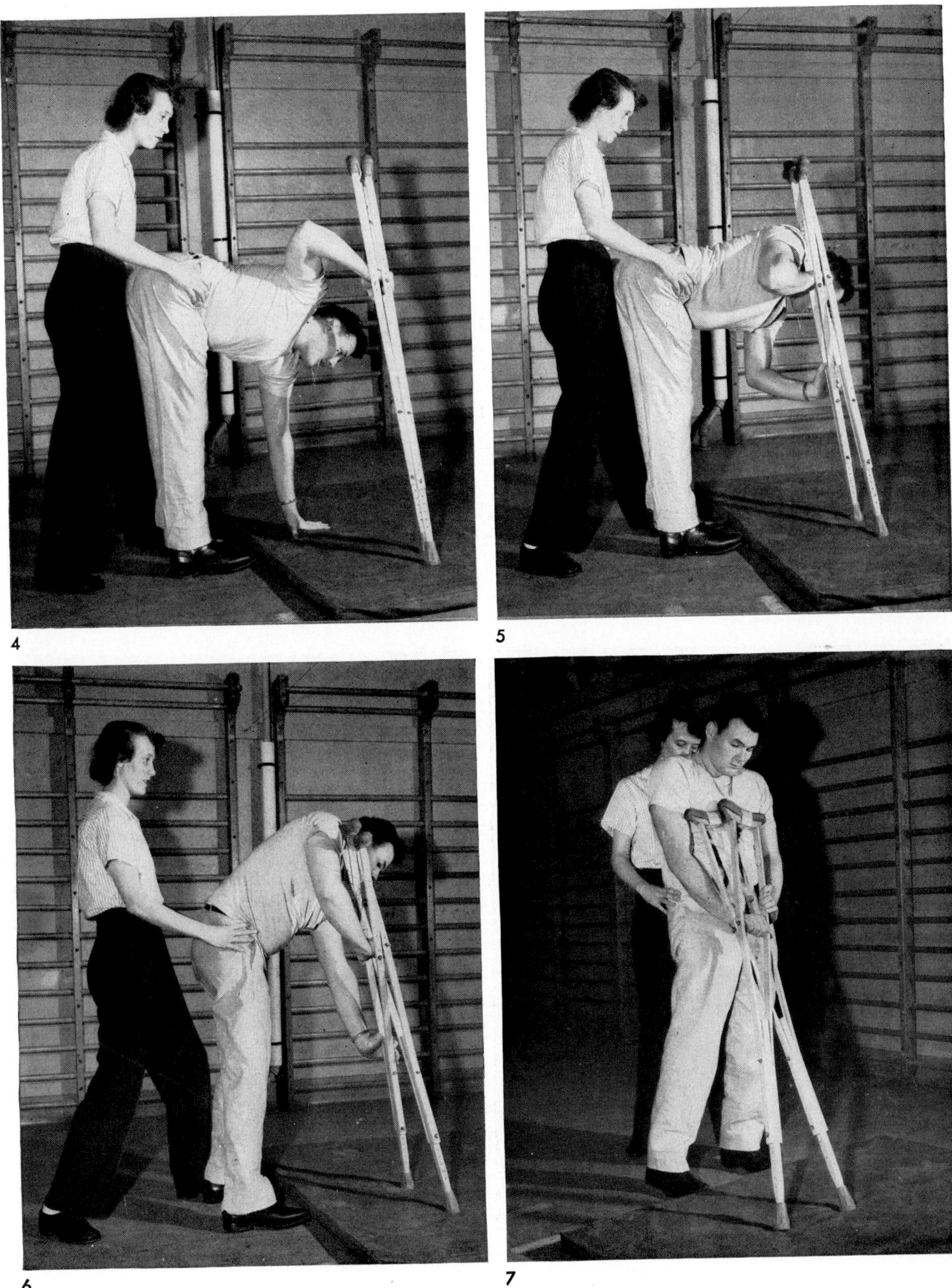

4

5

6

7

Fig. 49C. FALLING (for advanced crutch walkers only)

1. Tripod position
2. Turn crutches out from under arms.
3. Throw crutches sideways out of your way. At the same time let yourself . . .
4. fall forward . . .
5. . . . break the fall by bending sharply at waist, catching yourself on hands and bending elbows, then . . .
6. . . . walk forward with hands. Bend elbows slowly until you lie down.

Can be done only by patients who wear no hip locks.

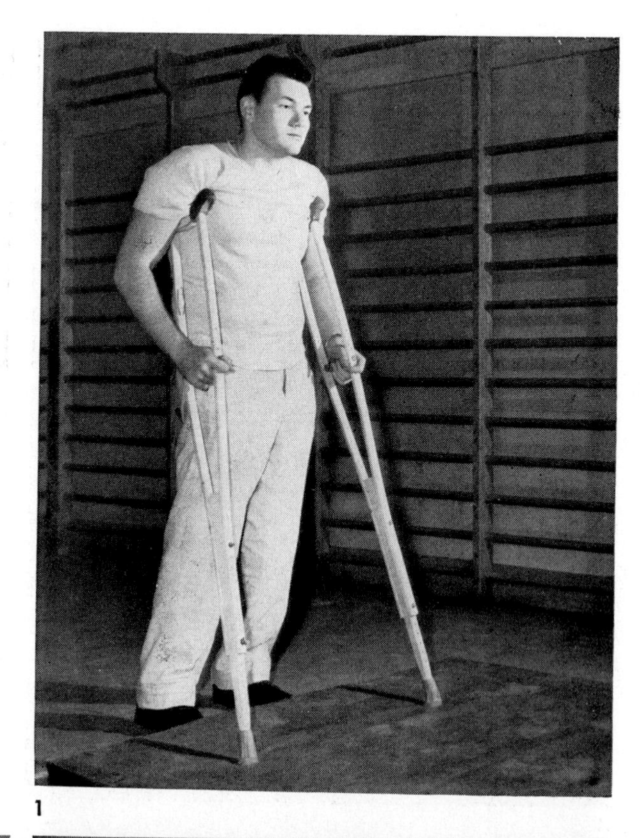

1

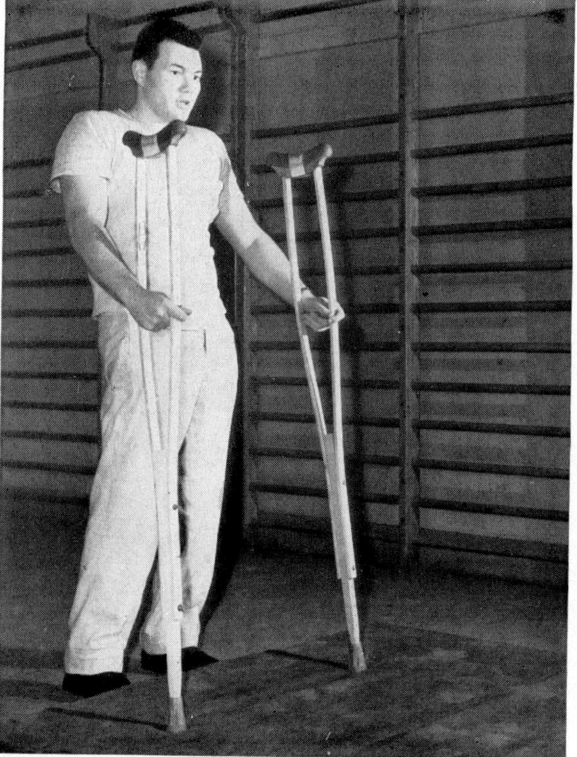

2

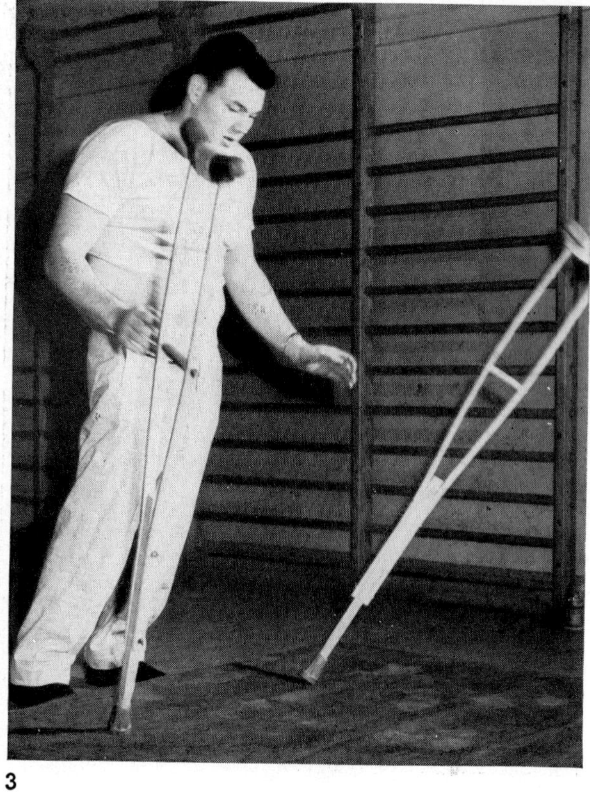

3

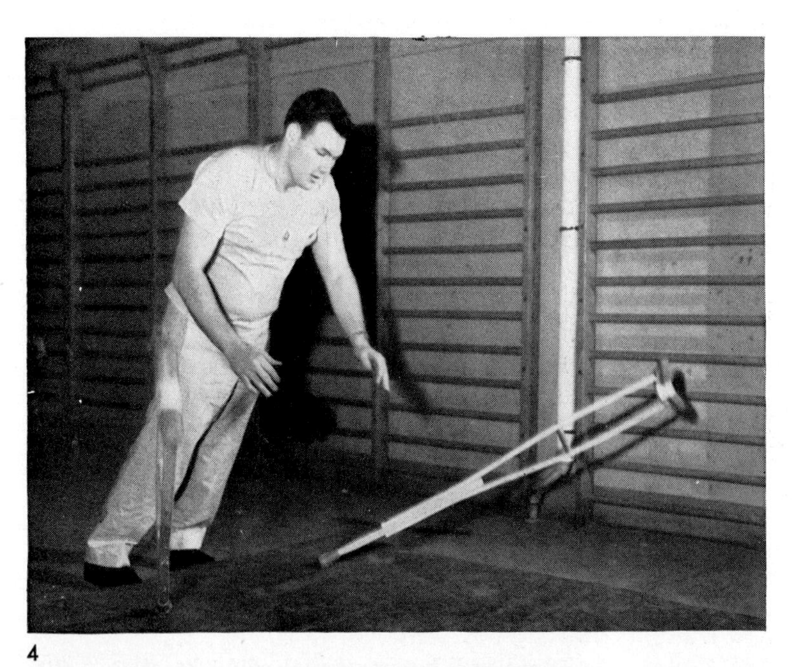

4

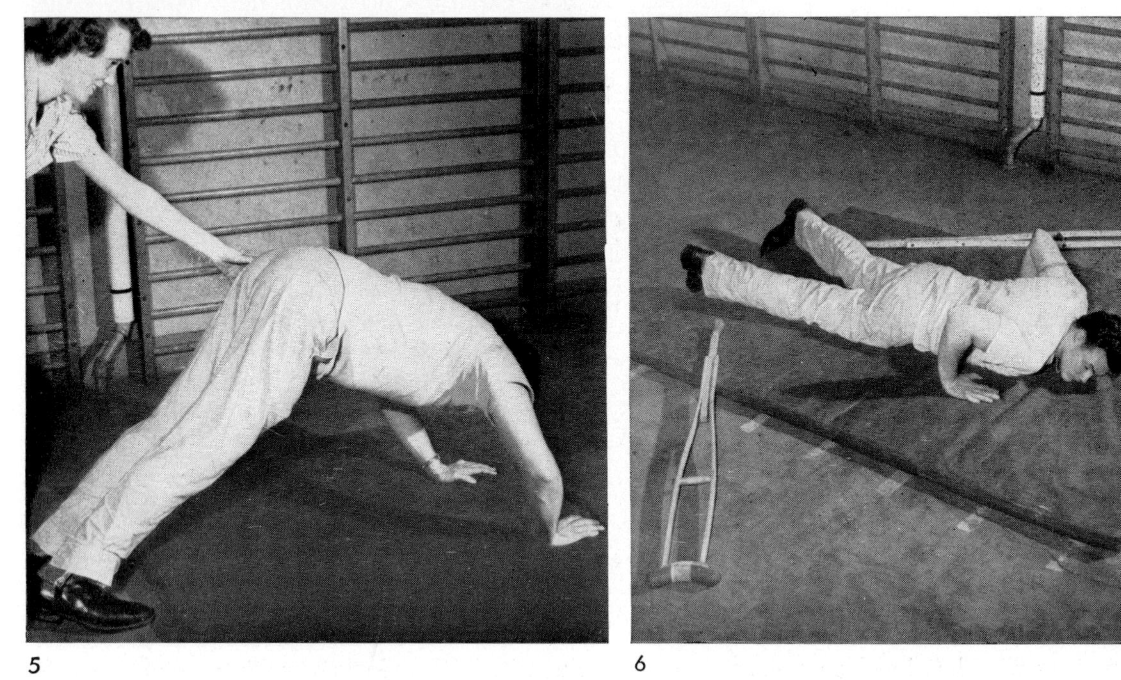

5

6

UP AND DOWN STAIRS

Going up the stairs backward is the easiest method, since catching of the toes on the edge of the steps is eliminated. Going up the stairs forward is more difficult because a much higher push-up is needed in order to clear the steps. Going down the stairs is usually done forward, although some patients find it easier to descend the stairs backward.

To avoid having someone carry one crutch for the patient, both crutches are placed under one arm and he grasps both hand bars with one hand. The other hand is placed on the railing. Extremely tall patients find it easier to grasp the top of the crutches instead of the hand bars. This method is suitable only for very advanced crutch walkers, since extraordinary skill and balance are necessary.

Because of the construction of the staircase in the picture, the patient places his right hand on the railing away from the wall when going up backward and down forward and his right hand on the railing next to the wall when going up forward. Since staircases have usually one railing either on the left or the right side, it is essential that the patient learns to push up with either the right or the left hand.

The patient practices on stairs of graduated heights. He will start out with steps 1 in. high and gradually learn to master higher and higher steps. The standard steps in houses are 8 in. high, the bus steps are 12 in. (see "Equipment" in Chap. VII).

Until sufficient skill and confidence are gained, one therapist walks in back of the patient or two therapists walk, one in front and one in back, ready to give support around the waist.

Fig. 50A. UPSTAIRS BACKWARD—DOWNSTAIRS FORWARD

Preliminary exercises: crutch walking in all directions; curbs in bars.

Upstairs backward:

Starting Position: Stand with back to staircase so that heels touch first step. Support yourself with right hand on railing away from wall and place both crutches under left arm. Stand as near to railing as possible and hold crutches closely under arm to ensure maximum lift.

Instructions:

1. Duck head and push up straight as high as possible; only then jackknife to gain more height so that you can clear first step and...

2. ...lower body by bending elbows slowly and place heels on first step. As soon as heels touch step, straighten up by bringing shoulders back so that pelvis tilts forward.

3. Place crutches with left hand on same step as feet. Slide right hand higher on rail so that both hands are approximately on one line.

4. Push on both hands again as above, until feet clear second step.

5. Lower body to next step and repeat entire procedure until you have reached the top.

Downstairs forward: Reverse entire procedure. (Read pictures in reverse sequence.)

Starting Position:

5. Stand well balanced with right hand on railing and crutches under left arm. Weight is on both hands as you...

Instructions:

4. ...lean forward so that head is approximately over step below. Push up so that feet clear step forward and...

3. ...bending elbows slowly, lower body and place heels on step below.

2. With left hand place crutches on step below. Slide right hand down on railing so that both hands are about on same line.

1. Push up on both hands as before until you are downstairs.

Helpful remarks: Unlocked hip locks make jackknife during push-up possible and thereby facilitate gaining height.

1. When hopping up or down first step, because of construction of most stair railings usually it will not always be possible to place right hand on same line with left hand when pushing. Therefore, body has to be twisted slightly away from wall for better mechanical advantage.

4. When hopping down or up all other steps, hand on railing should be on about same line with crutches so that body does not have to be twisted while pushing up.

2, 3, 5. Only heels land on step when hopping up or down. Toes are over edge of step.

Fig. 50A. UPSTAIRS BACKWARD—DOWNSTAIRS FORWARD

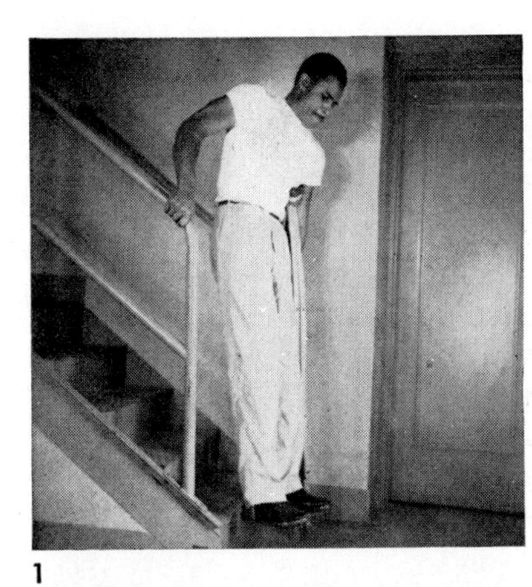
1

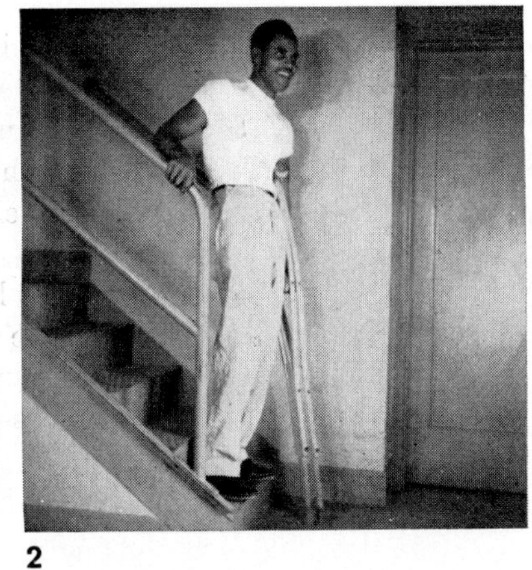
2

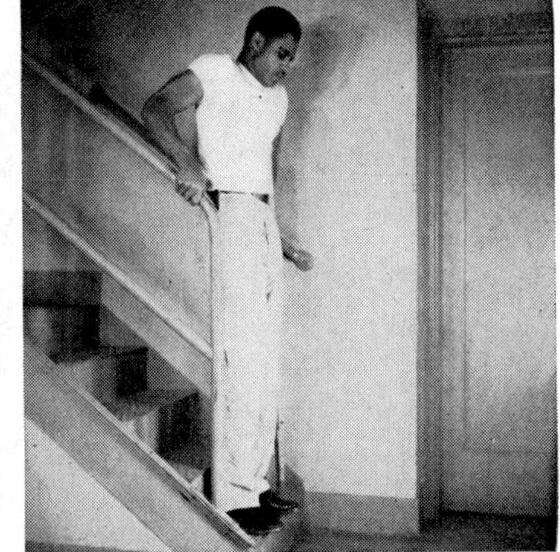
3

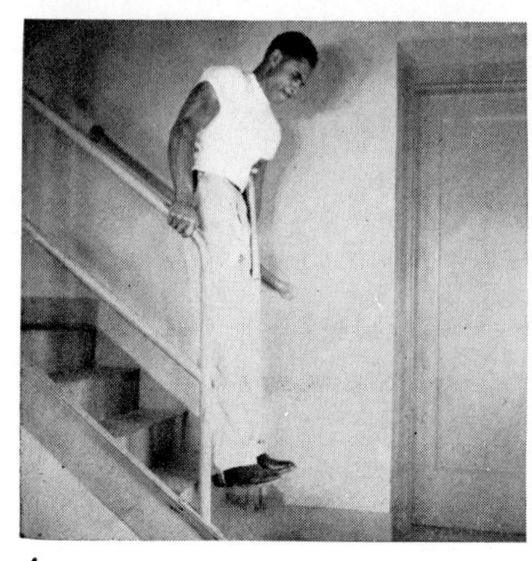
4

5

Fig. 50B. UPSTAIRS FORWARD—DOWNSTAIRS BACKWARD

Upstairs forward:

Starting Position: Stand at a slight angle facing stairs, right hand on railing next to wall, both crutches under left arm. Unlock hip lock(s).

Instructions:

1a. Place right hand fairly well forward on railing and jackknife while pushing up. Also twist pelvis slightly to prevent catching of toes on step. Push up somewhat higher than height of step and...

2a. ...let feet swing forward so that they land easily on next step. As feet touch step straighten up, bringing shoulders back and tilting pelvis forward.

3a. Lift crutches up to same step as feet. Place right hand well forward and push up, repeating whole procedure until you have reached top.

Downstairs backward: Reverse entire procedure. (Read pictures in reverse sequence.)

Helpful remarks: Unlocked hip locks make jackknife during push-up possible and thereby make it easier to gain height.

Fig. 50B. UPSTAIRS FORWARD—DOWNSTAIRS BACKWARD

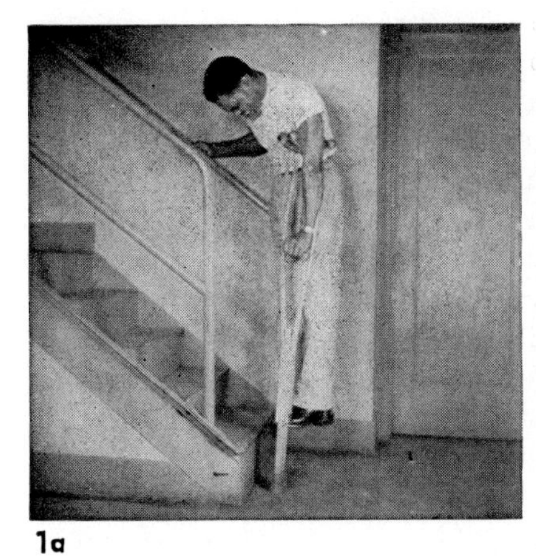

1a

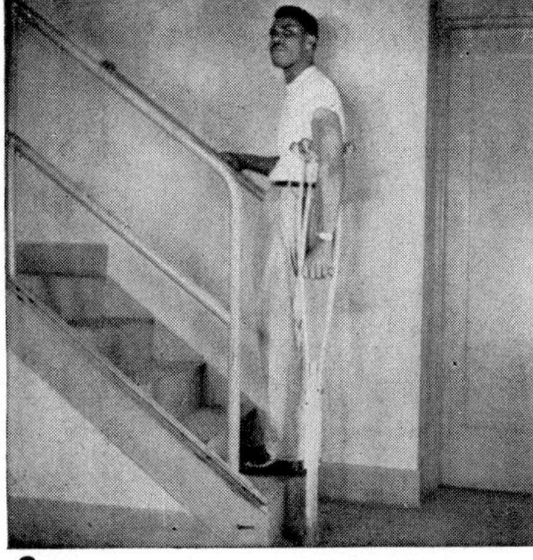

2a

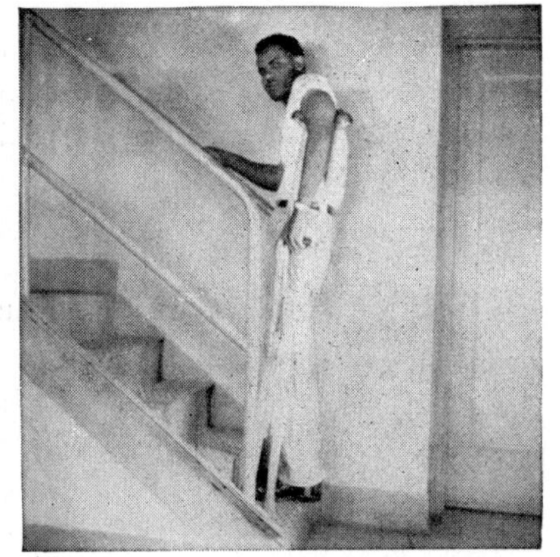

3a

Fig. 51A. UP AND DOWN CURB—one leg at a time

This method can be used only by patients who can move one leg at a time. To go up backward is easier than to go forward, since catching of toes on curb is eliminated.

Preliminary exercises: four-point gait in all directions.

Equipment: at first, curbs of graduated height are used in gym.

Up curb backward:

Starting Position: Back up to curb. Practice bringing leg back and up curb until you stand at right distance, so that heel will land on curb (Fig. 51A·1). Unlock hip lock(s).

Instructions:

1. Balance and support yourself on both crutches and right leg, bend slightly forward so that left leg can swing back and up and heel lands on curb. Continue to lean into...

2. ...both crutches and buckle so that weight is shifted over left leg in order to lift right leg back ...

3. ...and up. Bring shoulders back so that pelvis tilts forward. Hesitate slightly in this position to ensure good balance.

4. Lean on both crutches and move both feet backward. Move crutches same distance toward curb.

5. Balance and support yourself on both feet and right crutch so that you can lift left crutch up on to curb. Turn body slightly toward left, shifting weight to left crutch and lift...

6. ...right crutch up on to curb.

Down curb forward: Reverse entire procedure. (Read pictures in reverse sequence.)

Starting Position:

6. Stand near edge of curb.

Instructions:

5. Support yourself and balance on both feet and left crutch so that you can lift right crutch off curb and place it on street. Shift weight to right crutch and place...

4. ...left crutch on same line.

3. Lean into both crutches and move feet forward until toes are over edge of curb, move crutches same distance forward so that you are well balanced. Tall patients will have to buckle to maintain balance (see Fig. 51A·1).

2. Still leaning into both crutches, shift weight to left foot so that right foot can clear curb.

1. Lower foot and place it on street. Continue to lean on both crutches, shift weight to right foot, releasing left foot entirely from weight, so...

S.P. ...that it swings forward and place it next to right foot. As foot touches, straighten up.

Precautions: Until sufficient skill and confidence are gained, one therapist stands in back of patient or two therapists stand, one in front and one in back, ready to give support around waist.

Helpful remarks:

1, 2. There is a definite transfer of weight to one leg while strongly pushing on crutches. This and buckling will bring other leg up or down.

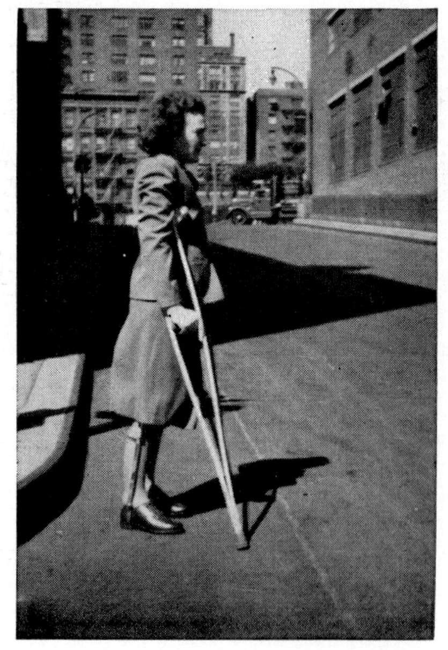

S.P.

Fig. 51A. UP AND DOWN CURB—one leg at a time

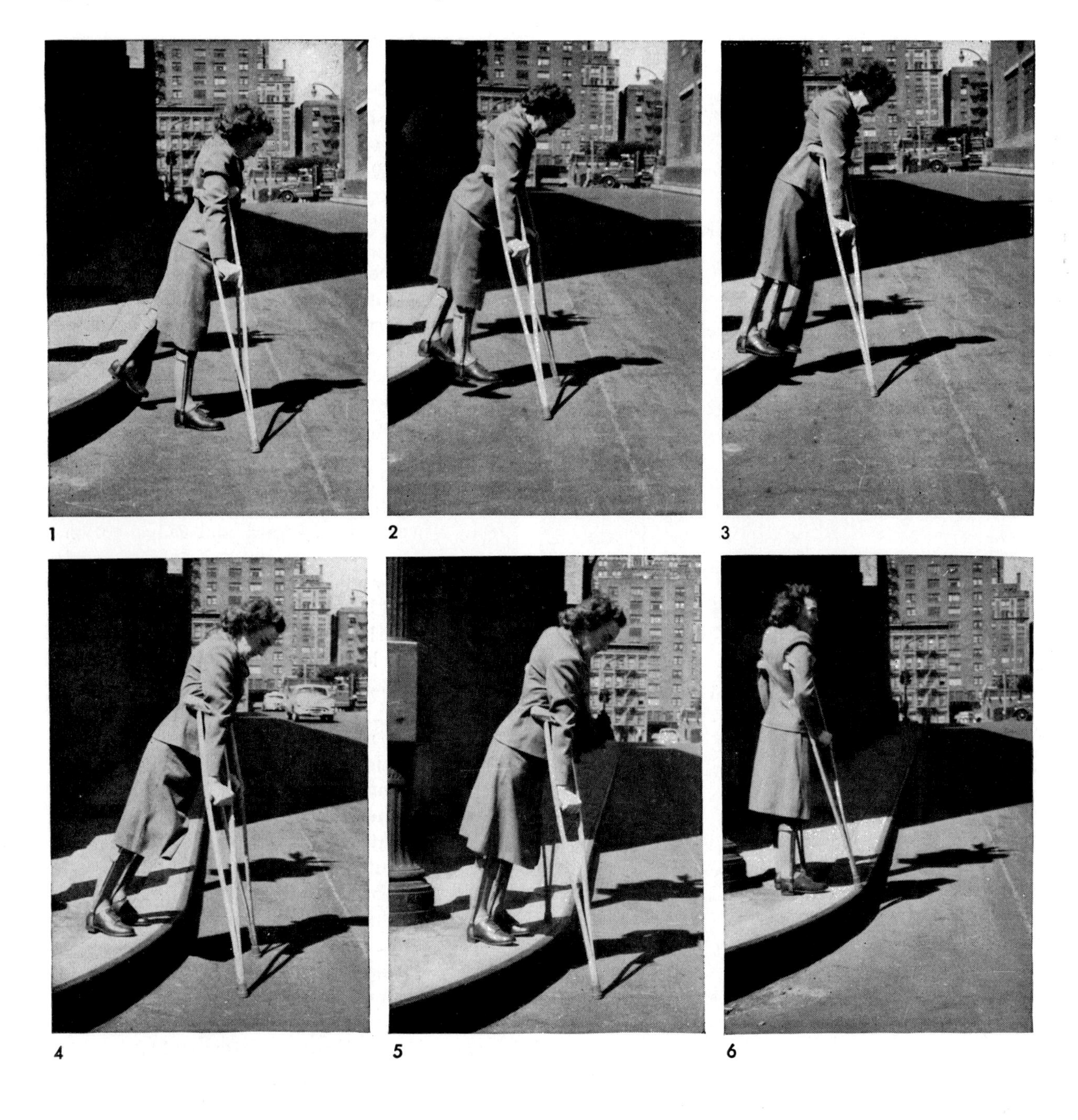

1 2 3

4 5 6

Fig. 51C. SWINGING UP CURB FORWARD

This method is only for very advanced crutch walkers who have extraordinary skill, sense of balance, and timing and who have mastered swing-through gait thoroughly.

Starting Position: Good tripod position. Distance from curb must be tried out so that when swing-through is completed (Fig. **51C**·2) feet will be well on curb. Lean into crutches...

Instructions:

1. ...duck head, push up, and jackknife (pull in abdomen) to gain sufficient height and...

2. ...swing through so that feet land (heels first) on curb. As heels land...

3. ...immediately bring shoulders back so that pelvis tilts forward. Weight is well distributed on hands and feet. Hesitate slightly in this position to ensure good balance and rhythm. Push up on crutches to start forward motion of trunk (and crutches) transferring weight from hands into feet. As body sways well forward lift crutches up...

4. ...on curb into a good tripod position with weight evenly distributed on hands and feet.

Precautions: Since this method is very difficult, it is imperative that in the beginning two therapists, one in front and one in back, assist patient. Later on, one therapist will be sufficient.
It is important that patient does not attempt to swing up onto curb without a trained therapist unless this method is mastered thoroughly.

Helpful remarks: Eventually patient should learn to perform swing-through gait and swing up onto curb in one continuous movement without stopping.

Fig. 51C. SWINGING UP CURB FORWARD

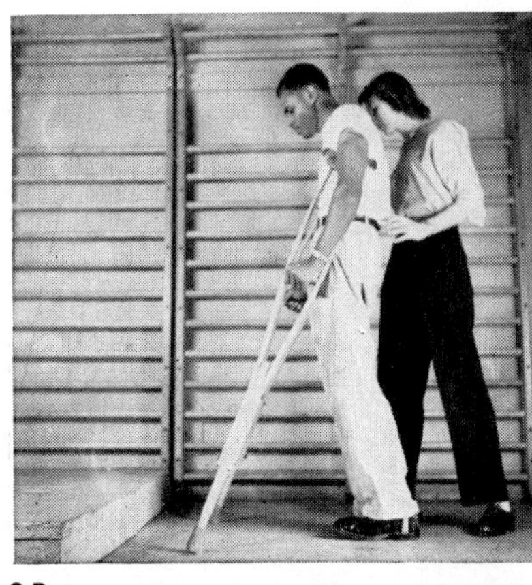
S.P.

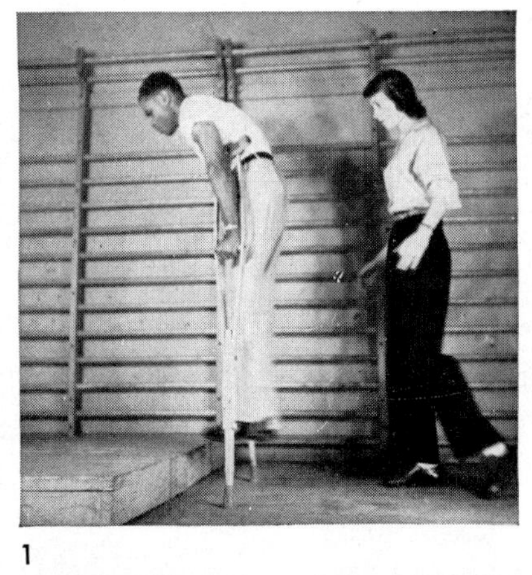
1

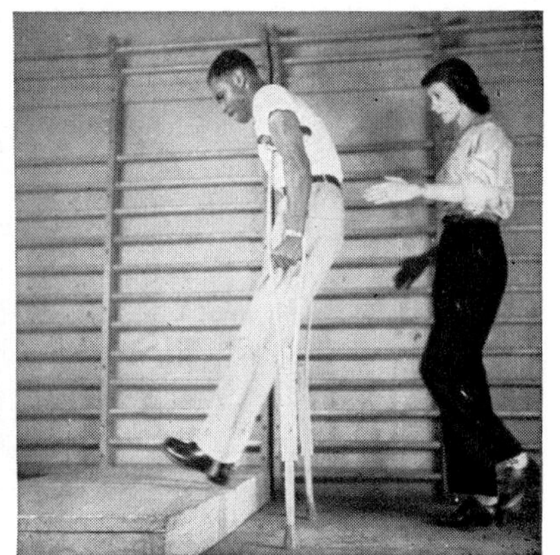
2

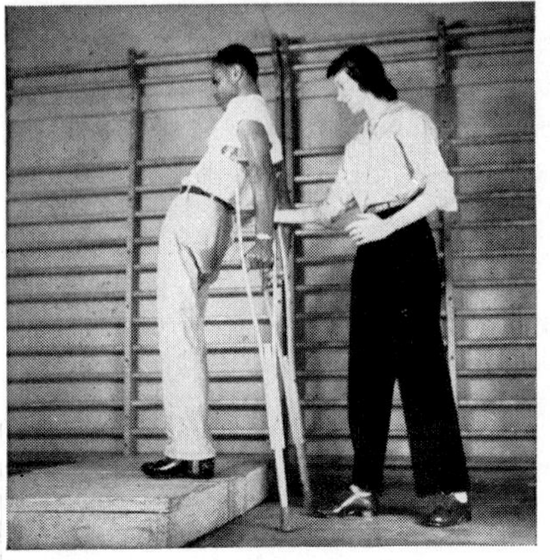
3

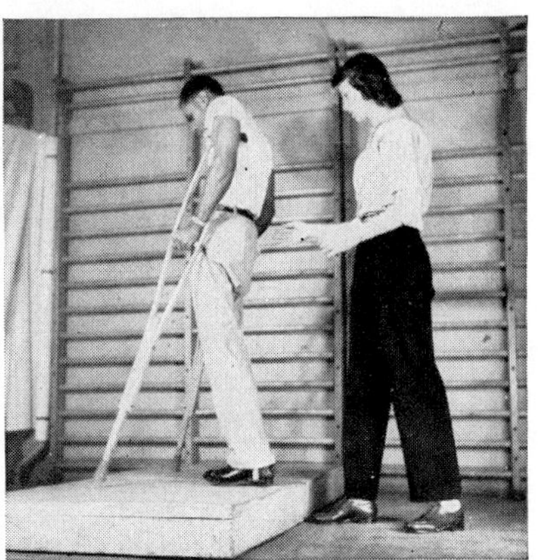
4

Fig. 51D. HOPPING DOWN CURB

Starting Position: Stand as near edge of curb as possible.

Instructions:

1a. Place both crutches, either alternately or simultaneously on floor (for details see Fig. **51A**). Walk crutches forward and shuffle (or walk) feet forward over edge of curb. Buckle pelvis so that you are well balanced in a jackknife position with weight distributed on crutches and feet.

2a. Lean well into crutches, bring shoulders back, let pelvis tilt forward as you straighten up, and push on both hands so that heels slide down from edge of curb...

3a. ...and nearly simultaneously place crutches more forward into an exaggerated tripod position.

Precautions: As soon as heels touch floor, crutches must be brought forward quickly to establish a wide base for good balance.

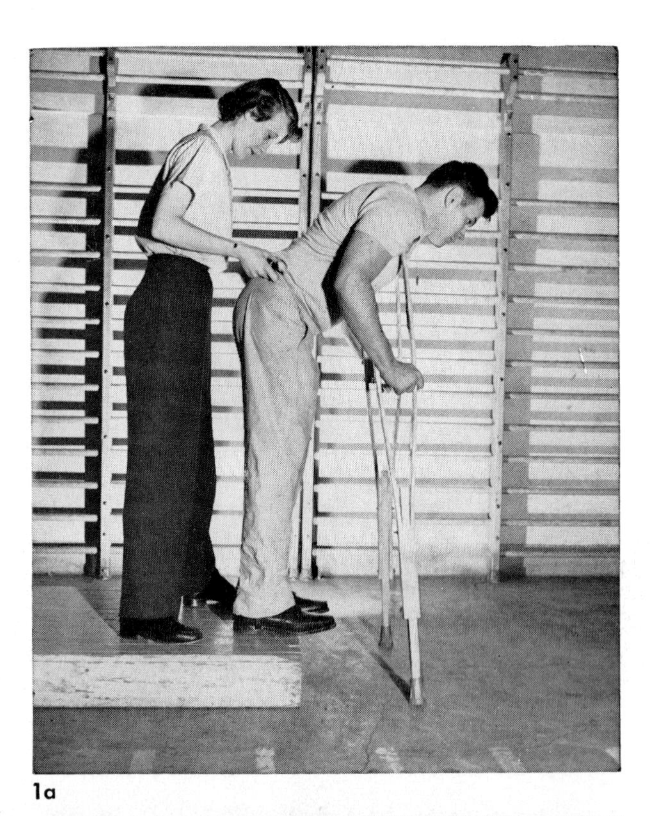

1a

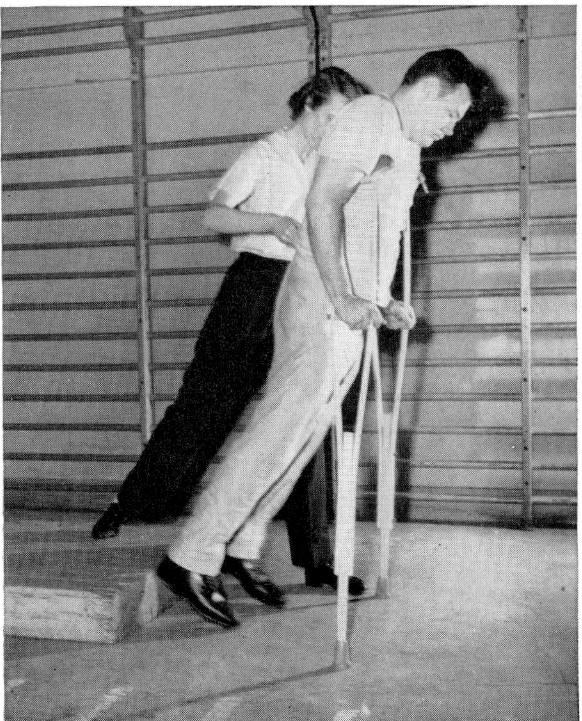

2a

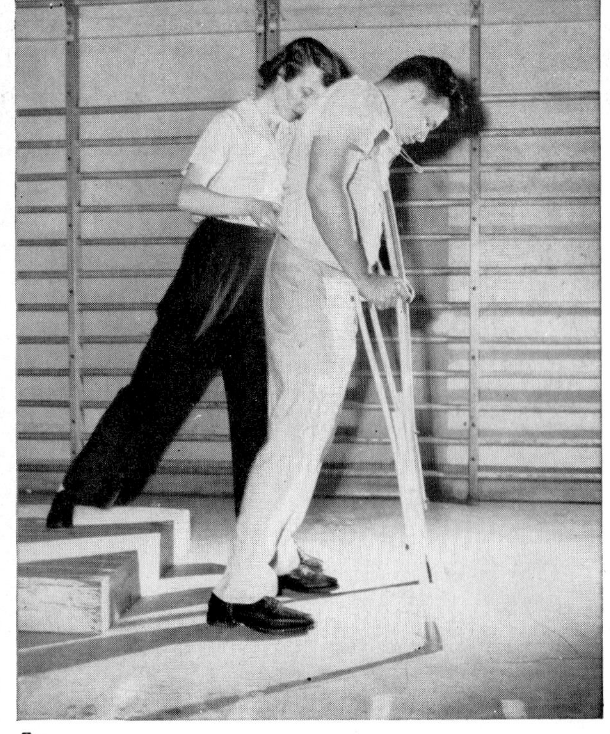

3a

Fig. 51E. SWINGING DOWN CURB

Starting Position: Same as in Figure **51D.**
Instructions:

1b. Same as Figure **51D**·1a. Come to a jackknife position with feet on curb and crutches on floor.
2b. Lean well into crutches, bring shoulders back, let pelvis tilt forward as you straighten up; keep head ducked as you push strongly on both crutches so that you lift body slightly off curb and feet swing through crutches until heels. . .
3b. . . . land in front of crutches.
3a. Bring crutches and body forward to an exaggerated tripod position as in swing-through gait.

Precautions: Same as for Figure **51D.**

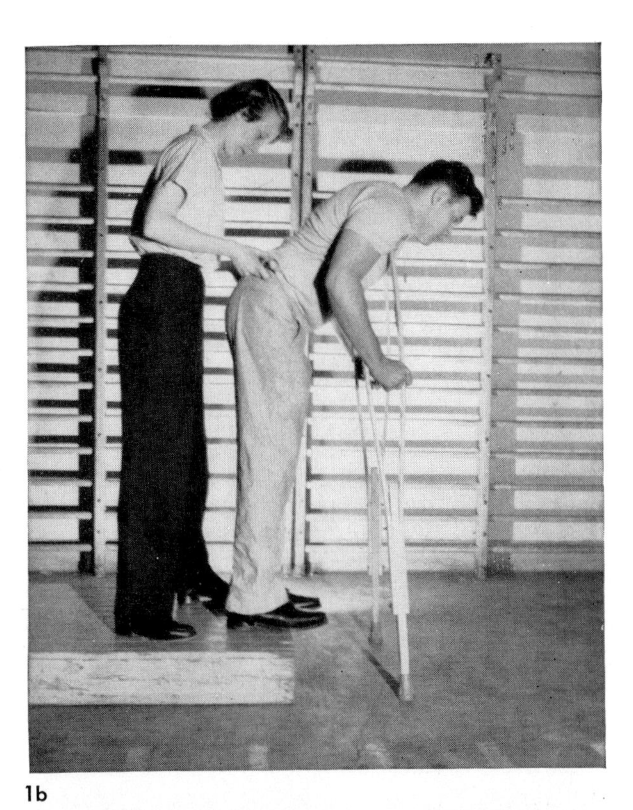

1b

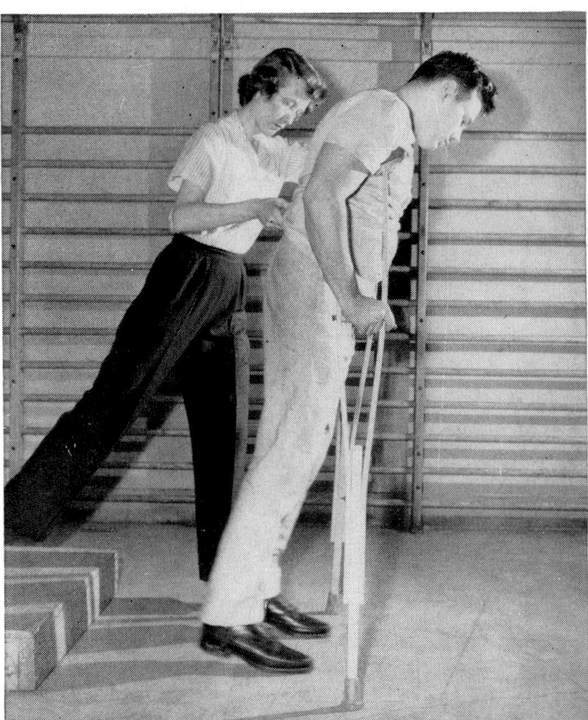

2b

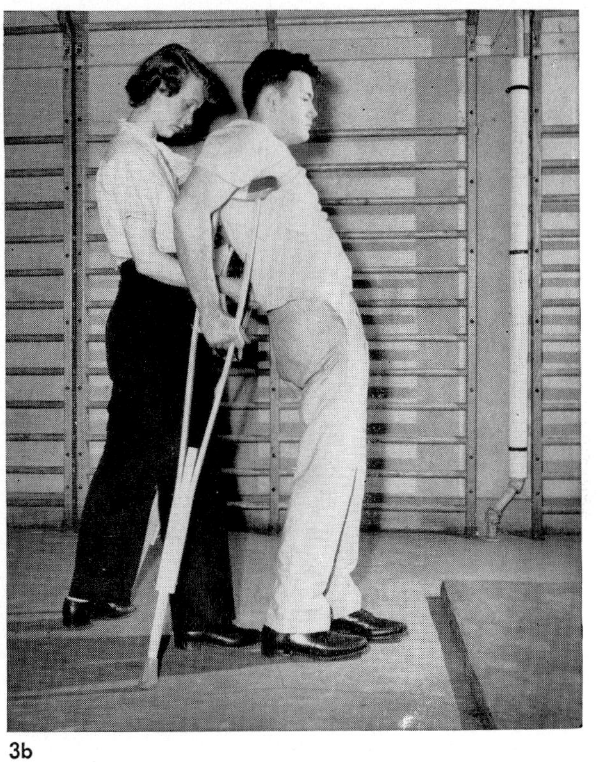

3b

Fig. 52. INTO AND OUT OF CAR ON CRUTCHES

Most patients find it easier to get on front seat. Same principles as described below hold for getting on back seat. Construction of car doors will determine choice. A four-door sedan allows more room and better approach to back seat.

Preliminary exercises: crutch walking in all directions; getting in and out of chairs.

Equipment: car in gym; later, car in street.

Into car:

Starting Position: Stand as near to car as possible so that you can easily unlock door with one hand while other hand rests on other crutch or car.

Instructions:

1. Open door as wide as possible, supporting yourself on both feet and holding on to car for balance. Roll window down so that you can hold on to window frame as you...

2. ...turn around, bringing your back against front seat to...

3. ...steady yourself. Hold on to window frame for balance and place both crutches toward your left against car.

4. Place left hand on back rest of front seat. Lean strongly on left hand, keeping door open with right hand, let pelvis buckle and slowly lower body (by bending left elbow) on to...

5. ...seat. Place both crutches in car. Adjust braces and legs and move over behind steering wheel.

Helpful remarks:

3. This is the position for unlocking hip locks.

4. Tall patients will unlock knee locks in this position, bracing themselves with buttocks against seat and then sit down.

Out of car: Reverse entire procedure. (Read pictures in reverse sequence.)

Starting Position:

5. Sit on front seat. Roll door window down and open door as wide as possible. Turn body so that you face street. Lock both knees. Place both crutches toward left against car.

Instructions:

4. Place left hand on back rest of front seat and right hand on window frame to keep door open. Push strongly on left hand so that you slide forward on seat until heels are on sidewalk, bracing yourself against seat with buttocks. Continue...

3. ...until you come to an erect position. Shift weight to feet, bring shoulders back so that pelvis tilts forward. This is the position for locking hip lock(s). Steady yourself with one hand on door or back rest of seat as you place...

2. ...first one then other crutch under arms, so that you stand in a good tripod position.

1. Turn around and...

S.P. ...roll window up and close door.

Precautions: To prevent closing of door against feet, no pull must be exerted on door at any time. Hand on door is for balance rather than support.

Fig. 52. INTO AND OUT OF CAR ON CRUTCHES

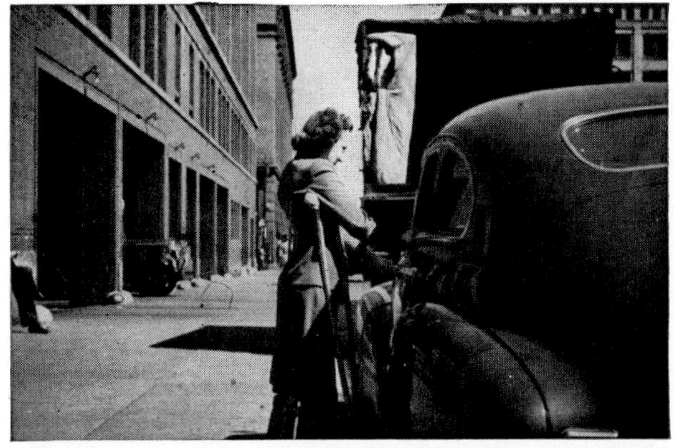
S.P.

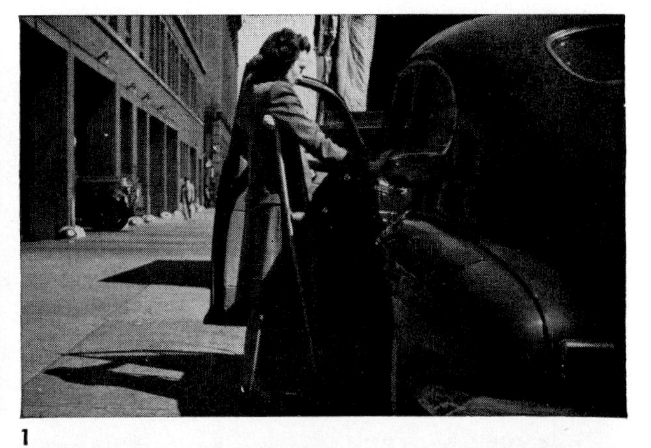
1

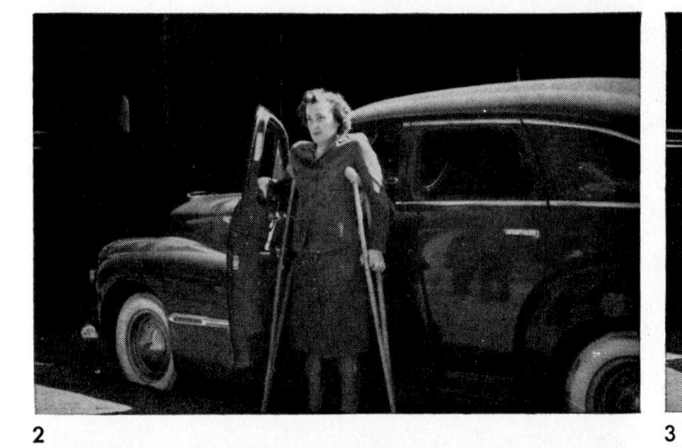
2

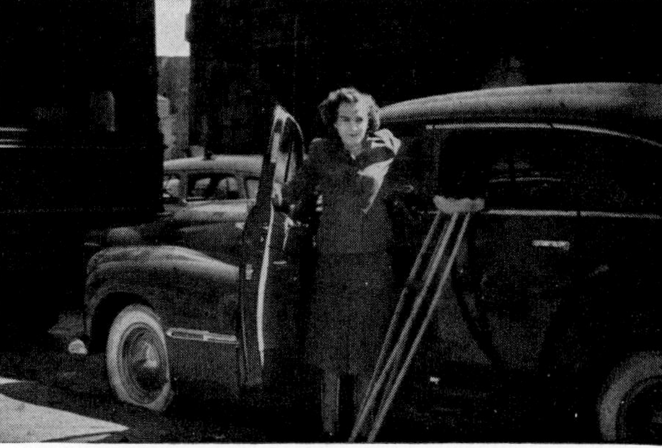
3

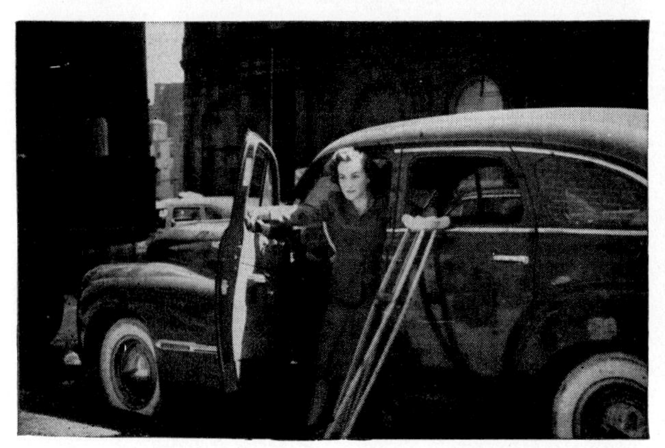
4

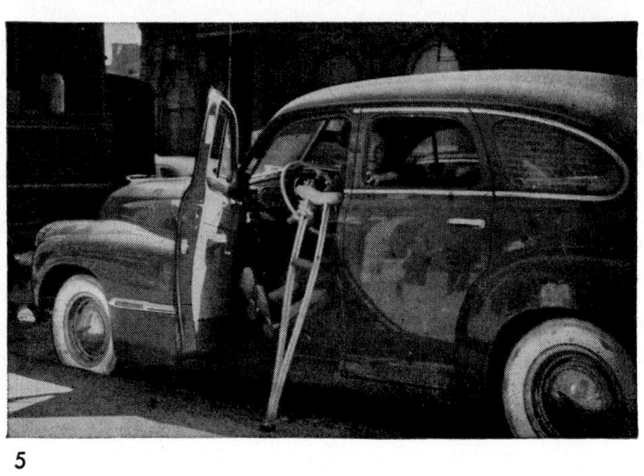
5

Fig. 53A. INTO AND OUT OF BUS FORWARD—one leg at a time

This method is possible only for patients who can move legs alternately.
Preliminary exercises: up and down stairs.
Equipment: bus in gym; later bus outdoors.

Into bus:

Starting Position: Stand in front of bus facing same. Hold on to front door with one hand while placing both crutches inside on step of bus. Move feet back sufficiently so that when leg swings forward toe will not catch. Unlock hip lock(s).

Instructions:
1. Hold on with each hand to one pole inside bus. Bend forward at waist and swing left leg up onto bus step.
2. Pulling with both hands, pull body weight up and forward over left leg so that right leg follows up onto step. When both legs are on step, be sure to bring shoulders back and arch back to tilt pelvis forward in order to straighten up. Place both crutches under one arm and grasp solid rail or handle with other hand for balance. Lock hip lock(s).

Getting out of bus is done forward with both legs simultaneously (Fig. **53B**).

Fig. 53B. INTO AND OUT OF BUS—both legs simultaneously

Preliminary exercises: crutch walking in all directions; stair climbing.
Equipment: bus in gym; later, bus outdoors.

Into bus backward: It is easier to mount bus backward. This will eliminate catching toes on edge of step.

Starting Position: Back up to bus steps and lean against them. Hold on with right hand to bar inside and place crutches to left of door outside.
Instructions:
1. Grasping bar inside with right hand and tops of both crutches with left hand, hoist body up into bus by pulling with right arm and pushing on left hand. Jackknife and pull abdominal muscles in so legs come forward and you gain height until...
2. ...feet land on bus step. Bring shoulders back, tilt pelvis forward and straighten up. Lift crutches in. Turn around, place both crutches under one arm, so that you can hold on to strap or solid bar with other hand.

Out of bus forward: Reverse entire procedure. (Read pictures in reverse sequence.)

Starting Position:
2. Stand on bus step with back to bus. Hold on to inside bar with right hand and place both crutches toward left of door, outside on street. Place left hand on tops of both crutches.

Instructions:
1. Pull with right hand and at same time push on left hand, lift your body off step, at same time jackknifing and pulling in abdominal muscles so that feet clear step forward...

S.P. ...lower body slowly by bending left elbow while still pulling strongly on bar with right hand.

Variation: Some patients, instead of pushing on crutches, hold on to bars inside of bus, pulling with both hands, in order to hoist body in.

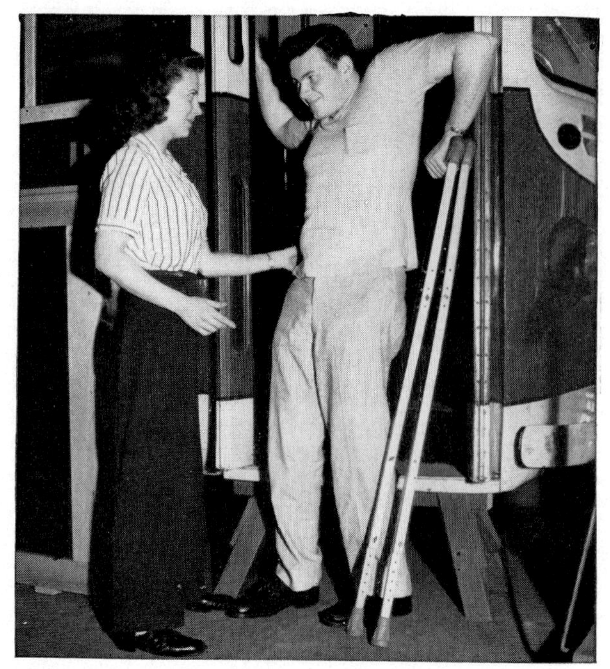

S.P.

Fig. 53A. INTO AND OUT OF BUS FORWARD—one leg at a time

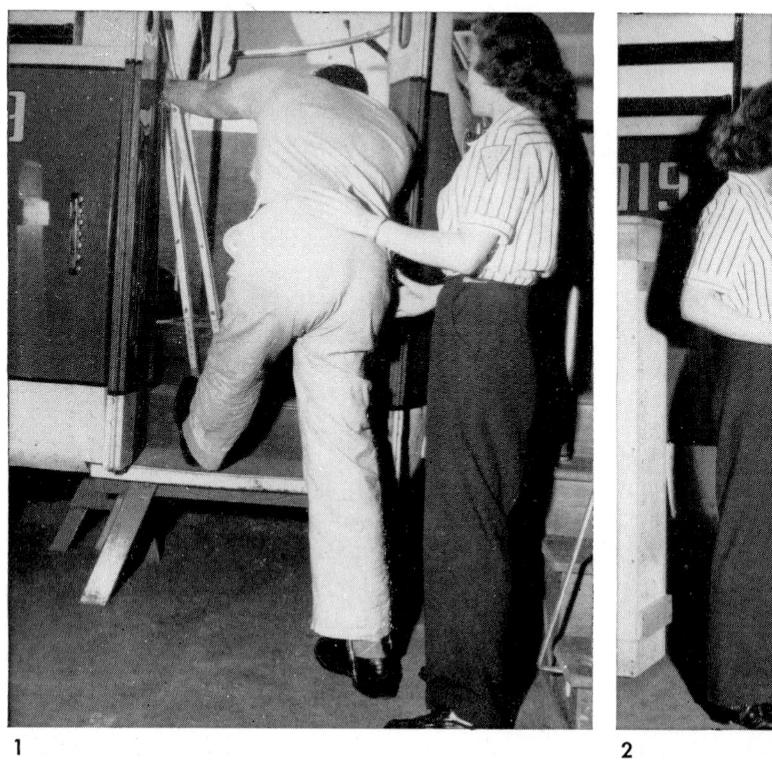

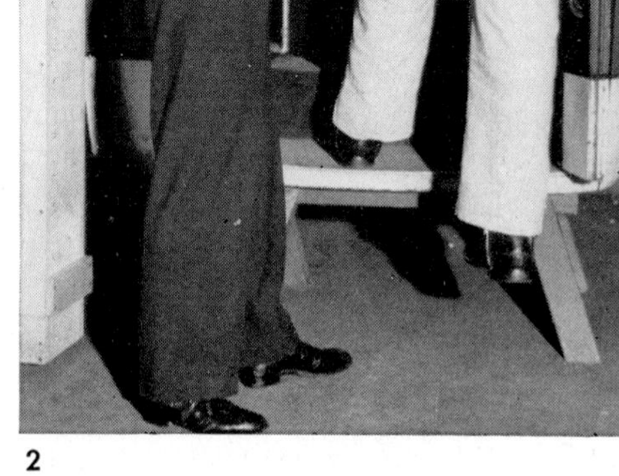

1

2

Fig. 53B. INTO AND OUT OF BUS—both legs simultaneously

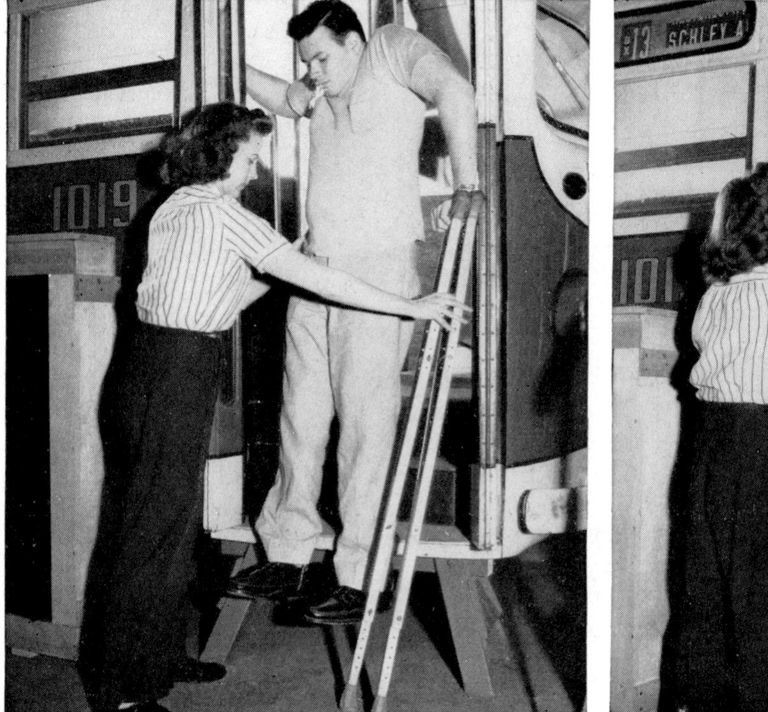

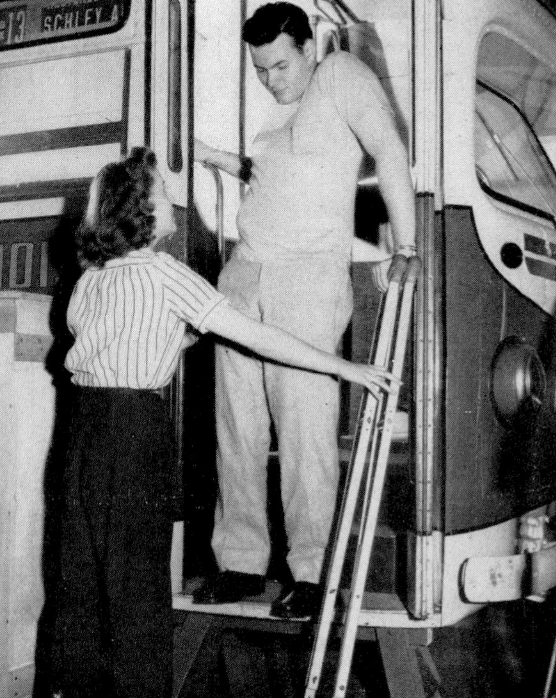

1

2

CHAPTER VII

Special Problems

Wheel Chairs*

The wheel chair best suited to meet the needs of a disabled person is the collapsible type which is made of light chromium-plated metal with back rest and seat of fabric or plastic, footboards, and large wheels which the patient can propel. These chairs are neat in appearance, are propelled with ease, give freedom of movement in relatively confined spaces, are easily folded for automobile transportation, and give a maximum of comfort. There are several stock models of collapsible wheel chairs, but modifications can be built into these standard-model chairs to suit the individual patient.

The first consideration must be given to the patient's convenience, for if he cannot use the wheel chair with some degree of comfort, it will be of little or no use. No two patients are of exactly the same height and weight or have the same disability; therefore, it is essential that a chair be selected according to the patient's needs.

For the purposes of this book, we will discuss only the models and modifications that meet the requirements of patients with involvement of the lower extremities.

Another important factor in the planning of a chair is the type of area in which it is to be used and the obstacles this area presents, *e.g.*, the width of a standard wheel chair including the wheels is 24 in. (folded 10 in.), height of seat from floor 20 in. The over-all length including the wheels is 39½ in. These measurements must be considered in relation to the passage space, bathroom fixtures, etc., in the patient's home or place of work.

* Adapted from G. G. Deaver, Wheelchairs, *Phys. Therapy Rev.*, Vol. 29, No. 11, November, 1949.

To meet the conditions under which the patient lives and works, the prescription of a wheel chair should specify in detail the wheel-chair parts and their necessary adjustments. The following outline will prove helpful when ordering a wheel chair.

I. Wheels
   A. Big wheels. The standard size is 24 in., but the wheels can be made bigger or smaller. They should be made 20 in. if the armrests are removable, so that they do not interfere when the patient slides sideways. Extra wheel sockets should be ordered. This will make it possible to change the size of the wheels without reconstructing the chair. A handrim is suggested for self-propulsion in order to protect the patient's hands.
      1. Big wheels in rear. These are most practical for all purposes. It is easiest to transfer from this type of wheel chair to furniture, car, etc.
      2. Big wheels in front. The advantage of this type of chair is that it will turn around in a small space.

   B. Small wheels. They may be in front or back (according to the position of the big wheels). The standard size is 5 in. Eight-inch front wheels are more practical since they roll easier over rugs, carpets or any small obstacles indoors as well as outdoors. The 8-in. front wheels increase the over-all length of the wheel chair about three inches. This should be remembered in relation to the area in which the wheel chair is used.

   C. Tires. Solid rubber is standard on stock models. Pneumatic tires may be ordered.

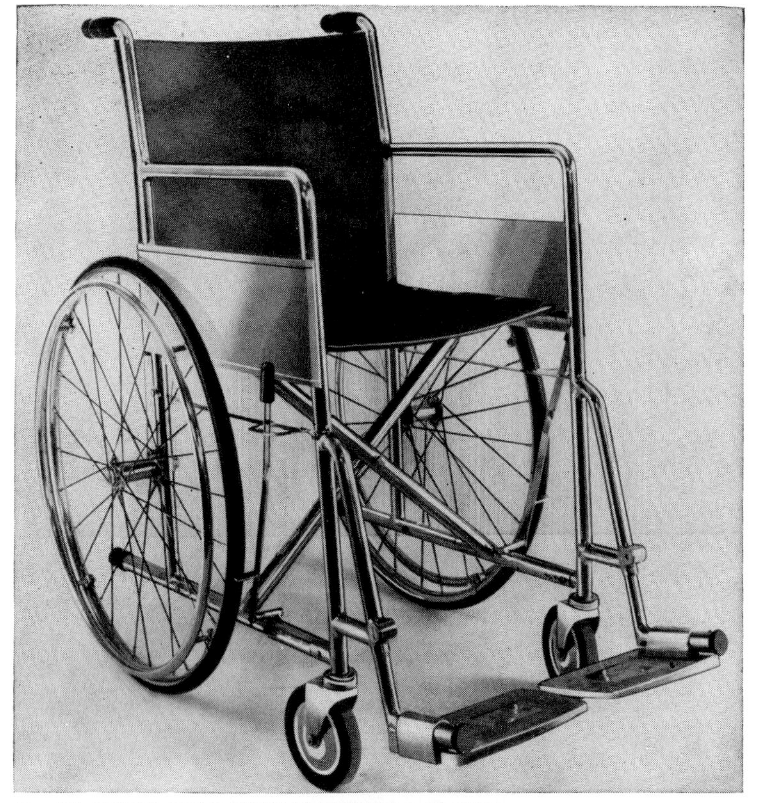

Fig. 54. WHEEL CHAIR WITH BIG WHEELS IN REAR

Figures 54 to 70 inclusive, courtesy of Everest & Jennings, wheel chair manufacturers, Los Angeles, California

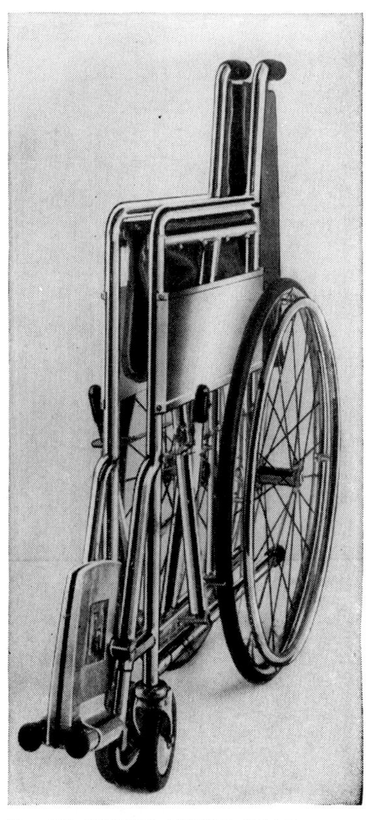

Fig. 55. FOLDED WHEEL CHAIR

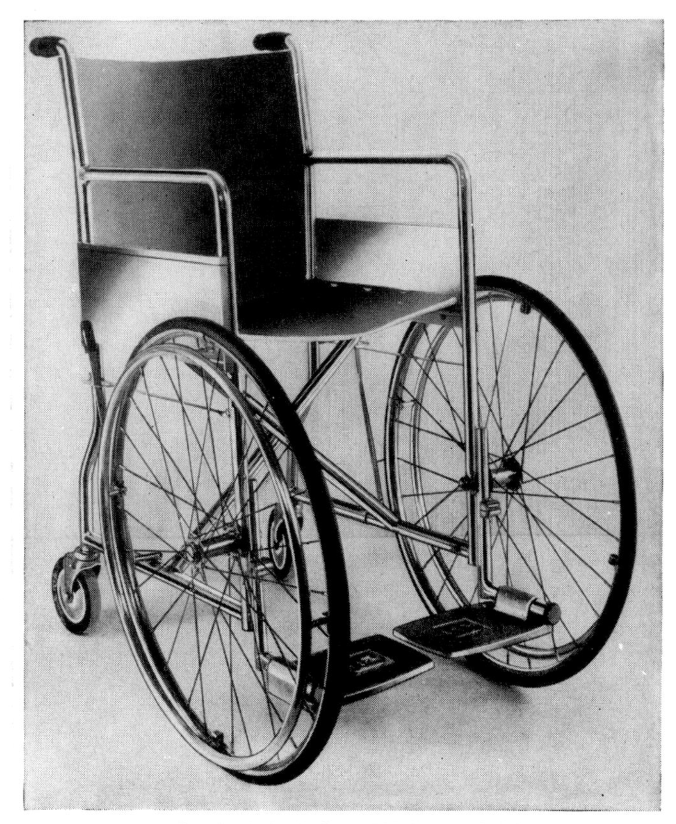

Fig. 56. WHEEL CHAIR WITH BIG WHEELS IN FRONT

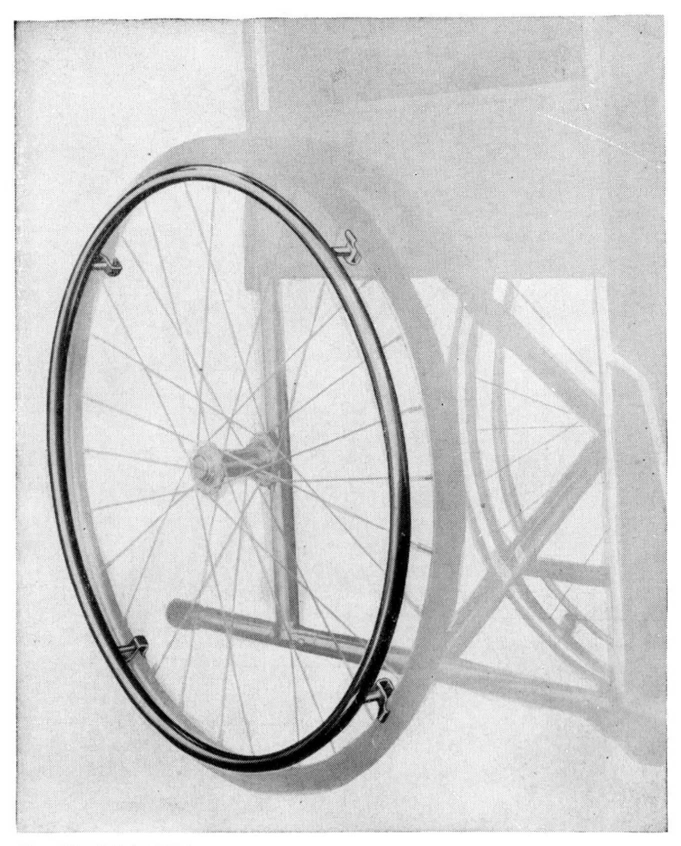

Fig. 57. HAND RIM

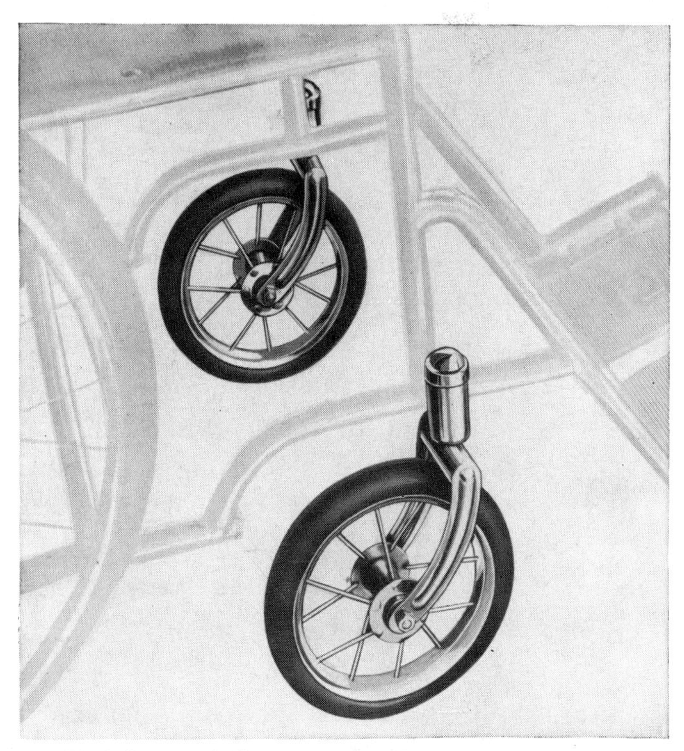

Fig. 58. FRONT WHEELS

II. Seat and footrests. The height of the seat from the footrests is adjustable. The distance between the footrests and the seat should be planned according to the length of the lower extremities of the individual patient. The thickness of the seat cushion must also be considered. The following footrest adaptations may be ordered:

A. Adjustable leg rests allow for adjustment in length. They can also be elevated to any desired angle.

B. Swinging footrests make it possible to roll chair closer to furniture, car, etc. They also reduce the over-all length of chair, *e.g.*, for use in home elevators.

C. Wooden leg rests (adjustable).

D. Fabric or plastic leg-rest panel.

Both *C* and *D* serve to support the lower legs and thereby ensure good alignment.

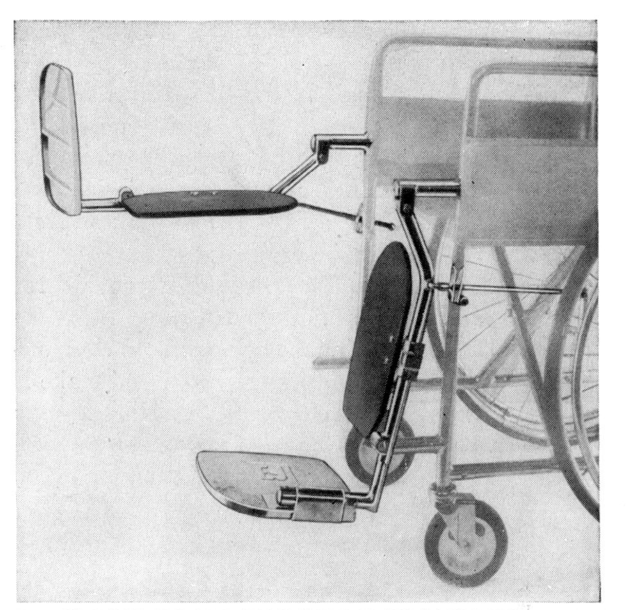

Fig. 59. BOLT-ON ADJUSTABLE LEG RESTS (WOODEN)

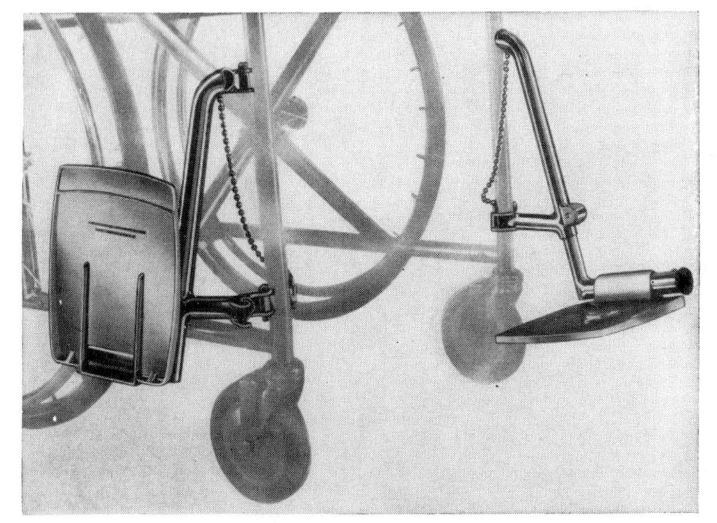

Fig. 60. SWINGING FOOTRESTS

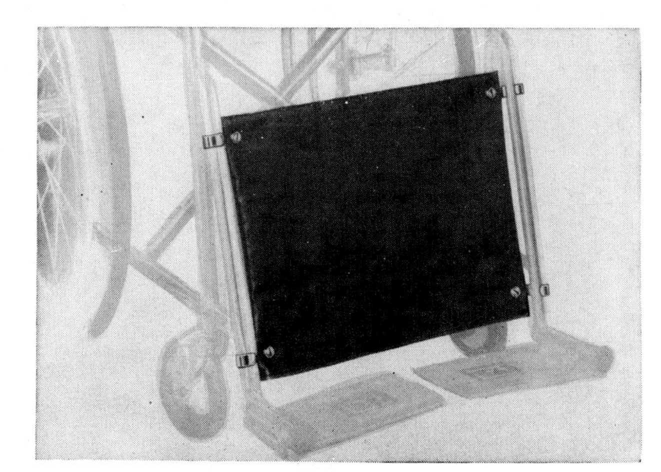

Fig. 61. PLASTIC LEG-REST PANEL

III. Seat and armrests. Width of seat: between front uprights—18 in.; at seat level—16 in. The depth and width of the seat must be considered in relation to the size of the patient. Additional width will be needed to accommodate braces or other appliances. To increase the width of the seat, the following armrest adaptations may be ordered:

- *A*. Offset arms. They will also provide for lowering seat and arms.
- *B*. Detachable arms. They facilitate close approach to furniture, car, etc., and make it possible for the patient to slide sideways when transferring from and to wheel chair. They also allow patient to sit close to table, desk, etc. Twenty-inch big wheels should be ordered with detachable armrests (see "Big wheels").
- *C*. Desk arms. Made removable or nonremovable, they allow close approach to low desk or table.

  It must be remembered that any increase in width of seat will also increase the overall width of the chair.

  Armrests may be uncovered, upholstered, covered, or wooden. Any addition to the uncovered armrest will increase its height.

IV. Stainless skirt guards: They are suggested to prevent clothes from touching wheels.

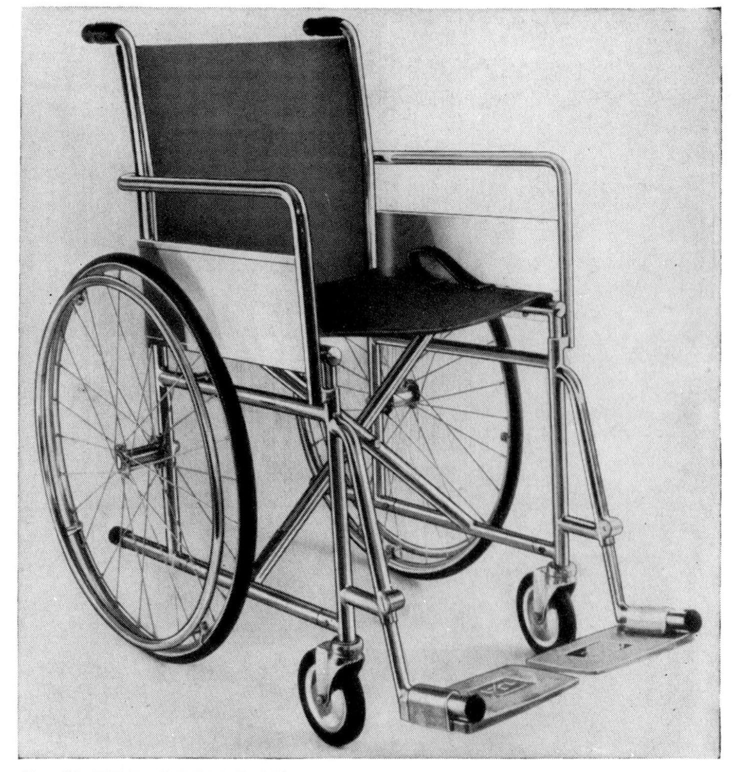

Fig. 62. FIXED OFFSET ARMS

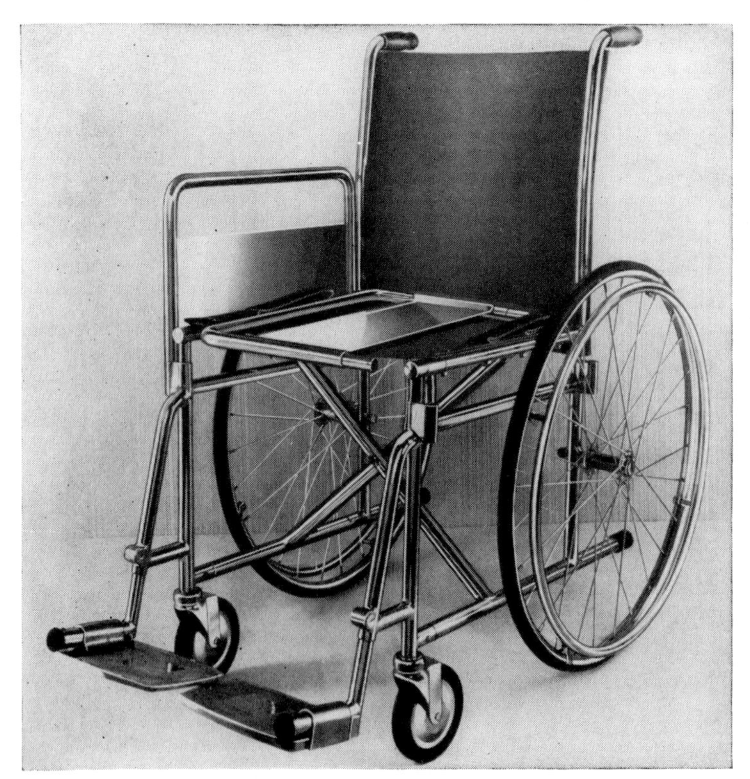

Fig. 63. DETACHABLE ARMS

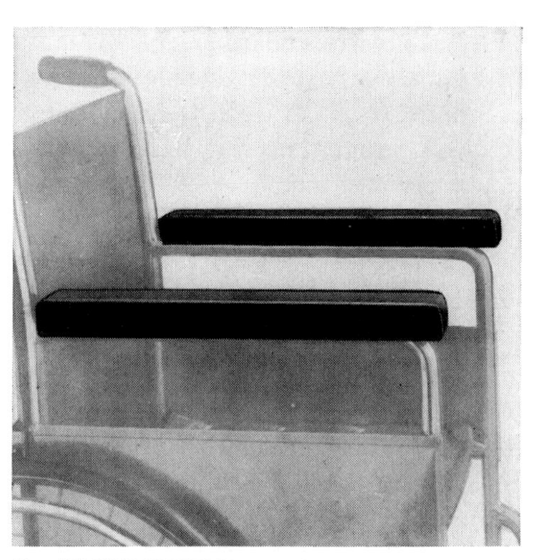

Fig. 65. UPHOLSTERED ARMS

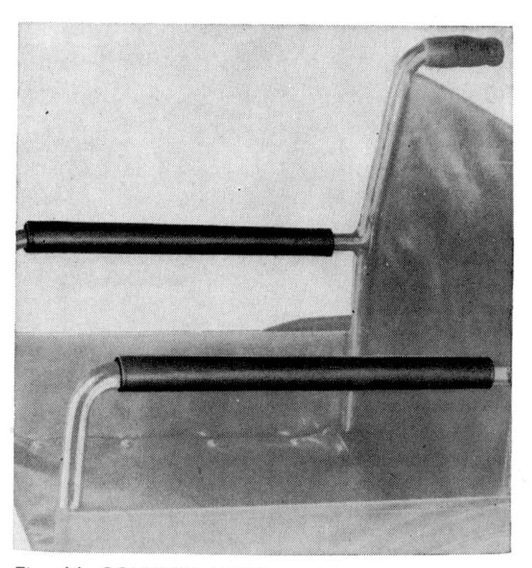

Fig. 66. COVERED ARMS

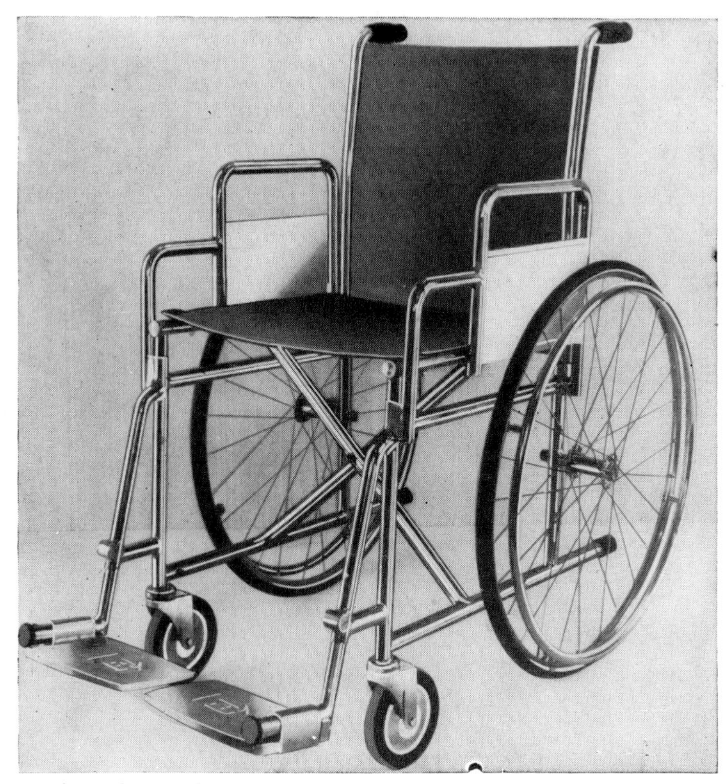

Fig. 64. DESK ARMS

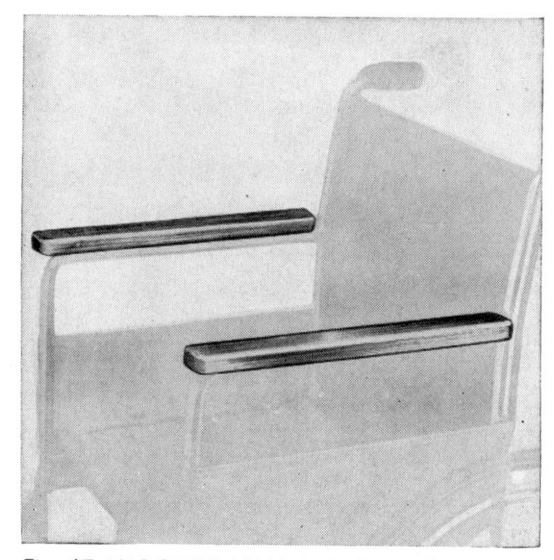

Fig. 67. WOODEN ARMS AND SKIRT GUARD

The *stirrup* attachment is placed on the shoe in front of the heel. The attachment makes the shoe part of the brace but allows for the use of the ankle joint at the proper place. In order to use this kind of brace for more than one pair of shoes, the stirrup attachment to the shoe can be made detachable from the brace by means of a special lock (French lock) at the ankle joint. If there is spasticity at the ankle joint, it is advisable to make a thin steel insole and rivet the stirrup to the plate. This acts like a foot plate.

The type of *shoes* the patient wears with his braces depends upon the purpose of the brace; the type of disability; and the age, sex, and occupation. Some general principles which should be considered are as follows:

1. If the brace is to be attached to the shoes, the leather must be of good quality and the sole of the shoe thick enough to hold the metal attachments.
2. A shoe that has a broad low heel is usually best for the attachment of the brace and walking. To avoid sliding, it has been found that genuine rubber heels (not synthetic rubber) are essential.
3. An oxford is the most desirable shoe to wear because it is easier for the patient to put on, neater in appearance, and less difficult to obtain in the color, size, and shape desired. The high shoe may be necessary when there is spasticity in the muscles of the leg and foot in order to prevent the heel from coming out of the shoe.
4. A larger shoe is necessary if a foot plate is used.
5. When there is no sensation in the feet, it is important to select the proper size shoes in order to prevent blisters and abrasions. The shoes should be of the blucher type, which have a soft leather vamp and no hard box to obstruct the movements of the foot and toes. There should also be no seam across the toes, to avoid any irritation of the skin.
6. If there is a difference in length of the lower extremities, a lift should be placed on the shoe of the short extremity. The height of this lift can best be obtained by taping pieces of wood to the sole of the shoe. These pieces of wood are shaped like the sole of the shoe. When the desired height is obtained, a permanent leather or cork lift can be substituted for the wood.

To avoid the appearance of too high a lift, the following procedure may be used: If in a given case the difference is found to be ½ in., then a ¼-in. lift is added to the shoe of the shorter extremity and ¼ in. is subtracted from the sole of the other shoe.

A simple way of testing whether the lower extremities are of equal length is the swing-through gait in parallel bars (Fig. **36E**) or on crutches (Fig. **42F**). If the right foot lands in front of the other, it is an indication that the right leg is shorter.

Ankle Stop and T or Y Strap. The purpose of the ankle stop and the straps is to control the movements of the ankle joint. In the lower leg the brace has two side bars (one lateral, one medial) that are jointed together at the top of the leg by a posterior cuff which is held in place by an anterior leather strap that is buckled in front. The height of the cuff should be such that it does not "pinch" when the knee is flexed. The side bars can be attached to a foot plate or to the shoe by a stirrup or caliper attachment (see above).

The joint can be free, limited by an ankle stop in dorsal or plantar flexion or fixed so as to allow one motion and prevent the other. By means of a T or Y strap, the foot can be prevented from supinating or pronating.

The following factors have to be considered when selecting the most suitable type of ankle stop or strap:

An ankle stop is used to limit plantar flexion to 90 deg. when there is weakness or flaccid paralysis of the dorsal flexors and normal or spastic plantar flexors.

To control the plantar flexion it may also be necessary to use a foot plate with a strap to hold the ankle joint at 90 deg. In extreme spasticity when the heel cord is pulling out of the shoe, the foot plate is held on the foot with a leather cuff around the ankle.

If a stirrup is used, a thin steel insole should be placed in the shoe and the stirrup riveted to the plate. The leather in the shoe is attached to a cuff around the ankle.

The single-bar wire night brace has proved most satisfactory in keeping the ankle at a 90-deg. angle during the night. The brace is made of wire and an old shoe in the following way: The heel of the shoe is removed, and a single outer (lateral) bar made of wire is attached with tubing to the bottom of the shoe. The upper part of the wire is connected to the side of a cuff which encircles the upper part of the leg. A small metal upright is attached to the bottom of the shoe to prevent plantar flexion of the foot.

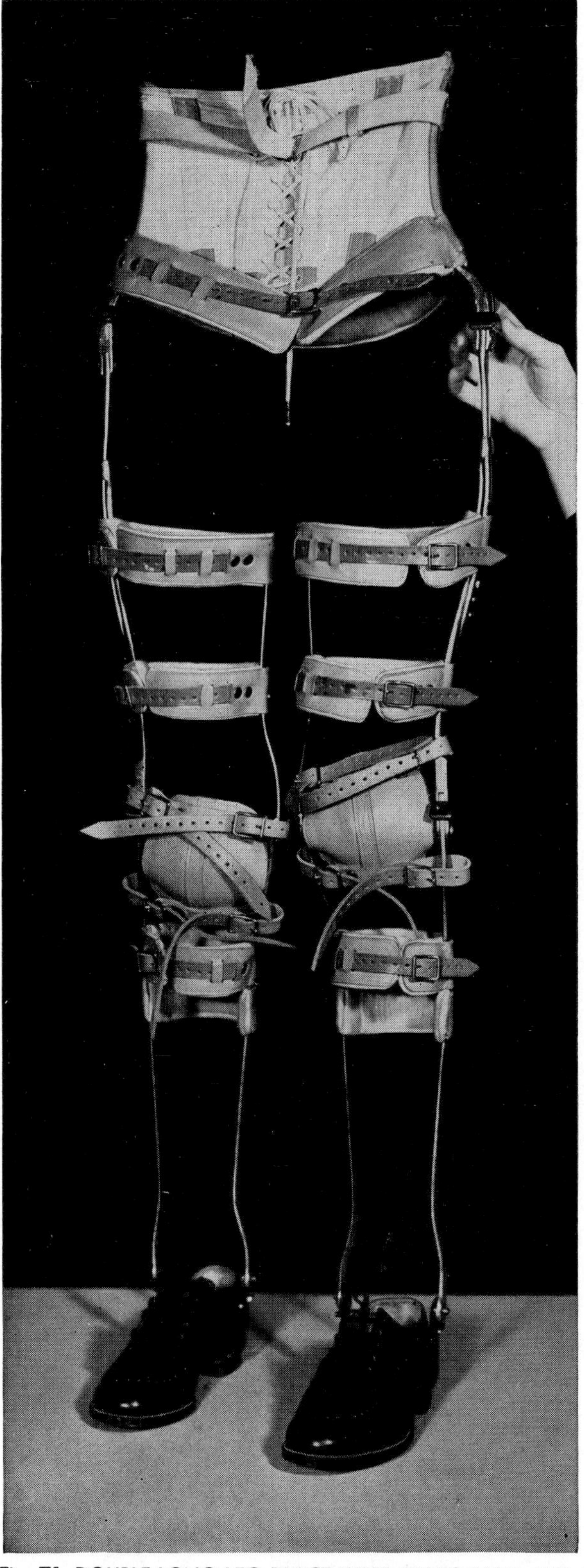

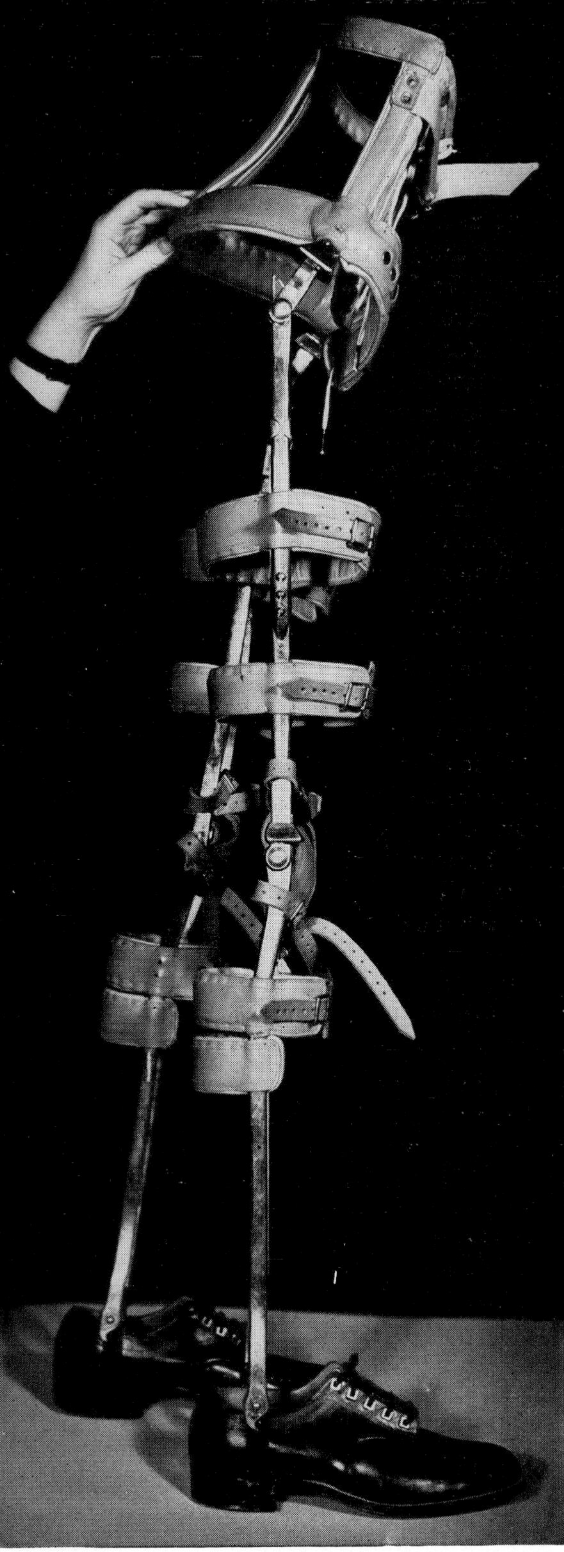

Fig. 71. DOUBLE LONG LEG BRACE WITH PELVIC BAND AND SPINAL BRACE

The leather covering the toes is removed to give freedom of movement to the toes. This brace has proved especially useful for growing children who have weak dorsal flexors.

When there is a flaccid paralysis of the dorsal and plantar flexors, the joint on the brace should limit the motion to about fifteen degrees in dorsal and plantar flexion.

When there is weakness or a flaccid paralysis of the plantar flexors and normal or spastic dorsal flexors, a reverse stop limits dorsal flexion to 90 deg.

It is necessary to use surgical-steel lateral bars when spasticity is present.

Duraluminum, because of its softness, should never be used at the joints. If duraluminum is used for the lateral bars, a steel or brass bushing must be used at the joint, so that the steel will not wear out the duraluminum.

If on movement of the foot or while weight bearing the foot pronates or supinates, it is necessary to use a T or Y strap to correct the turning of the foot in the following way:

1. To correct supination, the strap is sewed to the outside of the lateral aspect of the shoe, and the ends are buckled tightly over the inner (medial) bar.
2. To correct pronation, the strap is sewed to the outside of the medial aspect of the shoe, and the ends are buckled tightly over outside (lateral) bar.

The Knee Joint. The knee joint of the brace, with its lock, kneepad, straps or pads, controls the movements of the knee joint. The joint of the brace is placed at the height of the anatomical knee joint and is part of the lateral side bar. The side bars from the lower leg extend over the knee joint to the upper end of the thigh. The bars are joined together by two posterior cuffs. One about 4 in. above the knee, the second about 2½ in. below the groin. Similar to the cuff below the knee, the one cuff above the knee must be adjusted at such a height that it does not "pinch" when the knee is flexed.

The knee joint of the brace is a box joint which is locked by a ring lock. The ring lock fits around the box in such a fashion that there is just enough play for the ring to slide up and down easily. A screw on the top of the box prevents the ring from sliding up too high on the side bar.

In order to lock or unlock the brace, the knee must be fully extended and the side bars in perfect alignment, so that the ring can slide easily up for unlocking and down for locking the brace (see Locking and Unlocking Braces, Fig. **29**).

The knee is held in extension by locking the knee lock

1. If there is inability to extend the knee while weight bearing because of weak or paralyzed knee extensors and normal or spastic knee flexors, because of flexion contracture of the knee; when the hamstrings are so weak that the knee goes into hyperextension; when there is flaccid paralysis of both knee extensors as well as knee flexors.
2. If the heel cord is short because of tightness of the gastrocnemius.

The knee pad and the two cuffs, one above and one below the knee, provide three points of resistance to hold the knee in good alignment.

In the correction of knock-knees and bowlegs, a third strap on the kneepad or padding may be used. Since the strap has to be tightly buckled, continuous pressure on the soft tissues is exerted and also the blood supply is cut off. It therefore seems to be more feasible to use padding in the following way:

1. To correct bowlegs, padding is attached to the inside of the lateral bar above the knee joint.
2. To correct knock-knees, padding is attached to the inside of the medial bar of the knee joint.

The Pelvic Band. The pelvic band with the hip locks controls the movements of the hip joint and aids in maintaining correct alignment of the pelvis. (It is used, for example, for patients with spinal-cord lesions below T/10.) The pelvic band is attached with side bars to the side bars of the thigh. These bars are extension bars, so that they can be adjusted easily as indicated (see p. 171).

In order to avoid pressure areas, the pelvic band is shaped to fit snugly around the pelvic contour. It should not be possible to place a hand between the band and the patient's back. The pelvic band is curved downward over the lumbar region (not straight across the back) and tilted forward about twenty degrees. In this way the pressure of the band will be evenly distributed around the entire pelvis.

The hip joint of the brace is placed at the height of the hip joint of the extremity and is part of the lateral side bar. Like the knee lock it is a box joint and locked with a ring lock.

1. The pelvic band is used to prevent external rotation and abduction of the hip. (External rotation of the hip must be differentiated from eversion of the foot.)
2. The locking of the hip locks will hold the hip in extension if the ability of extending the hip while weight bearing is lost because of
   a. Weak or flaccid hip extensors with normal or spastic hip flexors; also if there is a hip-flexion contracture.
   b. When hip flexors and hip extensors are flaccid.
3. A butterfly (single or double) is used to prevent jackknifing if there is a pronounced lordosis.
4. The pelvic band also serves as an assistance for weak abdominal muscles.

A Thomas ring or ischial bearing is used if there is weakness or paralysis of the gluteus maximus and/or medius. It is often attached to a long leg brace (but seems to be more adequate when attached to a pelvic band).

The Thomas ring should be right under the ischial tuberosity. A simple test for good fitting is the following: The patient stands with his weight evenly distributed on both feet. If the ring fits adequately, it should not be possible to place a finger between the ring and the ischial tuberosity.

Since the well-fitting Thomas ring supports the ischial tuberosity, it acts as a seat for the patient and thereby helps in carrying the weight of the pelvis. It also prevents sideward falling and swaying of the trunk.

The Spinal Brace. This is used to support the abdomen rather than for support of the back, when the abdominal muscles are extremely weak or paralyzed (*e.g.*, for patients with spinal-cord lesions above T/10).

The spinal brace consists of an apron and steel ribbings and is just high enough to cover the lumbar spine. The steel ribbing is on each side against the ribs and also in back parallel with the spine. The apron is anchored in back to the pelvic band, to the steel ribbings on the side, and extends freely to about the pubic bone in front. In this way, the apron is pulled against metal when laced and thereby does not compress the soft tissue between the ribs and the pelvis, but lifts and holds the abdominal contents up and pushes the spine back. This aids in increasing the patient's endurance, since it provides resistance for the diaphragm when breathing. This resistance would normally be supplied by the tonus of the abdominal muscles.

The apron should be laced as tightly as possible, starting from the lower part up. This is best done in the supine position. Sometimes two straps, one across the lower and one across the upper part of the apron, are used to help in tightening it. A corset with or without steel ribbings does not seem satisfactory, since it only compresses the abdomen.

CORRECT FITTING OF BRACES

The brace has to be checked and adjusted carefully until proper fitting is ensured. The following points should be observed before the brace is put on:

1. The joint locks should slide easily up and down.
2. The ankle stop should be adjusted at the desired degree.
3. The knee joint should flex at 90 deg. (or less).
4. The pelvic band should bend at the hip joints at 90 deg. (or less, but not more).
5. The brace should "stand" alone.

Once the brace is put on, it has to be checked in the supine as well as sitting position. The final test is made in the standing position, which is most easily done with the patient standing in parallel bars.

The following factors must be considered:

1. The bars should be in correct alignment, so that the patient can stand in the best possible posture.
2. The joints of the brace should correspond with the anatomical joints and lock and unlock easily.
3. The ankle stop should be so adjusted that the toes do not drag.
4. When the cuff below the knee is unfastened, the knee should not move forward in the brace.
5. The soft tissues should not touch the metal, so that any pressure is avoided.
6. The leg length has to be checked (see Figs. **36E** and **42F**).
7. The patient should also be able to sit comfortably in his brace.

It is important to remember that the patient changes his body contour as well as his posture as he progresses with his walking and climbing activities, which in turn will make brace adjustments necessary. It cannot be emphasized too strongly how important it is to observe the fit of the brace continually.

D. *Dressing and Undressing Activities*

1. Put on underclothes
2. Removing underclothes
3. Put on buttoned shirt (zipper)
4. Remove buttoned shirt
5. Put on slip-over garment
6. Remove slip-over garment
7. Put on slacks
8. Remove slacks
9. Tying shoes (buckle, zipper)
10. Tying tie
11. Putting on hose
12. Removing hose
13. Put on braces or prosthesis
14. Remove braces or prosthesis

E. *Hand Activities*

1. Write name and address
2. Fold letter, place in envelope and seal envelope
3. Open envelope, remove letter
4. Use dial telephone
5. Turn pages of book
6. Wind wrist watch
7. Open and close cylinder lock
8. Open and close ice-box door
9. Open and close door lock with key
10. Open and close drawers
11. Open and close door hooks
12. Open and close window
13. Pull window shade
14. Push doorbell
15. Use workshop switch
16. Use work plug switch
17. Use work push button
18. Work key light switch
19. Work pull-chain light
20. Ring doorbell
21. Open and close cabinet lock
22. Turn four-pronged faucet
23. Turn circular faucet
24. Open and close medicine chest
25. Open and close bottle
26. Open and close safety pin
27. Strike match

F. *Wheel-chair Activities*

1. Bed to wheel chair
2. Wheel chair to bed
3. Raising and lowering foot rests
4. Propelling wheel chair forward 30 ft. and stopping
5. Propelling wheel chair backward 30 ft. and stopping
6. Locking and unlocking brakes on wheel chair
7. Opening and closing door in wheel chair and return
8. Wheel chair to chair
9. Chair to wheel chair

F. *Wheel-chair Activities (continued)*

10. Wheel chair to toilet
11. Toilet to wheel chair
12. Wheel chair to tub and/or shower
13. Bathtub or shower to wheel chair
14. Wheel chair to automobile
15. Automobile to wheel chair
16. Wheel chair to floor
17. Floor to wheel chair

G. *Elevation Activities*

1. Bed to erect position
2. Erect position to bed
3. Wheel chair to erect position
4. Erect position to wheel chair
5. Chair to erect position
6. Erect position to chair
7. Erect position to chair at table
8. Chair at table to erect position
9. Upholstered chair and/or sofa to erect position
10. Erect position to upholstered chair or sofa
11. Erect position to toilet
12. Toilet to erect position
13. Down to floor
14. Up from floor

II. *WALKING ACTIVITIES*

H. *Progressing Activities*

1. Walking forward 30 ft.
3. Walking backward 30 ft.
8. Opening and closing door, erect and return

I. *Gait* (Underarm crutches. . . . Lofstrand crutches. . . . . Wooden canes . . . . . Other support. . . . .)

1. Four-point alternate
2. Swing-to
3. Swing-through
4. Two-point alternate

J. *Climbing Activities*

1. Up 15-deg. ramp, 3 ft.
2. Down 15-deg. ramp, 3 ft.
3. Up 6 standard steps, one hand rail
4. Down 6 standard steps, one hand rail
5. Up 6 standard steps, no hand rail
6. Down 6 standard steps, no hand rail
7. Up and down one flight of stairs, one hand rail
8. Up and down one flight of stairs, no hand rail
9. Up curb
   a. 4-in. curb
   b. 6-in. curb
   c. 8-in. curb
10. Down curb
   a. 4-in. curb
   b. 6-in. curb
   c. 8-in. curb

with plastic. Measurements: length, 28 in.; width, 9½ in.; height, 18 in. (The highest bench is ½ to 1 in. lower than the wheel-chair seat. Each successive bench is 2 in. lower in height. There should be eight benches. The lowest bench is 4 in. high. Two boards 2 in. and 1 in. thick may be added to complete the ramp to the mat.)

2. Bus: model or standard bus in gym or out of doors. If this is not possible, 12-in. steps (height of bus steps) may be used (see "Staircase," below).
3. Car: model or standard car in gym or out of doors. Also taxi.
4. Curbs and ramps: for practice in gym (see Curbs, Fig. 51B). Material: wood. Measurements of curbs: 42 by 42 in. Standard curbs are 8 in. high; practice curbs should be graduated in height from 1 to 8 in. Each curb should be 1 in. higher than the preceding curb. Measurements of ramps: length, 41 in.; angle of incline, 15 deg.; height, from 0 to 8 in.; width, 42 in.
5. Crutches: extension crutches with tops and tips: (see "Crutches" in Chap. V). All sizes should be kept in stock.
6. Canes: different sizes.
7. Mats: for mat exercises (see "Bed and Mat Exercises," Chap. II). Standard gym mats with rubber or plastic cover. Measurements: length, 85 in. (7 ft. 1 in.); width, 60 in. (5 ft.) or 36 in. (3 ft.); thickness, 2½ in.
8. Parallel bars: (see "Ambulation," Chap. V). Should be adjustable in height and width. Material: metal pipes. Measurements: length, minimum 6 ft. (whole length of gym if possible); height, should be adjustable to height of 39 in. (minimum height 30 in.); diameter of pipes, 1½ in.; width, between uprights, minimum 23½ in.
9. Sandbags: for push-ups (Fig. 5); for positioning. Material: heavy canvas filled with sand and covered with plastic. Weight: 1 to 10 lb. (should be marked outside).
10. Stall bars: standard.
11. Staircase: (practice steps). Material: wooden steps, metal side railing. Measurements: height of railing, 32½ in.; diameter of pipe, 1½ in.; width of staircase, 43 in.; depth of step, 11 in. Standard steps are 8 in. high, bus steps are about 12 in. high, the practice steps should be graduated in height from 1 to 12 in. Each step should be 1 in. higher than the preceding step.
12. Wheel chairs: Several folding wheel chairs (big wheels in rear) should be available for testing and teaching. Standard measurements: height of seat from floor, 20 in., from foot rests, 18 in.; width of seat, 16 in., over-all width 24 in.; depth of seat, 16 in.; over-all length, 39¼ in.

INDEX